Sports Injuries

Acknowledgements

Thanks to Mark Sherman for the cover photograph and for those used in figures 1.1, 1.2, 1.3, 4.26, 4.27, 4.28, 4.29 and 4.30.

Sports Injuries

Causes, diagnosis, treatment and prevention

STEPHEN BIRD

Principal Lecturer, Department of Sports and Exercise Science, Canterbury Christ Church College, UK

NEIL BLACK

Director, Citisport Sports Injuries Clinic, Epsom, Surrey, UK

PHILIP NEWTON

Chartered Physiotherapist, Director, Lilleshall Sports Injury and Human Performance Centre, Newport, Shropshire, UK

Consultant Editor

JO CAMPLING

Stanley Thornes (Publishers) Ltd

First published in 1997 by:
Stanley Thornes (Publishers) Ltd
Delta Place
27 Bath Road
CHELTENHAM
GL53 7TH
United Kingdom

03 04 05 06 / 11 10 9 8 7 6

A catalogue record for this book is available from the British Library

ISBN 0 7487 3181 4

Page make-up by Pure Tech India Ltd

Printed in Great Britain by Ashford Colour Press

Contents

Preface

The contents of this text are arranged and indexed to make them as accessible as possible to the wide range of readers who may wish to consult it for a variety of reasons. For example, by referring either to a specific sport, a specific injury or a specific site of injury and then following the references to other sections within the text the reader should be able to acquire the relevant information s/he needs about the causes, diagnosis, treatment, rehabilitation and prevention of a particular injury.

An initial series of chapters provides the necessary background information on sports injuries, their causes, diagnosis, treatment, rehabilitation and prevention, including a number of specific common sports injuries. The following chapters then refer to specific sports and include within them examples of the types of injury that occur. In some cases where an injury is common to a number of sports and has been covered elsewhere in the text the reader will be directed to the appropriate section.

The guidelines provided on treatment and diagnosis should enable the therapist to make professional judgements about particular injuries or the particular set of symptoms s/he is presented with. This is important since no text of this type can be completely comprehensive in its coverage of all sports injuries, because of the vastness of the subject. However the information provided should enable the therapist to confidently make a diagnosis and prescribe an effective course of treatment and rehabilitation.

For those involved in sport as participants, coaches, administrators and managers the text will provide important information on the causes of injuries and their prevention.

Stephen Bird
Neil Black
Philip Newton

Canterbury, Epsom and Newport

List of abbreviations

ACJ	Acromioclavicular joint
ACL	Anterior cruciate ligament
ACS	Acute compartment syndrome
AL	Arcuate ligament
ATFL	Anterior talofibular ligament
CP	Chondromalacia patellae
CCS	Chronic compartment syndrome
CFL	Calcaneofibular ligament
CT	Computerized tomography
DOMS	Delayed-onset muscle soreness
ECRB	Extensor carpi radialis brevis
EMG	Electromyography
EMGBF	Electromyographic biofeedback
ES	Electrical stimulation
FCL	Fibular collateral ligament
GH	Glenohumeral articulation
ITB	Iliotibial band
LCLC	Lateral capsulo-ligament complex
LCNT	Lateral cutaneous nerve of the thigh
MCL	Medial collateral ligament
MCLC	Medial capsulo-ligament complex
ME	Myalgic encephalomyelitis
PEC	Parallel elastic component
PFJ	Patellofemoral joint
PCL	Posterior cruciate ligament
PEME	Pulsed electromagnetic energy
PFJ	Patellofemoraljoint
PFPS	Patellofemoral pain syndrome
PKB	Prone knee bend
PNF	Proprioceptive neuromuscular facilitation
PTFL	Posterior talofibular ligament
ROM	Range of motion
SA	Subacromial articulation
SCJ	Sternoclavicular joint
SEC	Series elastic component
SLR	Straight leg raise
SRC	Static resisted contraction
ST	Scapulothoracic
SWD	Short-wave diathermy
TA	Achilles tendon (tendo achillis)
TFJ	Tibiofemoral joint

TFL	Tensor fascia lata
TNS	Transcutaneous nerve stimulators
ULTT	Upper limb tension test
US	Ultrasound
VM	Vastus medialis
VMO	Vasus medialis oblique

1. An overview of sports injuries: types, causes and prevention

1.1 INTRODUCTION

With the increased number of people participating in sport and exercise the practitioner is increasingly confronted with what are often termed 'sports injuries'. Since such injuries occur through participation in sport the role of the good practitioner is not just to diagnose and treat the injury but also to rehabilitate the individual, provide advice on aspects of training, aid them on their return to fitness and help minimize the risk of further injury. With this in mind, sports injuries present the practitioner with a unique set of problems since not only do they have to contend with treating the injured tissue, but the individual is also likely to want to get back to playing sport again as soon as possible. Therefore in order to effectively fulfil their vital role, practitioners must have a good understanding of the physical demands placed upon the body by different sports, as well as the basic physiology of damaged tissue. Indeed this is central to the diagnosis and rehabilitation of any sports injury since individual sports will often possess their own characteristic set of common injuries, which are related to the demands of the activity. Therefore a practitioner who only treats the injury and does not adequately prepare the individual to play sport again is only fulfilling half his/her role.

The reasons why people participate in sport or exercise are many: for the professional sportsperson it represents a way of life and a means of income while for most others the reasons are likely to be health, fitness, recre-ation, the enjoyment of competition and the social interaction it facilitates. However regardless of the reasons why people exercise or their standard, participation in sport conveys a risk of injury to all, although some may be more vulnerable than others.

Some of the injuries that occur in sport, such as slight cuts or bruises, are relatively minor and can be dealt with by the individual him/herself or at least with basic first aid procedures that do not require any specialist knowledge. Conversely other injuries, such as those to the neck, spine and eyes, may be so severe that they require expertise in a specialist field of medical care, rather than that of the practitioner working in the general field of sports injuries. Fortunately these injuries are relatively rare and although the sports injury practitioner may encounter them from time to time they will usually be concerned with the kind of sports injuries that are not life-threatening or likely to result in permanent disability. Indeed, to anyone not involved in sport such injuries may almost go unnoticed or cause only minor inconvenience. However they are likely to prevent or inhibit the sports performer from training and competing to his/her full potential and hence assume greater significance. Typically such injuries include pulled muscles, sprained ligaments, overused tendons and damaged joints. The initial sections of this text outline the different types of injuries which fall into this category, their causes and how they may be prevented. Each individual injury encountered by the practitioner will be unique; however, by applying certain guidelines the practitioner can effectively diagnose, treat and help to prevent further injuries even though no case will present with exactly the same set of factors.

1.2   THE TYPES OF SPORTS INJURY

Sports injuries can be broadly categorized into two types, according to how they occur:

- Traumatic (Figure 1.1)
- Gradual overuse (Figure 1.2).

The cause of a traumatic injury can be located to a specific incident or event. Examples would be spraining an ankle when running over rough ground, dislocating a shoulder when colliding with an opponent, pulling a muscle, or bruising when being hit by a ball. Conversely, injuries that occur through gradual overuse develop slowly. They may develop during a match or race, or alternatively they may develop over a period of weeks. A typical scenario for this type of injury would be for a runner to feel slight tenderness in his/her Achilles tendon after a run. This often goes away overnight but returns after a subsequent training session. This cycle repeats itself with the injury getting progressively worse as time goes on until the soreness can be felt all the time, both during and after training, thereby preventing the athlete from running properly. It is about this time that the runner realizes that s/he has a problem and may seek help. However s/he

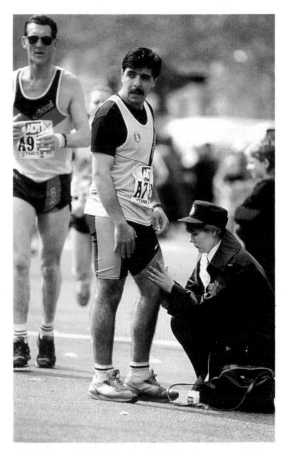

Figure 1.2   Overuse injury.

will not be able to locate the cause of the injury to a specific incident since it developed gradually from a slight, innocuous 'niggle'.

Both the traumatic and overuse types of injury may have external and internal contributing factors. For example, if a traumatic injury is caused by a collision with an opponent then the cause is obviously external. Conversely a pulled muscle often occurs through the mis-coordination of muscles which fail to contract and relax properly; hence the cause can be classified as internal. However a sprained ankle will often be caused by a combination of both external and internal factors. In the case of overuse injuries a poor racquet handle that results in blisters would be an external cause whereas

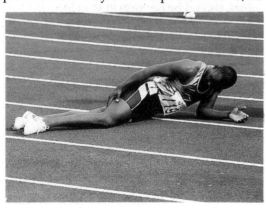

Figure 1.1   Traumatic injury.

too much jumping that resulted in an inflamed tendon would be an internal cause.

1.3 SPORT-SPECIFIC INJURIES

Since different sports and different forms of exercise such as jogging, cycling or aerobics place different demands upon the participants each will have a characteristic profile of common sports injuries. For example, most of the injuries that occur in contact sports such as rugby or American football are caused by collisions and hence are 'traumatic'. Conversely in an activity such as marathon running most of the injuries will be caused by the excessive repetition of a particular movement and the resultant gradual overuse. Furthermore, in addition to each sport possessing a specific injury profile, even within a sport it is quite common for different playing positions to be susceptible to different injuries. For example in the game of soccer the goalkeeper is more likely to suffer from kicks to the upper body than the other players as s/he dives for a ball. In the later sections of this text this will be looked at in more detail. Individual chapters are devoted to specific types of sport and their associated injuries, with details of their causes, diagnosis and treatment, suggestions for rehabilitation and recommendations for prevention.

1.4 THE CAUSES AND PREVENTION OF SPORTS INJURIES

The general causes of sports injuries are set out below. Considering these factors and taking appropriate action can help to prevent many injuries, or at least minimize their occurrence and severity.

- Lack of warm-up
- Inadequate fitness and physical weakness
- Inappropriate training
- Lack of recovery
- Biomechanical imbalances and anatomical factors

- Inadequate skill/technique
- Inappropriate footwear
- Inappropriate clothing
- Lack of protective safety equipment
- Inappropriate environment
- Breaking the rules
- Inappropriate opposition
- Prior injury.

1.4.1 Warm-up before sport and strenuous exercise

The reduction in the risk of injury is just one of the benefits of a warm-up. The others include preparing the body for physical exertion, preparing the heart for the physical activity, rehearsal of the movements and skills needed and mental preparation for the event. A warm-up should be undertaken prior to any form of strenuous physical activity. It should normally consist of four stages:

1. gentle loosening exercises;
2. some form of aerobic activity such as jogging;
3. static stretching;
4. sport- or activity-specific exercise.

Performing gentle loosening exercises in the initial stages of a warm-up is important, especially if the individual has been relatively sedentary for some time, e.g. sitting at a desk or in a car. These exercises, such as gentle rotations of the ankle, hip, wrist and shoulder joints, should be performed in a slow and controlled manner. Gentle jogging on the spot can also help to start warming up the leg muscles and Achilles tendons.

The aerobic component of the warm-up should be related to the activity. In most cases this would mean some form of jogging, swimming or cycling. It should be commenced at a gentle pace and gradually increased as the body responds to the physical demands placed upon it. This aspect of the warm-up enhances the flow of blood to the muscles by increasing the heart rate, the stroke volume of the heart and the circulation of blood to the muscles via the selective dilation and constriction of appropriate blood vessels. Commencing strenuous exercise without such a warm-up can put unwanted strain on the heart as well as the muscles. The aerobic warm-up will also help to increase the temperature of the muscles, which facilitates the transmission of nerve impulses, increases the speed of the chemical reactions used to release the energy needed by the muscles and enhances the overall process of muscle contraction. Therefore the effects of this part of the warm-up are to gradually prepare the body for the physical demands that will be made upon it during the subsequent more strenuous activity and should be undertaken for 10–20 minutes, depending upon the individual and the activity. In the case of someone going out running this aspect of warming the body up may be incorporated directly into the run by simply ensuring that the runner starts slowly and increases speed gradually over a period of minutes.

Following the aerobic component of the warm-up a series of static stretching exercises should be completed. Those out running should pause for a few minutes to complete these before resuming at their full training pace. These should be used to stretch all the major muscle groups of the body but will tend to concentrate on those muscles most used in the activity. Hence the precise composition of the stretching routine will depend upon the sport or activity being prepared for. This component should last for at least 5–10 minutes, each stretch being held for a minimum of 10–15 seconds. In activities requiring a high level of flexibility, such as gymnastics, the martial arts and hurdling, the stretching component of the warm-up is likely to take far more than 5–10 minutes, with each stretch being held for longer, possibly more than 60 seconds in some cases.

The content of the final stage of the warm-up will depend upon the activity. In team or racquet games it is likely to involve the practice of skills such as shooting, passing or hit-ting the ball. In other activities it may involve practice throws, hurdling, practice vaults or working through a routine.

Throughout the warm-up routine appropriate clothing which helps to keep the body warm should be worn. A consistent warm-up routine will also help to prepare the individual mentally for the training or competition.

Specific research into the benefits of warming up in reducing the risk of injury is difficult. One of the reasons for this is because of the ethics associated with getting individuals to exercise without warming up (with the expectation that they are more likely to suffer from an injury). Hence experimental evidence on the subject is scant. However despite this there is general agreement that an appropriate warm-up will greatly reduce the likelihood of injury. This is based upon the knowledge that cold muscles, tendons and ligaments are less elastic than warm ones and hence are more likely to tear when stretched. Conversely, the additional elasticity of warmed-up tissues reduces the risk of both traumatic and over-use injury. Remember that it is not just the elite sportsmen and sportswomen who are prone to injury: a warm-up is important for all.

1.4.2   The importance of fitness

If individuals are not fit enough for their chosen sport or activity then the physical stresses that they experience during it may cause injury. A lack of strength, speed, flexibility or endurance can all contribute towards injury. If a person tries to run a marathon with very little training then his/her body will not be used to the repeated movements and pounding experienced by the legs and this can cause injury. Conversely a fit marathon runner will have a body that is well conditioned for the activity and should not experience such problems. In many sports a lack of flexibility can cause injury, one of the most common injuries being 'pulled' hamstring muscles due to short or 'tight' hamstrings. A lack of endurance can cause players to tire in the later stages of a match; this may affect their coordination, reduce their level of skill and cause them to lose concentration and make mistakes, all of which may make them or their opponents more vulnerable to injury.

Fitness is also specific to the sport itself and being fit for one activity does not necessarily make a person fit for another. For example a very fit fencer may be fit to fence but not fit for the marathon or a game of rugby; likewise a fit swimmer may not be fit to play squash. Always remember that each sport has its own fitness requirements, which must be trained for. If a person attempts a sport for which they are not fit then they are risking injury. This is exemplified by the commonly used adage: 'Get fit to play sport, don't play sport to get fit'.

1.4.3   Training

The correct training and level of fitness will reduce the risk of injury by making the participant's body more able to withstand the physical demands of the activity. However, inappropriate training can cause injury. When considering a person's training programme a number of factors need to be considered. These include the type, duration, intensity and frequency of the exercise they are doing along with their capacity to cope with the physical stress it places upon their body. If a person attempts to do too much, too often, of too high an intensity, then they are likely to suffer from overuse injuries and their training must be modified. What is appropriate for one individual is not necessarily so for another, since it depends upon their physical capacity to train and their level of fitness. In this context it is also important to mention the aspect of progression. The body adapts gradually to appropriate training loads; therefore training should commence at a relatively easy level initially and progress with an increase in intensity, duration and frequency over a period of weeks. Attempting to progress too rapidly will not give the body time to adapt and overuse will occur. This is especially relevant to the beginner and the sports performer who has had to stop training through injury. Often these individuals are prone to try and get back into full training too soon without realizing that their bodies have lost a certain amount of fitness and cannot cope with the training loads they were using before the injury. Therefore gradual progression is essential in any rehabilitation programme.

Undertaking the wrong type of exercise or using a poor technique can also cause injury. This is most obvious in areas such as weight training, where lifting weights with a poor technique can cause strain to areas such as the back.

1.4.4   Recovery between exercise sessions

Sport and physical activity in general places physical stresses upon the body. If given adequate time to recover these stresses will act as a stimulus and cause the body to adapt to the stresses in a positive manner, making it fitter: this is the training principle. However if adequate recovery time is not allowed between training sessions or matches then the body is unable to recover fully. This can result in any minor damage to tissues not being fully repaired and as a consequence of this it will be damaged further during subsequent exercise sessions; this is how overuse injuries are caused.

An additional consequence of hard training is a depletion of the muscles' glycogen stores. Muscle glycogen is an essential fuel during strenuous exercise, the depletion of which causes fatigue and inhibits performance. Glycogen stores are replenished by eating plenty of carbohydrate in the form of bread, pasta, potatoes, rice and, where appropriate, energy replacement drinks. However, with prolonged or repeated hard training these stores may not fully recover despite eating the right things. This means that the individual may start the next session in a semi-depleted state, causing him/her to fatigue quickly, a factor that may make him/her more vulnerable to injury. The same may also be true of dehydration and fluid replacement after exercise. So eating and drinking regimens must be considered as an integral part of a training programme at all times.

It is therefore important to ensure that adequate recovery time is included in any training programme and many top coaches advocate rest days for their performers. These help to ensure that potentially vulnerable tissues are not overstrained and the body has the chance to make any minor repairs. They also facilitate the replenishment of energy stores and fluid levels. An alternative way of providing a means of recovery is to work alternately on hard and easy sessions or to work on different aspects of fitness on alternate days. For example those undertaking weight training will often train the muscles of their upper and lower body on alternate days.

1.4.5   Biomechanical imbalances and anatomical factors

An imbalance between muscle groups or bone lengths, or the mobility at joints, can sometimes cause excessive stress to be placed on particular parts of the body, resulting in injury. Furthermore, this can then cause the individual to compensate for a problem in one part of the body, such as the knee, which can then result in problems in other areas, such as the back. In addition to this, aspects of the individual's basic anatomy may also cause him/her to be prone to particular injuries. For example those who excessively pronate while running are vulnerable to knee injuries, as are those who have relatively wide hips, since this can cause the patella to track across the knee at an angle, which causes it to rub and become inflamed. Assessing the individual for these imbalances is a

skilled process and is discussed later in this text.

1.4.6   Skill and technique

A lack of skill can contribute to the risk of injury to the individual and his/her opponents. In the game of squash players who do not control their racquet swing are likely to hit their opponents with it. Likewise a player who lacks skill and makes clumsy tackles in games such as rugby and soccer is more likely to cause injury. Even in sports like basketball a lack of skill can contribute to injury.

1.4.7   Wearing the appropriate footwear

Since different sports and forms of exercise place different stresses upon the body the footwear worn in each activity must be appropriate. The physical demands of basketball, which requires a lot of rapid turning, abrupt stops and changes in direction, are very different to those of road running, in which the legs are repeatedly subjected to the stresses of the feet striking a hard surface. Therefore the footwear worn for sport must be comfortable, provide appropriate traction, cushion the impact of the foot striking the ground and be designed for specific movements such as changes in direction. So it would be inappropriate to wear a pair of running shoes for a game such as tennis, since they are not designed to protect the wearer from the stresses of rapid changes in direction or sideways movements.

On occasions the practitioner or coach may be required to advise an individual on the choice of footwear and, if suitably qualified, the possibility may exist of modifying his/her footwear through the use of insoles and supports. In some sports the footwear should also provide specific support and include features that reduce the risk of injury. For example, some shoes are designed for specific running gaits with considerations for those who experience excessive foot pronation or supination. Conversely, poorly designed shoes can contribute to injury, causing blisters or the inflammation of tissues. Likewise, shoes with inadequate cushioning or those that are worn out can lead to injuries of the foot, knee, hip and back. This is also true if the shoe becomes excessively worn in one place. When looking at a pair of worn sports shoes it is not just the amount of wear on the sole that is important. View them from the back to see if they still provide the relevant support or if they are misshapen and collapsing.

1.4.8 Appropriate clothing

In some activities there are rules governing the wearing of items of clothing in order to reduce the risk of injury. This includes items such as rings, earrings and necklaces, which are not permitted in games such as basketball. Loose clothing which may catch on apparatus and equipment is also of concern in some activities such as gymnastics. In orienteering full arm and leg cover is often insisted upon to reduce the number of cuts, scratches, stings and insect bits that may occur when running though rough undergrowth. In general terms each sport has its own set of expectations of what is appropriate clothing and standards of dress may be specified. Often this is for the general safety and wellbeing of the participants, as is the use of appropriate protective equipment and clothing.

1.4.9 Protective clothing and safety equipment

Protective clothing and safety equipment (Figure 1.3) is used to reduce the risk of injury.

In some sports its use is compulsory; in others it may be recommended. For example, in sports such as American football padding and helmets must be worn, whereas in cricket their use is advised. Likewise, the use of safety goggles in badminton and squash is also advisable to prevent eye injury from the shuttlecock or ball. Shin pads are needed in

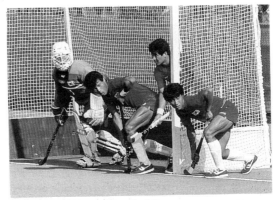

Figure 1.3 Protective clothing.

sports such as hockey and soccer, with the goalkeeper in hockey and the goalminder in ice hockey requiring additional specific protection because of their vulnerability to certain forms of injury.

1.4.10 The environment

In some instances the environment can contribute to the incidence of injury. Rough playing surfaces may increase the risk of sprained ankles or injury due to the unpredictable movement of a hard ball, as in hockey or cricket. In games such as rugby where collisions with the goal posts are possible these should be padded to cushion any impact. In addition to this any unnecessary equipment, such as unwanted benches or spare posts should be removed from the playing area to prevent collision and injury.

1.4.11 The rules

In sports some of the rules are there to reduce the likelihood of injury to players (e.g. rules on tackling, the positioning of players and general conduct on the field of play). In addition to this some rules also concern the age of the participants. For example there are rules governing the age at which children are permitted to run in races of certain distances. This is set out to prevent young children, whose bodies are not yet fully matured, from getting overuse injuries through running too far. The rules in some sports will also be modified according to the age of the participants, again in order to reduce the risk of injury. Therefore any rules that apply to a particular sport should be strictly adhered to.

1.4.12   Inappropriate opposition

In some cases the risk of injury is increased if the opposition is inappropriate. This may be the case in sports that involve physical contact or in the case of cricket, where an inexperienced batsman is unable to avoid a very fast ball or 'bouncer'. Problems with inappropriate opposition are even more likely to occur with children, where there is often a large difference in terms of physical size and maturity among children of the same age.

1.4.13   The implications of prior injury

With appropriate training and rehabilitation it is usually possible for the sports perfor-
mer to get back to full fitness. However the progression back to fitness needs to be carefully planned and gradual. A rehabilitation programme which does not do this is likely to leave the individual vulnerable to a repeat injury. A torn muscle must be gradually returned to its previous levels of flexibility and strength before it can be subjected to the full rigours of competitive sport. A muscle which is still weak, tight and contains the remnants of an injury is likely to tear again.

In this context the good practitioner who is treating an injured performer will also seek to eradicate the cause of the initial injury, if possible. This may be through advising on equipment, clothing, footwear, training, warm-up and safety. Such advice is essential if the practitioner is to be fully effective and forms the foundation of the practitioner's reputation; differentiating between those who know how to treat the sports performer and sports injuries and those who just treat the injury.

2. The physiological basis of injuries to muscles, tendons, ligaments, bones and joints

2.1 INTRODUCTION

It is a fact that any part of the body can be injured while playing sport. However the tissues and structures most likely to be damaged and subsequently treated by the practitioner are the muscles, tendons, ligaments and joints. Injuries to these structures can occur either through overuse or from a 'traumatic' incident. In the case of the latter, if the injury is relatively minor, the practitioner could be the first qualified professional to deal with it. Conversely, if it is relatively severe the injury may require immediate specialist medical treatment prior to the later involvement of the sports injury practitioner. Likewise, traumatic injuries to structures such as the head, eyes, bones and internal organs will often require specialist medical treatment and are likely to be dealt with by a casualty department rather than the sports injury practitioner. Therefore, in general, the practitioner will usually be involved with the treatment of less severe, non-life-threatening injuries.

In some situations the practitioner may be present when an injury occurs if, for instance s/he is providing medical support for a team or at an event, in which case s/he will be able to take immediate action. However it is far more common for the practitioner to be presented with an injury a number of hours or even days after it happened. This difference in the amount of time which has elapsed since the incident took place can make a significant difference to the diagnosis, treatment and time required for complete recovery.

In order for the practitioner to effectively diagnose and treat injuries to the muscles, tendons, ligaments and joints a good understanding of their basic structure is essential. This knowledge will provide him/her with a fuller appreciation of the physiological basis of the injury and its implications. Furthermore, an understanding of the various stages of the healing process and the ways in which the tissues respond to treatment will provide a foundation for prescribing an effective treatment programme. In addition to this a knowledge of the ways in which the tissues adapt to appropriate physical stress should also enable the practitioner to give advice about a progressive return to training and ultimately competition. Since most practitioners and other readers of this text will already possess a sound understanding of basic physiology, this chapter will provide only a brief general overview of the structure of these tissues in relation to their implications for injury and treatment. It will then review the nature of the common injuries that afflict these tissues and outline how they respond to treatment.

2.2 MUSCLES

2.2.1 The general structure of skeletal muscles

The general structure of skeletal muscle is illustrated in Figure 2.1.

The cells of a skeletal muscle are known as muscle fibres and are specialized for the

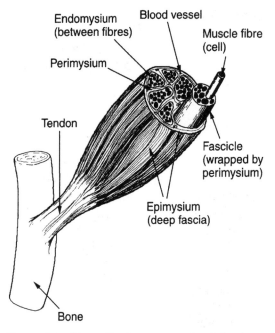

Endomysium
(between fibres)   Blood vessel

Perimysium

Muscle fibre
(cell)

Tendon

Fascicle
(wrapped by
perimysium)

Epimysium
(deep fascia)

Bone

Figure 2.1 Generalized structure of a skeletal muscle and sarcomeres.

process of contraction. They are long thin cells (approximately 20–80μ m in diameter) that contain many nuclei and are composed of smaller units called **myofibrils** (approximately 1–1.5μ m in diameter). Each myofibril is made up of filaments of contractile proteins whose organization provides it with the capacity to contract. There are two kinds of contractile filament: thick filaments made of myosin protein and thin filaments made of actin protein. These filaments are arranged to form **sarcomeres**, which are approximately 2.5μ m in length and are repeated along the length of the myofibril. These thick and thin filaments slide past each other during the process of muscle contraction.

Also contained within the muscle are various forms of collagenous connective tissue (fasciae), which serve to hold the different components in place and attach the numerous structures. For example, each muscle fibre is surrounded by a membrane called the **sarcolemma** and a sheath of connective tissue called the **endomysium**. Within the muscle

the fibres are grouped in bundles called **fasciculi**, which are themselves surrounded by a sheath of connective tissue called the **perimysium**. Each muscle is made up of a number of these fasciculi and the whole muscle is surrounded by an outer covering of connective tissue called the **epimysium**. While each skeletal muscle has this overall arrangement there are variations in the shape of skeletal muscles and the alignment of the muscle fibres within each muscle. These variations relate to the position of the muscle and its function and are discussed in sections 2.2.2 and 2.2.3. A knowledge of each muscle's arrangement of fibres can be important to the practitioner, especially if s/he is attempting to use treatments such as cross-fibre frictional massage.

Within each muscle are numerous blood vessels. These include the larger blood vessels, which are situated in the perimysium, and the smaller blood capillaries, which provide the site of exchange with the muscle fibres and are situated in the endomysium. It is calculated that in some muscles there are about 3000 capillaries in every square millimetre. During exercise the muscles require a greatly increased blood supply in order to deliver the additional oxygen and nutrients that are needed, as well as to remove any excess heat and the products of metabolism. In some individuals the flow of blood through the muscles may increase from resting levels of about 1 litre per minute to over 25 litres per minute. This increased blood flow has significant implications if a muscle is damaged during exercise. This is because the increased blood flow can result in far more bleeding into the muscle and the formation of haematoma as a result.

Also found within skeletal muscles are various neurones. These include the motor neurones, which transmit nerve impulses from the central nervous system to the muscle fibres and stimulate them to contract. Others are the sensory neurones, which transmit information from the muscles to the central nervous system informing it of the current state of the muscle. This includes information on whether the muscle is contracted, stretched, relaxed, fatigued or rested. Muscle injury can include damage to the nerves, which will affect the signals sent to and received by the brain. This has implications for both sensory and neuromuscular coordination of the injured region. Conversely, damage to or the irritation of a nerve at some other point in the body may cause referred pain, which is felt within the muscle despite its origin being elsewhere.

Towards the ends of the muscle the connective tissue that runs throughout its length becomes more abundant and forms a **tendon** or **aponeurosis**, which attaches the muscle to a bone. A tendon is a ribbon or cable-like structure while an aponeurosis is a sheet of connective tissue. The detailed structure of these, along with the injuries that can occur to them, is discussed in section 2.4.

2.2.2 The alignment of muscle fibres within a muscle

Each muscle within the body fulfils a number of roles, which may sometimes place conflicting demands upon it. The general shape of the muscle, its alignment of fibres and the type of fibres it contains are related to these roles and are sometimes a compromise between the demands for strength, amount of shortening during contraction and the limitations upon the size of the muscle. For example, in order to generate a large amount of force a muscle needs to contain a large number of muscle fibres. However there are limitations on the size to which the muscle can develop and hence the number of fibres it can contain. But if the muscle fibres within the muscle are arranged at an angle to the axis of the muscle (Figure 2.2), rather than along its length, then more fibres can be packed into the same volume of muscle.

This makes the muscle stronger without an increase in size. However this form of align-

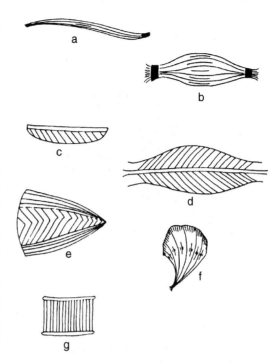

Figure 2.2 Differing alignments of muscle fibres. (a) Longitudinal fusiform, e.g. sartorius. (b) Spindle-shaped fusiform, e.g. biceps brachii. (c) Unipennate, e.g. tibialis posterior. (d) Bipennate, e.g. rectus femoris. (e) Multipennate, e.g. middle deltoid. (f) Triangular, e.g. pectoralis major. (g) Quadrate, e.g. rhomboid.

ment reduces the amount of shortening which is possible. Therefore muscles which are required to shorten by a considerable amount tend to have their fibres aligned along the long axis of the muscle but this makes them relatively weak for their size. The overall structure of the muscle is therefore often a compromise between the conflicting requirements of its roles. Other factors which influence the strength of a muscle are related to the stimulation it receives from the nervous system, the size of the individual fibres and the type of fibres. In this context it is important to note that while the overall alignment of fibres cannot be altered through training the size and quality of the fibres can, along with the neurological aspects of contraction.

For the practitioner it is important to appreciate the different possible alignments of fibres within muscles when treating an injury. This is especially so if the treatment requires massage, since the direction of massage may be influenced by the alignment of the fibres. In summary, muscles which have their fibres arranged parallel with the long axis of the muscle are capable of a considerable amount of shortening and are referred to as **fusiform muscles**. Examples of these are rectus abdominis and sartorius, which are long, strap-like muscles, and the spindle-shaped brachialis. Triangular-shaped muscles such as pectoralis major also have a parallel arrangement of fibres but, because one point of attachment is very small compared with the other, the muscle has an overall triangular shape. When this type of muscle contracts it is capable of exerting a large amount of force at a small point of attachment.

Muscles whose fibres are arranged across the long axis of the muscle are generally described as being **penniform** or **pennate**. Pennate muscles are further divided into those which are unipennate, bipennate and multipennate, according to the number of directions in which the fibres are arranged. **Unipennate muscles** have their fibres arranged in a single direction across the muscle: an example is the extensor digitorum longus of the leg. **Bipennate muscles** have their fibres orientated in two directions; an example is rectus femoris at the front of the thigh. **Multipennate muscles** have their muscle fibres arranged in several directions, an example of this type of muscle being the deltoids.

2.2.3   The different muscle fibre types

All muscle fibres have the same general structure. However, research has indicated that there are a number of different types of muscle fibre and these are classified into two broad groups, Type 1 fibres and type 2 fibres. **Type 1 fibres** have a relatively high aerobic capacity and are fatigue-resistant. They are sometimes referred to as **slow twitch** or **red fibres**. **Type 2 fibres** are larger, stronger and more anaerobically orientated. They are also referred to as **fast twitch** or **white fibres**. The overall ratio of type 1 to type 2 fibres within a muscle may depend upon inherited factors and the training of the individual, although this is an area of controversy that is currently open to debate. In general, however, it is suggested that a high proportion of type 1 fibres endows the muscle with endurance properties while a high proportion of type 2 fibres makes it stronger and faster, at the expense of endurance. However this is again an area of debate, as some of the research is contradictory. Further research has suggested the additional division of the type 2 fibres into the subclasses of type 2a, type 2b and type 2c. Of these, the type 2a fibres are the most aerobic, type 2b the most anaerobic and type 2c intermediate to the other two.

The implications of these differences for the practitioner relate to the way in which these fibres are recruited. The type 1 fibres tend to have a low recruitment threshold, which means that they are involved in most if not all of the contractions made by that muscle. Conversely, the type 2 fibres are less easily recruited and tend to become involved only when the amount of force required by the muscle rises above a certain level. This means that in rehabilitation programmes light exercise involving weak or moderate contractions will help to recondition the type 1 fibres, but to restore the condition of the type 2 fibres more forceful contractions must be employed. These must therefore be included as part of a progressive reconditioning scheme.

2.2.4   The types of injury that occur to skeletal muscles

Injuries to skeletal muscles may occur either through a traumatic incident or through overuse (repetitive strain injury – RSI). The physiological aspects of such injuries are described in this section and will then be referred to in later sections on sport-specific injuries. This should help the practitioner to appreciate the implications of such injuries to the performer and the basis of any treatment process.

The types of injury that occur to muscles are:

- Traumatic:
  - Pulled, torn or strained muscle – caused by overstretching;
  - Bruised muscle – caused by the impact of an external force pressing the muscle against the underlying bone;
  - Some forms of acute compartment syndrome, where bleeding in the muscle causes a build-up of pressure;
- Overuse:
  - Myositis – inflammation of the muscle caused by overuse;
  - Some forms of chronic compartment syndrome, where the muscle expands without the necessary expansion of the surrounding fasciae.

(a) Traumatic injuries

Pulled, torn or strained muscles

Pulled, torn or strained muscles are caused by the rapid overstretching of the muscle. This often occurs when the muscle is forced to lengthen while it is still tense. In coordinated movement some muscles must relax and lengthen (**antagonists**) while others (**agonists**) contract. If an antagonist does not relax and lengthen sufficiently then the tense fibres will be forced to stretch and may be pulled apart by the action of the agonist. This can occur when accelerating rapidly, changing direction or performing explosive movements such as jumping. A common example of this affects the hamstrings when sprinting: as the thigh moves upwards and forwards due to the contraction of the hip flexors the ham-

string muscles at the back of the thigh must relax and lengthen. If they do not, the action of the hip flexors at the front of the thigh will force them to lengthen even if some of the fibres are still contracted, thereby resulting in torn fibres. Another cause is simply overstretching when reaching for a ball or trying to make a tackle. In either case fatigue is sometimes a contributing factor to torn muscles, since the accumulation of lactic acid can inhibit the required coordination between the muscle groups. Sports performers with short or 'tight' hamstrings that lack adequate flexibility are especially vulnerable to this type of injury.

When a muscle is torn in this manner it is not just the muscle fibres that are damaged. The associated connective tissue and the blood vessels in this region are also torn. This results in bleeding in the area and the formation of haematoma. The severity of a pulled muscle can vary greatly, from the tearing of a few fibres to a complete rupture. While complete rupture is relatively uncommon, when it does occur it tends to be in the region of the muscle–tendon junction, although the reason for this is unclear. The extent of the damage within the muscle will affect the amount of bleeding that occurs in the region and hence the size of haematoma. This will have implications for the recovery process and the length of time needed before the individual can return to competition.

In the case of some muscle tears the epimysium that surrounds the muscle remains intact. This confines the bleeding to within the muscle and results in the formation of an intramuscular haematoma (Figure 2.3(a)).

This causes a build-up in pressure within the muscle, and pain, which further inhibits its activity. If, however, the epimysium is also torn, the bleeding can leak into the spaces between the muscles, forming an intermuscular haematoma (Figure 2.3(b)). This leakage can result in discoloration under the skin, but because of the leakage there is less of a build-up of pressure within the muscle. It

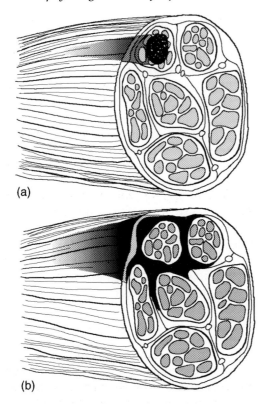

(a)

(b)

Figure 2.3   (a) Intramuscular haematoma. (b) Intermuscular haematoma.

should be noted, however, that because of the effects of gravity the discoloration may sometimes appear below where the actual tear has occurred.

Bruised muscle

A bruised muscle is caused by a blow to the muscle, which crushes it against the underlying bone. The overall effects of this are similar to that of a pulled muscle, with resultant torn fibres, damaged connective tissue, bleeding and the formation of haematoma. The treatment and repair process for such injuries are therefore similar.

The repair process for torn and bruised muscles

The repair of torn and bruised muscles involves two separate processes. These are (1) the formation of scar tissue in the form of non-contractile collagenous tissue and (2) the regeneration of the contractile muscle fibres.

Immediately after injury and for about the first 24 hours the site of damage is invaded by **macrophages**, a type of white blood cell. In the presence of damaged tissue these are converted into **fibroblasts**, which multiply and produce a precursor form of collagen protein. This continues over a period of days, with the fibroblasts maturing to form **fibrocysts** and in doing so shortening. The effect of this is the formation of a region of short, tight scar tissue, which can then be strengthened over a period of months. It creates connections within the damaged area, enabling the muscle's contractile fibres to function around it. However because this region of scar tissue is short, relatively inelastic and non-contractile it can inhibit the activity of the muscle and is vulnerable to further injury.

As the damaged tissue is removed the second process is initiated and new fibres are regenerated about a week after injury. These fibres are, however, relatively small and will take several months to enlarge and strengthen. This fact should always be remembered when designing any rehabilitation programme, as a graduated return to exercise is essential, with the muscle fibres being gradually exposed to greater amounts of stress. Additionally, appropriate stretching exercises need to be incorporated to regain the full length of the damaged, tight and potentially vulnerable region. Although exactly which exercises, their intensity and when they are introduced will depend upon the injury, since stretching the region too soon may cause further injury.

Acute compartment syndrome

When a muscle is damaged and an intramuscular haematoma forms it causes swelling within the muscle and a build-up of pressure. While this may not have significant effects at rest, during exercise it can inhibit the flow of blood into the muscle. This will deprive the muscle fibres of oxygen and result in the accumulation of lactic acid. This can cause more fluid to pass into the fibres causing additional swelling (oedema). The overall result is a cramping sensation within the muscle.

Complications to traumatic muscle injuries

Complications to muscle injuries can include infection through a wound or the formation of serum-filled cysts caused by the incomplete reabsorption of the haematoma. These require surgical drainage. An additional complication can occur when the injury has been caused by a blow or kick. In such cases the muscle will have been crushed against the underlying bone and if some bone cells (**osteoblasts**) from the periosteum flake off into the haematoma they may begin to develop and calcify (**ossify**). This will result in the formation of a small area of bone within the muscle (myositis ossificans). This causes pain that is aggravated by further exercise or massage.

(b) Overuse injuries

Compared with other tissues such as tendons, bursae, joints and the periosteum, overuse injuries of the muscles are relatively rare. However such injuries do include some forms of compartment syndrome and myositis.

When any body tissue, including muscle, experiences excessive pressure, friction, repeated overload or trauma, one of the consequences is inflammation. This is accompanied by swelling and pain, which impairs the action of the tissue. If this is not treated effectively then scar tissue can result, which will delay the recovery process. In the case of muscles, compartment syndrome may develop when the muscle swells without the necessary expansion of its surrounding connective tissue. This may be caused by a traumatic injury, as described previously, where the swelling is due to haemorrhage within the muscle or an expansion of the muscle with training. In the latter case the problem may only become apparent during strenuous exercise when the increased blood flow causes a further expansion of the muscle. If the expansion is inhibited by the surrounding connective tissue then the muscle fibres will be deprived of oxygen and the resultant accumulation of lactic acid may cause oedema, further swelling of the fibres and cramp within the muscle.

Inflammation of the muscle (**myositis**) due to overuse is rare compared to the incidence of inflammation in associated tissues such as the tendons, periosteum and bursae. Recovery from myositis requires rest followed by the gradual resumption of training loads.

Delayed-onset muscle soreness (DOMS)

Following excessive or unfamiliar training it is not uncommon for individuals to report muscular soreness 24–48 hours after the activity. This can also occur if an athlete returns to a training programme after a lay-off. The reason for this soreness is reported to be the unaccustomed stress that has been placed upon the muscles, although the specific causes of the resulting soreness remain unclear. DOMS is most common following eccentric muscle work, particularly downhill running or plyometric exercises.

Research into the causes of DOMS has identified increased levels of certain muscle enzymes and the presence of myoglobin in the blood (**myoglobinaemia**) indicating structural damage to the muscles. This is supported by electronmicrographs showing muscle fibres with ruptured sarcolemmas and damage to the Z disks, particularly in marathon runners.

Another contributing factor to DOMS is the general inflammatory response, with an increase in the number of circulating white blood cells being observed to accompany the soreness.

The factors that appear to accompany DOMS are:

- structural damage, releasing intracellular proteins into the blood;
- disturbed calcium homeostasis, resulting in cell necrosis;
- an inflammatory response involving macrophages, histamine, kinins and potassium ions, which irritate the free nerve endings.

For further reading on DOMS see the list of references at the end of this chapter.

2.3 FASCIAE AND INJURIES OCCURRING TO THEM

Fasciae are sheets of connective tissue which serve a number of functions in the body. Within the muscles they divide the muscle fibres into groups while thick sheets of fascia form the palmar and plantar fasciae of the hands and feet. These can be damaged through trauma or overuse, resulting in tears and/or inflammation. The plantar fascia, which forms a sheet of connective tissue under the foot, is a common site for injury in runners: explosive movements or overuse can cause **plantar fasciitis**. The specific site for this injury is commonly close to its attachment with the calcaneum bone of the heel (Figure 2.4).

2.4 TENDONS AND APONEUROSES

2.4.1 The structure and function of tendons and aponeuroses

In order for muscles to function they need to be attached to bones or, in a few cases, to other muscles. This is achieved through specialized connective tissue in the form of tendons or aponeuroses. **Tendons** are ribbon or cable like structures which attach muscles to bones. They are made of collagenous connective tissue continuous with that forming the epimysium, perimysium and endomysium of

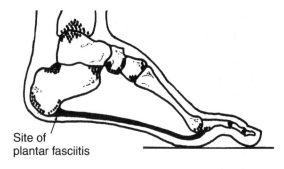

Figure 2.4 Plantar fasciitis.

the muscle. The region where the muscle and tendon join is referred to as the **musculotendinous junction**. At the other end of the tendon the connective tissue fuses with the connective tissue covering the bone (the **periosteum**), forming the region referred to as the **tenoperiosteal junction**. Tendons are made of collagen fibres, which are arranged in a parallel manner in order to withstand the tension they experience when the muscle contracts. The tissue is relatively strong and possesses only slight elasticity. Among the collagen fibres are fibroblasts and elastin protein which gives the tendon its limited elasticity.

An **aponeurosis** is similar to a tendon but is in the form of a sheet of connective tissue. This gives the muscle a broader area of attachment and may be used to attach muscle to bone or one muscle to another. The connective tissue within a muscle is similar to that of tendons and aponeuroses but the collagen fibres that make up the fasciae are arranged into an irregular network rather than being parallel.

In general, tendons have a relatively poor blood supply which, in the case of the Achilles tendon, is reported to deteriorate with age. The elasticity of the tendons is also reported to diminish with age, which can make them more vulnerable to damage in older individuals, especially when recommencing sport after a prolonged lay-off.

Many tendons are surrounded by a sheath made up of two layers, an inner **visceral layer**, which is situated next to the tendon, and an outer **parietal layer** (Figure 2.5).

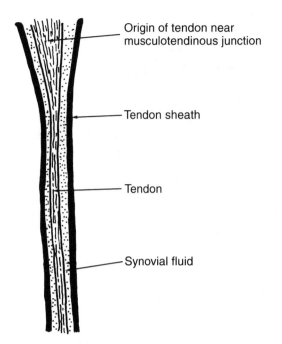

Figure 2.5   A tendon sheath.

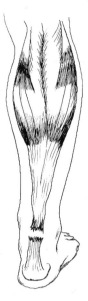

Figure 2.6   Achilles tendon rupture.

The space between the two contains a lubricating fluid which is similar to the synovial fluid found in joints. This protective sheath permits the tendon to move without causing excessive rubbing and friction with the surrounding tissues. However two of the largest tendons in the body, the Achilles and patellar tendons, do not possess this sheath but are in contact with the surrounding connective tissue.

2.4.2   Tendon injuries

Tendons may be damaged either through a traumatic injury or by overuse, which results in a repetitive strain injury. In some situations the repetitive strain placed upon a tendon may cause a number of microscopic tears in a localized area. This is known as **focal degeneration** and weakens the tendon, making it more vulnerable to rupture. Other degenerative disorders of the tendons include **tendinosis** while general inflammation of the tendon due to overuse is referred to as **tendinitis**.

Traumatic injuries to tendons include ruptures (strains) which result in a number of fibres being torn. These occur when the tendon experiences excessive strain during explosive movements such as sprinting or jumping. The degree of rupture can vary from the tearing of just a few fibres, which may go virtually unnoticed, to a complete rupture (Figure 2.6).

The latter may be heard as a snap and results in the loss of function of the tendon's associated muscle. Any degree of rupture will result in bleeding in the tendon, which must be minimized in order to facilitate the subsequent recovery process. Partial ruptures may be acute or chronic. In the case of the former the time of the rupture can be located to a specific incident whereas in the latter the state of partial rupture develops slowly. Here the onset of pain or discomfort is gradual and although present before exercise will often diminish when warming up only to return later. Continued, repeated bouts of exercise may cause a further deterioration of the condition of the tendon until the pain is persistent. However, there is a certain amount of debate about the classification of this chronic injury.

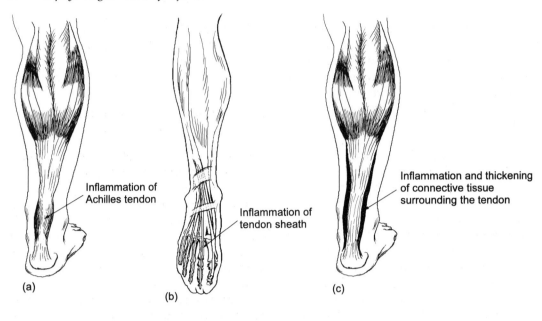

Inflammation of
Achilles tendon

Inflammation of
tendon sheath

Inflammation and thickening
of connective tissue
surrounding the tendon

(a)

(b)

(c)

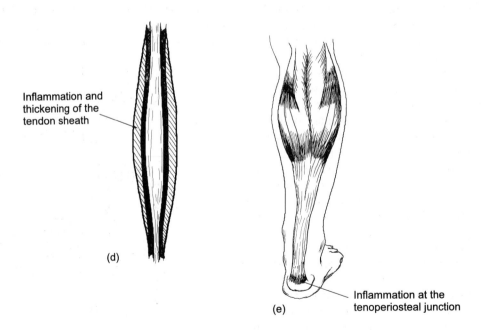

Inflammation and
thickening of the
tendon sheath

(d)

Inflammation at the
tenoperiosteal junction

(e)

Figure 2.7   Tendon pathologies. (a) Tendonitis or tendinitis.
(b) Tenosynovitis. (c) Paratendinitis or peritendinitis.
(d) Tenovaginitis. (e) Tenoperiostitis.

Overuse injuries to the tendon result in inflammation due to excessive friction, pressure or overload. This can result in inflammation of the tendon itself, the tendon sheath, the surrounding connective tissue and the attachment between the tendon and bone.

Injuries that result in the degeneration and/or inflammation of the tendon and/or its associated tissues can be classified in a number of ways. However it should also be remembered that it is possible for an injury to be complicated by involving a number of structures and therefore being in effect a mixed lesion. A variety of terms have been used to describe the different pathologies that affect tendons and the practitioner should be aware of the use of these different terminologies. A general description of the different tendon pathologies is given below and is illustrated in Figure 2.7.

- **Tendinitis** – inflammation of the tendon fibres. High heel tabs are often blamed for causing this in the Achilles tendon. In some cases a slight partial rupture of the tendon may be diagnosed and classified under this heading.
- **Tendinosis** – a degeneration of an area of the tendon caused by overuse.
- **Tenosynovitis** – inflammation of the tendon sheath. This sometimes occurs in the sheaths of the long tendons, such as those of the extensor carpi radialis of the forearm or the dorsiflexors of the foot. The latter is commonly caused by sports performers lacing their shoes too tightly, which results in excessive friction as the tendon moves.
- **Paratendinitis** – inflammation of the connective tissue that surrounds the tendon. This may occur in the tendons that lack a surrounding fluid-filled synovial sheath and is a relatively common overuse injury of the Achilles tendon where the surrounding paratenon becomes inflamed.
- **Tenovaginitis** – inflammation and thickening of the tendon sheath.

- **Tenoperiostitis** – inflammation of the attachment of the tendon to the bone in the region where the tendon joins the periosteum (tenoperiosteal junction).

2.5 THE PERIOSTEUM AND INJURIES TO THE PERIOSTEUM

The periosteum is a sheet of connective tissue that covers the bone. Its collagenous fibres are continuous with those of the tendon and the two combine to form the tenoperiosteal junction. When a muscle contracts the force is transferred to the bone via the tendon and periosteum. The pulling action of the muscle is therefore transferred to the periosteum, which can become inflamed (periostitis) through excessive strain or repeated overuse. In some cases damage to the underlying bone is also reported. A relatively common injury of this type in juniors is Osgood–Schlatter's disease (Figure 2.8).

This is caused by the repeated strain placed on the periosteum by the patellar tendon, which joins the tibia in the region of the growth plate. The repeated pulling of the

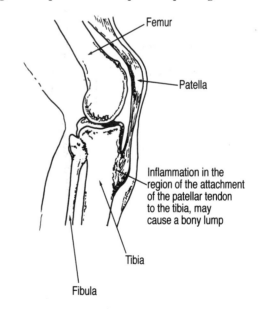

Femur

Patella

Inflammation in the region of the attachment of the patellar tendon to the tibia, may cause a bony lump

Tibia

Fibula

Figure 2.8 Osgood-Schlatter's disease.

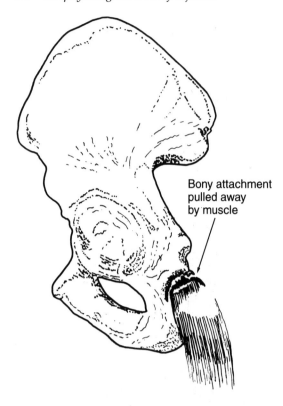

Figure 2.9   Avulsion fracture.

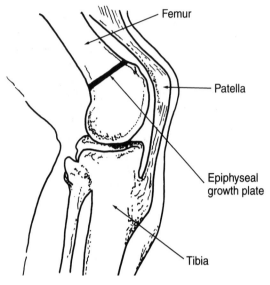

Figure 2.10   Epiphyseal fractures.

tendon in this region can damage the bone, causing inflammation, tenderness, swelling and the development of a bony lump.

However, in some cases when excessive force is experienced in the tenoperiosteal region, the tendons and periosteum are of sufficient strength for it to be the bone itself that breaks away, resulting in an avulsion fracture (Figure 2.9). Avulsion fractures occur in juniors rather than adults because of the relative strengths of their tendons, muscles and bone, the immature skeleton of juniors being relatively weak compared to the mature adult skeleton.

2.6   BONES AND BONE INJURIES

Bones provide the body with support and protect vital organs. The joint system of the body enables the bones to act as levers for movement and to absorb the forces of impact when performing activities such as running.

Like the other tissues of the body the bones may be damaged through a traumatic injury or overuse. A fracture that results from a collision, violent impact or shearing force will require immediate medical treatment. The exact nature of the fracture or avulsion fracture (where the force of contraction has resulted in the tendon pulling away a small piece of bone) will depend upon a number of factors. In children fractures may also occur in the region of the epiphyseal growth plates (Figure 2.10) which is an area of relative weakness.

Here, a blow to the side of the bone, perhaps through tackling in soccer or rugby, may cause the bone to shear at the growth plate. However in the case of any traumatic fracture the obvious need for medical attention makes such injuries beyond the scope of this book.

On the other hand, overuse injuries, which develop more slowly are commonly presented to the physiotherapist who must diagnose them and treat them. Any coach must likewise be aware of the potential for these

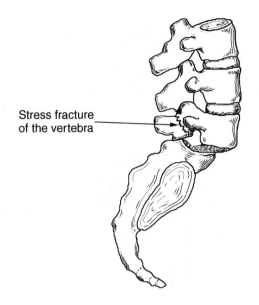

Stress fracture
of the vertebra

Figure 2.11 Spondylolysis.

seemingly insidious injuries to develop in
his/her performers.

Repeated stress on the bones can result in
stress fractures. For example, activities that
require repeated hyperextension of the spine,
such as gymnastics, can result in stress fractures of the vertebrae such as **spondylolysis**
(Figure 2.11), while endurance runners and
those who experience a lot of impact from
hard surfaces such as squash players may
develop stress fracture in the bones of the
legs and feet.

In these cases the most common sites for
stress fractures are the tibia, fibula, calcaneum
of the heel and the third and fourth metatarsals. Such injuries are often the result of
increasing the amount of training or competition too rapidly.

In young children whose bones are not fully
mature, additional injuries may occur to the
epiphyseal growth plates of the long bones
(Figure 2.12).

Since these areas are made of cartilage in
the immature skeleton, they are more vulnerable to injury. At maturity these growth plates
ossify into bone and are therefore not a problem for adults. Epiphyseal plate overuse

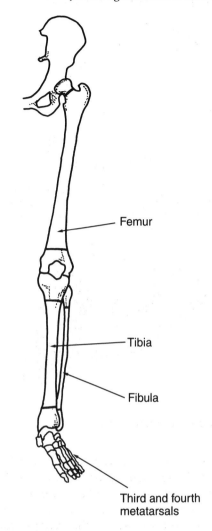

Femur

Tibia

Fibula

Third and fourth
metatarsals

Figure 2.12 Epiphyseal growth plate injuries.

injuries include premature epiphyseal closure, where the growth plate ossifies prematurely due to repeated stress. This prevents
the bone from lengthening any further and
may therefore stunt its growth.

2.7 JOINTS, LIGAMENTS AND BURSAE

2.7.1 The general structure of joints

While there are several types of joint in the
human body, including synovial, fibrous and

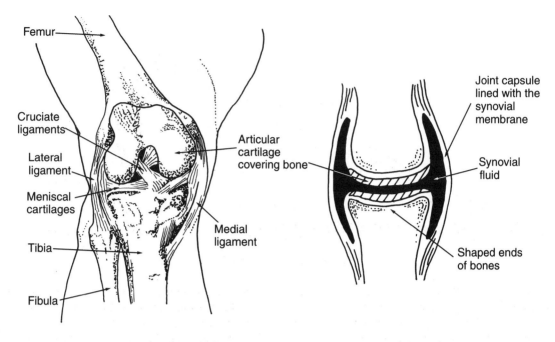

Figure 2.13   General structure of a synovial joint.

cartilaginous, it is the **synovial joints** that are usually the concern of the practitioner. These joints permit movement between adjoining bones, the direction and range of permissible movement being determined by factors such as the shape of the bones, the joint capsule, associated ligaments and the muscles that work across the joint. The general structure of a synovial joint is illustrated in Figure 2.13.

A synovial joint possesses a cavity containing **synovial fluid**, which lubricates it. The cavity is enclosed by a **joint capsule**, which is lined with a **synovial membrane** that produces the synovial fluid. Within the cavity the articulating bones are shaped and covered with a layer of articular cartilage (**hyaline cartilage**). This is hard-wearing and prevents excessive wear on the bone. Other cartilage within the joint can act as cushioning and provide the bones with greater stability when they move. **Ligaments** within and around the joint provide further stability and prevent excessive or unwanted movement, while permitting movement in the desired directions.

Ligaments are made of collagen protein and are relatively inelastic. **Bursae** are fluid-filled sacs found around joints and other moving structures. They prevent friction occurring when structures move across each other. For example, if a tendon was to move across a bone it would soon become inflamed and damaged by the repeated friction. However, the presence of a bursa situated between the two structures limits the amount of friction experienced. The functioning of the bursa can be imagined as being like a fluid-filled balloon one side of which can move while the other remains stationary.

2.7.2   Ligament injuries

Ligaments are damaged when they are overstretched. This occurs when a joint is forced beyond its normal range of movement in a particular direction. A sprained ankle is an example of this: the ligaments on the lateral side of the ankle are overstretched (Figure 2.14). Ligament injuries can range from a

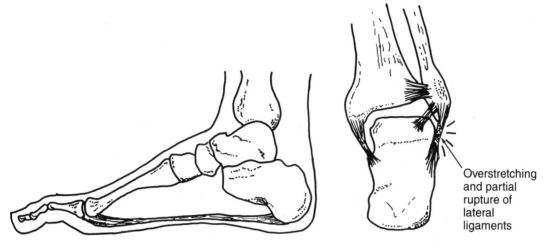

Figure 2.14   Sprained ankle.

slight overstretching to a complete rupture (Figure 2.15). Ligaments can also be damaged by overuse: for example, the elbow is a common site of injury in javelin-throwers.

2.7.3   Bursa injuries

The function of the bursae is to minimize the amount of friction experienced by moving structures and hence prevent inflammation, but with repeated overuse they can become inflamed (**bursitis**) (Figure 2.16).

They can also be damaged by a blow that causes the overproduction of fluid and swelling, which results in them pressing too firmly on the surrounding tissues. This then causes additional friction and inflammation.

2.7.4   Joint injuries

A sudden impact on a limb or a violent twisting action can damage a joint by stretching the

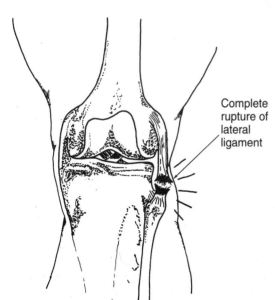

Figure 2.15   Ruptured ligaments.

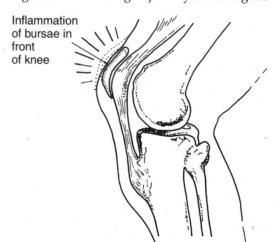

Figure 2.16   Bursitis.

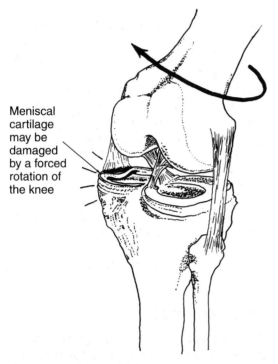

Figure 2.17   Meniscal injuries.

Meniscal cartilage may be damaged by a forced rotation of the knee

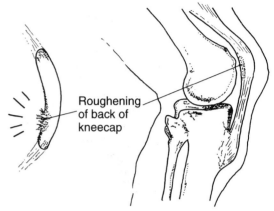

Roughening of back of kneecap

Figure 2.18   Chondromalacia patellae.

It is also possible in some injuries for pieces of bone to flake off into the joint cavity. This is the condition of **osteochondritis dissecans** (Figure 2.19), which can cause pain and locking of the joint if the bony flakes become trapped.

ligaments. This can also result in the overproduction of fluid within the joint, which causes it to swell. Bleeding into a joint also causes swelling and will require drainage. Other structures that can be damaged within a joint are the **cartilages**. For example, the meniscal cartilages of the knee can be pinched and frayed by an inappropriate movement such as twisting the knee (Figure 2.17).

Joints are also prone to overuse injuries. The cartilages of the joint are again vulnerable, as are the articular cartilages, which can degenerate through overuse. Examples of these include chondromalacia patellae, in which there is a roughening of the back of the kneecap (Figure 2.18), and osteoarthritis of the articular cartilage.

Contributing factors causing chondromalacia patellae are a malalignment of the kneecap, muscular imbalance and a large Q angle caused by relatively wide hips (more common in females), each of which can result in the patella tracking across the head of the femur.

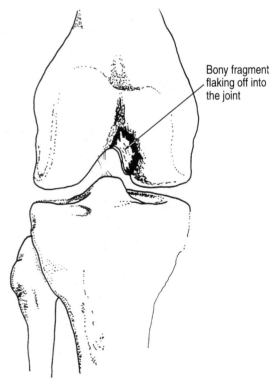

Bony fragment flaking off into the joint

Figure 2.19   Osteochondritis dissecans.

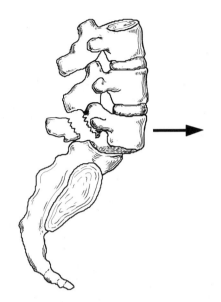

Figure 2.20 Spondylolisthesis.

swimmers, is **spondylolisthesis**. This is caused by repeated hyperflexion of the back and results in the vertebrae being moved out of alignment, most commonly in the region of the fifth lumbar vertebrae (Figure 2.20).

A blow to a joint, or overuse, such as excessive running on a hard surface, may cause **synovitis**, which is the overproduction of synovial fluid by the synovial membrane, causing the joint to swell. A very severe blow to a joint may cause its dislocation (Figure 2.21).

This may be partial (**subluxation**) or complete (**luxation**). In either case there is likely to be damage to the associated joint capsule, ligaments and other joint structures.

Another overuse injury, which is quite common among female gymnasts and butterfly

2.8 CONCLUSION

Having briefly reviewed the types of tissue injuries which can occur through participa-

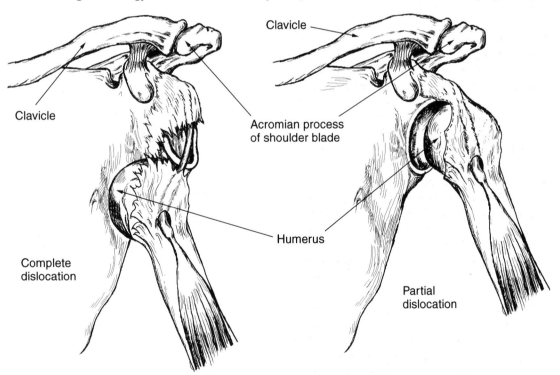

Figure 2.21 Joint dislocation.

tion in sport, in the following chapters we shall describe the procedures that may be employed during the processes of diagnosis, treatment and rehabilitation. The remaining chapters then discuss the injuries commonly associated with particular sports and refer these injuries back to the sections on diagnosis, treatment and rehabilitation.

2.9   FURTHER READING

2.9.1   Delayed-onset muscle soreness (DOMS)

Cleak, M.J. and Eston, R. G. (1992) Delayed onset muscle soreness: mechanisms and management. *Journal of Sports Sciences*, 10(4), 325–341.

Gleeson, M., Almey, J., Brooks, S. *et al.* (1995) Hematological and acute phase responses associated with delayed-onset muscle soreness in humans. *European Journal of Applied Physiology and Occupational Physiology*, 17, 137–142.

Hagerman, F.C., Hikida, R.S., Staron, R.S. *et al.* (1984). Muscle damage in marathon runners. *Physician and Sportsmedicine*, 12, 39–48.

Kuipers, H. (1994) Exercise-induced muscle damage. *International Journal of Sports Medicine*, 15(3), 132–135

McIntyre. D.L., Reid, W.D. and McKenzie, D.C. (1995) The inflammatory response to muscle injury and its clinical implications. *Sports Medicine*, 20, 24–40.

Pyne, D. (1994) Exercise induced muscle damage and inflammation: a review. *Australian Journal of Science and Medicine in Sport*, 26, 49–58.

Schwane, J.A., Johnson, S.R., Vandenakker, C.B. and Armstrong, R.B. (1983). Delayed-onset muscular soreness and plasma CPK and LDH activities after downhill running. *Medicine and Science in Sports and Exercise*, 15, 51–56.

Schwane, J.A., Watrous, B.G., Johnson, S.R. and Armstrong, R.B. (1983). Is lactic acid related to delayed-onset muscle soreness? *Physician and Sportsmedicine*, 11(3), 124–131.

Smith, L.L., Fulmer, M.G., Holbert, D. *et al.* (1994) The impact of a repeated bout of eccentric exercise on muscular strength, muscle soreness and creatine kinase. *British Journal of Sports Medicine*, 28(4), 267–271.

Talag, TS. (1973) Residual muscular soreness as influenced by concentric, eccentric and static contractions. *Research quarterly*, 44, 458–469.

2.9.2 Muscle fibre type

Bar-Or, O., Dotan, R., Inbar, O. *et al.* (1980) Anaerobic capacity and muscle fibre type distribution in man. *International Journal of Sports Medicine*, 1(2), 82–85.

Costill, D.L., Daniels, J., Evans, W. *et al.* (1976) Skeletal muscle enzymes and fibre composition in male and female track athletes. *Journal of Applied Physiology*, 40, 149–154

Flynn, M.G., Costill, D.L., Kirwan, J.P. *et al.* (1987) Muscle fiber composition and respiratory capacity in triathletes. *International Journal of Sports Medicine*, 8(6), 383–386.

Geraerd, E.S., Caiozzo, V.J., Rubin, B.D. (1986) Skeletal muscle profiles among elite long, middle and short distance swimmers. *American Journal of Sports Medicine*, 14(1), 77–82.

Gollnick, P.D. and Matoba, H. (1984) The muscle fibre composition of skeletal muscle as a predictor of athletic success. *American Journal of Sports Medicine*, 12(3), 212–217.

Hickson, R.C., Hidaka, K. and Foster, C. (1994) Skeletal muscle fiber type, resistance training and strength related performance. *Medicine and Science in Sports and Exercise*, 26(5), 593–598.

Mero, A., Jaakkola, L. and Komi, P.V. (1991) Relationship between muscle fibre characteristics and physical performance capacity in trained athletic boys. *Journal of Sports Sciences*, 9(2), 161–171

Mikesky, A.E., Giddings, C.J., Matthews, W. and Gonyea, W.J. (1991) Changes in muscle fiber size and composition in response to heavy resistance exercise. *Medicine and Science in Sports and Exercise*, 23(9), 1042–1049.

Miller, A.E., MacDougall, J.D., Tarnopolsky, M.A. and Sale, D.G. (1993) Gender differences in strength and muscle fiber characteristics. *European Journal of Applied and Occupational Physiology*, 66(3), 254–262.

Tesch, P.A., Wright, J.E., Vogel, J.A. *et al.* (1985) The influence of muscle metabolic characteristics on physical performance. *European Journal of Applied Physiology and Occupational Physiology*, 54(3), 237–243.

3. *The immediate diagnosis of an injury and appropriate action*

3.1 INTRODUCTION

As mentioned earlier in this text the immediate actions taken by the practitioner when presented with an injured sports performer will depend upon a number of different factors. Obvious differences will depend upon whether the practitioner is in attendance and observes the occurrence of the injury or conversely whether s/he first sees the person/injury a number of hours or even days after its occurrence.

3.2 DIAGNOSIS AND ACTION IF DEALING WITH AN INJURY IMMEDIATELY AFTER ITS OCCURRENCE

If the practitioner is in attendance and is the allocated person to take control of the situation then the following guideline procedures should be followed if possible. Unfortunately the real world of sports medicine often prevents things from happening this way, but despite any restrictions the practitioner must always be striving to achieve as close to the ideal as possible.

1. Identification as to whether the injury is life-threatening or otherwise. The required action in the case of life-threatening injuries will include standard medical procedures which are beyond the scope of this text.
2. If the injury is not considered to be life-threatening then the practitioner must decide whether it is feasible for the person to continue playing/competing in the event. This decision will also require considerations of whether they may recommence playing/competing immediately or whether some form of treatment is required before they can do so.
3. If it is likely that the person will be able to continue participating in the event the practitioner has to then consider whether any treatment will be performed on the spot or whether it is necessary to move the individual to another area. For example the application of strapping or stitches would normally be applied off the field of play in order to permit the game to continue with the injured player returning once the treatment had been completed.
4. If the practitioner considers that the injured person is not going to be able to continue participating in the event or expresses his/her belief that the individual should not carry on, then s/he must again consider where any treatment should take place or indeed whether any further investigation is required prior to the commencement of treatment – e.g. an X-ray where a fracture is suspected or a medical consultation where there has been a laceration or momentary loss of consciousness.
5. If the practitioner considers that no further investigation is required then any treatment must begin as quickly as possible or practical – a light compressional support or cold pack may be applied on the field and maintained in place while the player is carried off the pitch and back to the dressing room. Facilities

within the dressing or treatment room should be arranged so that the sportsperson is positioned comfortably with the limb in elevation. The practitioner should work quickly and efficiently, asking questions about exactly what happened, what the person felt immediately and how it feels now, prior to the removal of the support or cold application. Only when all relevant questions have been asked should the injured area be exposed and diagnosis attempted or treatment progressed.

3.3 GUIDELINES FOR IMMEDIATE TREATMENT AT THE SITE OF THE INCIDENT

Immediate treatment always begins with an attempted diagnosis. 'Attempted' is the correct word to use as it is often difficult to be sure, even if the cause of injury was witnessed by the practitioner. Experience is obviously valuable, but even the most experienced practitioners can find an initial on-site diagnosis very difficult. Fractures or dislocations are often obvious but meniscal or ligamentous lesions are likely to be more difficult to identify because of their initial symptoms. At this stage the aim is to decide how best to minimize the inflammatory reaction with immediate first aid measures, thereby giving more time for non-pressurized thought. Myofilament (muscular) damage develops and reaches its maximum after 2 hours, cellular damage and cell death continue for at least a further 22 hours in the absence of any further trauma to the area. Trauma must therefore be minimized. For example it is not necessarily an overreaction to carry a player from the field who has 'sprained' his/her ankle, or for a competitor to be stretchered out of the arena after falling from a trampoline when s/he could probably walk.

During these initial stages the practitioner will be assessing the emotional state of the person. Care must be taken when dealing with the injured performer. S/he may be devastated at having sustained the injury in the final of a competition for which s/he had been preparing for months or even years and the wrong words or an apparent lack of understanding at this time could destroy the early treatment programme. Indeed there is a growing body of evidence to support the importance of applied psychology in the treatment of any sports injury; which, if used correctly, can enhance the treatment programme and improve the injured sports performer's attitude to the recovery process and his/her return to competitive sport.

Following an injury the immediate physical treatment modalities will tend to be based broadly around the RICE principles – rest, ice, compression and elevation.

3.3.1 Rest

It is generally assumed that 'rest' does not require any real discussion; unfortunately this is a mistake that is often made. The extent of the rest needs to be identified and may include:

- rest from the activity during which the injury occurred;
- rest from irritable sporting activities;
- rest from sport generally;
- rest from normal functional activities;
- rest that involves little physical activity and generally keeping the feet up;
- total rest, i.e. staying on or in bed!

The practicalities of any advice concerning rest need to be taken into consideration: for example, whereas it may be feasible for a professional sportsperson to rest in bed for 24 hours it could be totally impractical for someone else who has no choice but to go to work the next day. Often the best approach is to explain the reasons behind the ideal circumstances, then discuss the practicalities and see how close to the ideal can be achieved. It is also necessary to discuss time scales at this stage. People generally need a reasonable indication of how long they may have to spend on total rest or similar. However it is often difficult to be sure about time scales at this stage so the reasons for this should be explained and an indication of time given, e.g. 'at least 2 days' or 'until there is no pain when you sit up' or 'until there is no pain when you put your foot on the floor'.

Testing the injury is something that should be avoided at this stage. People generally seem to have a desire to regularly 'see how it feels'. Often it is necessary to explain that *testing* the injury means further trauma and that it will only prolong the time away from training or competition.

3.3.2 Ice or cold therapy (cryotherapy)

Although it seems to be generally accepted that ice is an unquestionable element of immediate treatment there are some queries about its use that do need to be considered seriously. These include:

- the type of injury;
- the method of application;
- the timing and frequency of application.

Individual practitioners may also differ in their use of ice, some applying it in the treatment of 'acute' injuries while others use it in the more 'chronic' phases of injury rehabilitation. Indeed some use ice in the same way for both acute and chronic problems.

In general there seems to be agreement that cold:

- is analgesic;
- reduces tissue metabolism;
- reduces spasm and hypercontraction;
- minimizes secondary cell death.

There is however some controversy over the effects of cold on the local circulation. The basic issue is whether cold increases or decreases local blood flow. Most theories on this are based around personal interpretations of the 'hunting response', which is a cyclical response to cooling. In the 'hunting response'

the application of ice or cold causes an initial vasoconstriction of the blood vessels in the superficial tissues. This is then followed some time later by a reflex cyclical vasodilation, the effect of which is to reduce the likelihood of frostbite and serious damage to the tissues. These changes in blood flow to the superficial tissues are repeated in a cyclical manner and can be observed with changes in the colour of the skin. However in the deeper tissues it appears that there is a much more gradual and less marked cooling effect which does not produce such dramatic cyclical responses.

In practical terms it seems to be generally accepted that the sooner the cold is applied the better and wherever possible it should be applied in elevation. There may also be an additional advantage in maintaining compression simultaneously. Cold application should be maintained in place for 20–30 minutes and in an ideal world this would be repeated every 2 hours for the first 24–48 hours.

If the injury involves minor superficial bleeding or haematoma within the tissues then care must be taken not to create a dramatic cyclical response as this could increase rather than decrease the bleeding within the tissues. In these cases it is therefore important to avoid severe cold by having a number of layers of damp towelling or similar between the cooling medium and the skin, as well as reducing the timing of application to perhaps only 10–15 minutes, although it could be performed more regularly.

There is no evidence to suggest that cold therapy is of direct value in reducing a joint effusion once it has already formed. However this does not mean that it is of no value; indeed it may be used as an analgesic, or as a means of reducing spasm or tissue metabolism, and in these circumstances it could be of great benefit.

Practitioners have to form their own views on which of the many different methods of cold application are the most practical and effective, although as a guide most research seems to show that ice in a crushed form is generally a very acceptable method. However, care should be taken with the application of ice directly on to the skin as it can result in ice burns, and therefore at least one layer of damp towelling or protective oil should be applied to the skin.

3.3.3   Compression

The use of compression is generally advocated for the following reasons:

- to limit the available space for the progression of 'swelling' or haematoma formation – this applies particularly to the extremities of both upper and lower limbs where gravity related to anatomical relationships inhibits fluid removal;
- to improve the muscle pump mechanism, encouraging more efficient fluid removal;
- to provide comfortable support, thereby reducing the pain/spasm component of the injury.

Points to remember when applying compression are as follows.

- Wherever possible remove and re-apply in elevation.
- Pad around bony or 'lumpy' prominent areas.
- Compression should be applied from distal to proximal, i.e. from the bottom towards the top.
- Make sure the compression is not too tight. The person should not leave for at least 10–15 minutes so that you can check the circulation at that stage and ensure that he/she is informed about removing the strapping if they experience any more than 'mild' compressional circulatory discomfort.
- Make sure the person has no allergies to the adhesive element of the tape or bandage

used and that any cuts or grazes are cleaned and covered as appropriate.

One of the most questionable elements about compression is the subjectivity based around strapping being 'too tight' or 'too loose'.

3.3.4   Elevation

Unfortunately most sportspeople seem to think that elevation involves simply 'putting their feet up' or 'resting their arm/hand on a pillow'. It therefore needs to be explained to them that elevation is about comfortably supporting the limb in a position so that there is minimal resistance to venous and lymphatic drainage from the injury site back to the heart. This means that sitting with the foot on a stool when they have an acutely swollen ankle or knee is not the most effective form of elevation (Figure 3.1). To be effective the limb must be raised above the level of the heart and maintained there if practically possible.

3.4   OTHER FACTORS TO BE CONSIDERED DURING THE ACUTE PHASE

During the 'immediate diagnosis and treatment' phase the practitioner may use any of the previously mentioned techniques and is also likely to discuss with the sportsperson the plan for the next 24–48 hours, or until the person is to be seen again. Depending on the relationship between the practitioner and injured person numerous practicalities will

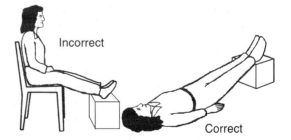

Figure 3.1   Correct and incorrect elevation.

need to be considered and/or discussed. These include the following.

- Can the person be 'trusted' to rest or do they need to have some form of strapping that does not allow him/her to move the injured area? Sometimes it is necessary to 'overimmobilize' the injured area in order to prevent the person from going out, drowning his/her sorrows and ending up at the local disco, the result of which could be a considerable amount of additional trauma to the injured site.
- Does the person with an acute ankle or knee ligament 'sprain' need to be strapped and put on crutches despite the fact that they can walk, albeit with a painful limp? Struggling along with a limp may cause further damage; remember that the aim is to minimize further irritation and thus encourage a speedy resolution.
- Non-alcoholic fluid intake should be maximized, as should the maintenance of a nutritious diet, bearing in mind that the body's systems need fluid, nutrients and energy to heal and rebuild the damaged tissues. Unless it is contraindicated for some reason it is not unreasonable to allow the individual to partake of some alcohol if s/he would normally do so. Being injured can be pretty miserable and there is no real value in depriving the individual of other pleasures.
- Since it is generally accepted that the injury will heal more efficiently with the positive stimulus of pain-free muscular activity and its associated biophysiological effects, the individual should be encouraged to perform any pain-free exercise as regularly as possible. It is often best to write these down for him/her and to practise all the exercises to be performed with him/her so that you can be fairly sure that they will be done correctly and that there is no possibility of the exercises causing further irritation.

- The use of oral anti-inflammatories and painkillers needs to be considered during this period. The thing to remember about anti-inflammatories is that they inhibit the naturally occurring prostaglandin response to injury and thus inhibit platelet aggregation, which can lead to prolonged bleeding and bruising. In practical terms they are probably safe to use where there is an inflammatory reaction with no bleeding in the tissues, but where there is any possibility of tissue trauma and associated haematoma it is best to avoid anti-inflammatories or painkillers for at least the first 24 hours following the injury.

3.5 INVESTIGATIONS OR CONSULTATIONS FOLLOWING ON FROM IMMEDIATE DIAGNOSIS AND TREATMENT

As previously mentioned, suspected fractures may need X-ray investigation, dislocations may need manipulation with or without general anaesthesia and then to be monitored for signs of neural compression. The rapid development of swelling at a joint may well be caused by haemarthrosis, which would be best treated by early aspiration. The complete rupture of certain ligaments may best be treated by early surgery or will at least require a surgical opinion. Any trauma to the head that led to a loss of consciousness or concussion will also require a medical or neurological assessment. During the immediate assessment period all these possibilities must be considered and action taken where appropriate.

3.6 DIAGNOSTIC CONSIDERATIONS AT THE SCENE OF INJURY

Chapter 6 deals with the specific diagnostic, assessment and treatment principles related to particular body parts. This is followed by sections later in this text that are devoted to considering the injuries that commonly occur in specific sports and a list of these injuries is given at the end of each section. Organizing the text in this manner should enable the reader to cross reference between these sections for more complicated differential diagnostic procedures. This particular section is therefore limited to 'on site' diagnostic considerations.

3.6.1   The diagnosis of bone injuries

The majority of injuries caused to bone are a result of:

- direct trauma caused by contact;
- severe excessive movement;
- movement in an unusual direction;
- repetitive trauma caused by overuse.

Direct trauma does not have to involve a blow, kick or contact with another sports performer. It is often the result of a fall on to an outstretched arm or similar incident. The practitioner will come across a variety of bony injuries that will have been caused by numerous factors. These include fractured fibulas caused by kicks, fractures to the arm from falls, stress fractures of the tibia, fibula or metatarsals in runners and stress fractures of the carpal bones in young gymnasts. Adolescents in particular can also suffer from avulsion fractures in the absence of any direct trauma and this has to be considered, especially when the pain relates to the ischial tuberosity or anterior superior iliac spine at the front of the pelvis.

Osteochondritic lesions also occur in the adolescent age group and involve a softening of the bone, which may be related to a temporary interference of its blood supply. Diagnostically, when a young or adolescent sportsperson presents with bony soreness, with or without obvious trauma, particularly around the foot, knee, wrist or elbow, osteochondritis has to be a consideration.

Osteoporosis, which can affect both males and females of all ages but especially women, will increase the likelihood of both stress and traumatic fractures. Dietary deficiencies and menstrual abnormalities, particularly in female athletes, increase the risk of these fractures because of hormonal imbalances which prevent the normal deposition of calcium in the bone, causing it to become weakened.

If the practitioner is presented with an individual suffering from local, palpable bone pain where there has been considerable local trauma or a severe excessive movement the possibility of fracture has to be considered and an X-ray investigation should be initiated if possible. How the practitioner explains the need for this to the injured person is critical, particularly if there is going to be an overnight delay for any reason. Stress fractures rarely show up on a 'normal' X-ray, particularly in less than 3 weeks. In fact it is only the newly developing callus around the site of injury that becomes evident. A radioisotope scan is therefore a necessary procedure in the investigation of a possible stress fracture.

3.6.2   The diagnosis of dislocations with or without fracture

With most dislocations there is a severe loss of function and an associated altered anatomical contour compared to the opposite side of the body. In such cases there is always the possibility of an associated avulsion fracture so an X-ray should be performed. Subluxations (partial dislocations) where the joint moves 'out of place' then relocates are usually picked up by the sportsperson's description of what they felt and observation of the incident, or alternatively a description of what occurred. However, there is still the possibility of an avulsion fracture, with the severity of the symptoms determining whether an X-ray is required. In these injuries there can also be severe trauma to the supportive tissue which will require immediate treatment. This is usually followed by a lengthy rehabilitation period which will attempt to stabilize the traumatized joint. Practitioners should always be on the look out for signs of associated neurological injury which can be caused by compressional trauma at the time of the injury and afterwards.

3.6.3 The diagnosis of injury to joint-related structures (joint capsule and ligaments)

Excessive or unusual movements with or without contact or direct trauma can put an excessive strain on to the supportive joint capsule and ligaments. These movements will lead to local inflammation causing pain, limitation of movement, sometimes swelling and a possible redness of the skin. A capsular effusion with relatively minor ligamentous damage may be quite painful from the onset but the swelling will develop relatively slowly, i.e. over a few hours or overnight. More severe ligamentous damage involving partial or complete rupture will lead to the development of swelling very quickly in the form of haemarthrosis and will occur in the region of 30–45 minutes. Therefore to a certain extent the speed and type of swelling can go some way towards indicating the severity of the injury and the structures involved. A knowledge of the mechanism of injury will obviously be very important in the diagnosis along with the local palpation of specific structures, assessment of the range of irritation-free movement and the reaction to the resisted action of related neuromusculotendinous units. This therefore highlights the need to have very good anatomical knowledge of the injured part.

3.6.4 The diagnosis of meniscal (fibrous cartilaginous) lesions

By far the commonest site of meniscal lesions is the knee joint, although similar problems occur in the wrist and even occasionally in the elbow. A common cause of such injury is femoral internal rotation on a fixed foot

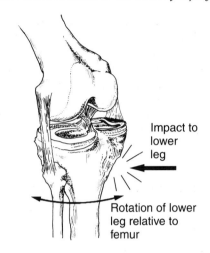

Impact to lower leg

Rotation of lower leg relative to femur

Figure 3.2 The causes of meniscal damage.

while weightbearing on a semiflexed knee (Figure 3.2).

Since the tibial collateral (medial) ligament is attached to the medial meniscus it is quite common to damage both structures simultaneously. Therefore in the early stages following injury any attempted stress tests for the meniscal structures are quite likely to traumatize the tibial collateral ligament and could possibly give a false impression of the injury. What this basically means is that it may be impossible to be sure of the extent of any meniscal damage until other structures become more settled, or at least a couple of days have passed, which will enable an observation of the injured part's reactions to time and treatments. At this stage a full explanation of the relationship between the structures is necessary, along with an indication of the likelihood and extent of meniscal and ligamentous damage.

Sometimes there is obvious meniscal damage which will lead to a locking of the joint, making the person unable to bend or straighten the knee past a certain point, as well as an associated clicking/bulging. This is a very definite sign and one that should merit the seeking of an orthopaedic opinion as quickly as possible. However it should be remembered that other loose or foreign bodies within the joint can also mimic a meniscal lesion.

Finally, it is worth noting that it is possible to damage the meniscal tissue without any major or obvious trauma. Previous injuries or trauma are often forgotten about, resulting in a situation where only a very minor twist or strain is necessary to extend a minor tear into a lesion that interferes with 'normal' joint mechanics.

3.6.5   The diagnosis of injury to muscles and tendons

The majority of injuries to musculotendinous structures involve **strains** or partial tears, as stated in Chapter 2. Complete muscular ruptures are relatively rare and usually occur with severe trauma or laceration, e.g. running into a sharp object or similar. However, moderate to severe blunt trauma to a muscle quite commonly initiates myositis ossificans, as discussed in section 2.2.4(a) (see Chapter 6 for an explanation of treatment procedures for this condition).

Partial or complete ruptures of tendons are more common, although thankfully still rare. When they occur the sportsperson will commonly describe a feeling of being 'shot' in the back of the leg when the Achilles tendon ruptures. These ruptures most commonly occur in people whose tendons have lost some of their tensile strength and elasticity because of either a previous injury or a period of relative inactivity followed by the introduc-

tion of a new fitness drive or a sudden increase in exercise intensity.

Complete ruptures are also seen in the body-building and weight-lifting groups: massive weights are used, putting the musculotendinous, tendon and tendon insertion components under enormous stress, which can lead to complete tears. In some cases there may also be a link with the use of anabolic steroids, which result in a rapid gain in muscular size and strength without the same rapid changes in the tensile strength of the associated tendons, whose structure may be adversely affected by the use of steroids, the overall effect of which is the overloading of these tissues and their subsequent rupture.

When testing for the complete rupture of a tendon there will often be a palpable gap at the site of the rupture, which may or may not be painful to pressure. Above the rupture there will be some 'bunching' of the muscular fibres and it may be a lot more painful at that point. Occasionally, complete ruptures of the tendon are misdiagnosed as severe muscular lesions because of the pain in the lower muscular area. Active movement may be pain inhibited or impossible if there is no other muscle capable of producing the same or a similar movement. Often there is no reaction of the distal element of the limb when the muscle belly is squeezed passively: for instance, when the Achilles tendon is ruptured, squeezing the gastrocnemius will produce no or minimal plantarflexion of the foot compared to the other side (see Chapter 6 for more details).

4. The assessment of the sports performer in the context of the causes and prevention of overuse injuries

4.1 INTRODUCTION

This chapter will attempt to define 'overuse injuries' and then devote a number of specific sections to the general causes of sports injuries, as outlined in Chapter 1. Within these sections examples will be given of assessment and the investigative procedures to be carried out when dealing with these types of injury.

4.2 OVERUSE INJURIES

In general terms an overuse injury is one that transpires without any specific direct or obvious indirect trauma. They tend to occur in activities that involve the repetition of similar actions or postures over a prolonged period of time. Sports with a relatively high incidence of overuse injuries are running, swimming and cycling. Similarly, other sports such as tennis, gymnastics, golf, weightlifting and javelin throwing, which require the repetitive practice of one element of the activity, also carry a high risk of overuse injuries. However this does not mean that all the injuries occurring in the above or similar sports are overuse injuries, since those of a traumatic nature can also occur. Likewise, overuse injuries can occur in sports such as rugby, soccer and hockey although they tend to appear less frequently than the more traumatic injuries associated with these sports.

4.3 THE CAUSES OF OVERUSE INJURIES

The general causes of overuse injuries are listed below; considering these factors and taking appropriate action where required will considerably reduce the risk of injury occurrence.

- Inadequate fitness and physical weakness (Chapter 1)
- Inappropriate training (Chapter 1)
- Lack of recovery (Chapter 1)
- Somatotype, postural and anatomical factors
- Muscular imbalance and weakness
- Biomechanical factors and gait analysis
- Neuro-muscular skeletal imbalance
- Prior injury
- Overloading due to repetition of specific action.

4.3.1 Somatotype, postural and anatomical factors

(a) Somatotype

It is well known that different sports place different physical stresses upon the participants' bodies: for example the stresses of marathon running are very different to those of javelin-throwing. It is also a fact that particular body types and body shapes are more or less able to tolerate these stresses. A consequence of this is that if an individual participates in a sport

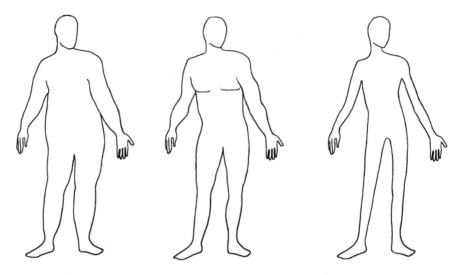

Figure 4.1   Extreme somatotypes. **(a)** Endomorph. **(b)** Mesomorph. **(c)** Ectomorph.

to which his/her body is not suited they will be more susceptible to injury. An individual's body type (**somatotype**) is largely determined by his/her genetics and can only be altered to a limited extent. An individual's somatotype is described by rating the preponderance of three components: endomorphy, mesomorphy and ectomorphy, which can be assessed using a number of scientific methods. The higher the rating for each of these the greater its preponderance in the individual's somatotype. Where individuals are predominantly of one component, i.e. they are rated highly on that component but very low on the others, they may be described as being a classic endomorph or mesomorph or ectomorph (Figure 4.1).

Each of these components can be described as follows:

- **endomorphy** – the roundness and fatness of the individual;
- **mesomorphy** – the muscularity of the individual;
- **ectomorphy** – the linearity of the individual.

Individuals with particular body types tend to gravitate towards the sports to which they are most suited, examples of which are given below:

- **mesomorphs** – male gymnasts, javelin-throwers, body-builders;
- **ectomorphs** – marathon runners;
- **endomorphs** – Often a feature of weight lifters and throwers although the additional fat may not necessarily be an advantage and therefore most top class sports performers tend to have a low endomorphy rating. However at a lower standard there is often an increase in the body fat component of the participants and hence his/her endomorphy rating.

Some sports require a high preponderance of more than one component; for example basketball players tend to have somatotypes that are both mesomorphic and ectomorphic. Team games and racquet players also tend to have a mixed somatotype and in sports where skill is the key component a greater variation of somatotypes is observed.

However, while generalized surveys in the past have shown a high degree of conformity between participants in the same event, or in the same team playing positions in team games, the advent of mass participation in activities such as marathon running and aerobic-type exercise classes has resulted in less conformity. This means that it is not so unusual for a very heavy mesomorph or endomorph to run in a marathon for which his/her body is less well suited, hence considerably increasing the potential for overuse injuries in these activities. This increased risk could be multiplied many times if they also possess any biomechanical anomalies. The details of these are discussed later in this chapter.

(b) Postural factors

The posture shown in Figure 4.2(a) is thought to be anatomically the most efficient, creating minimal joint and skeletal stress while maximizing muscular function. Deviations and anomalies, as indicated in Figure 4.2(b), either create an overworking in 'normal' functional circumstances that is taken into the sporting activity, or increase the likelihood of

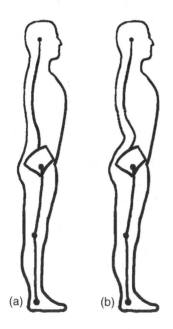

Figure 4.2 **(a)** Anatomical efficient posture. **(b)** Inefficient posture.

injury due to repetition of an inefficient or incorrect action.

(c) Anatomical factors

Specific sporting actions require certain ranges of motion at relevant joints to be able to perform the movement correctly and efficiently. For example, to run one needs more than $10°$ of ankle dorsiflexion and up to $15°$ of hip internal rotation and extension. Any inherited developmental or trauma-related anomaly that restricts the range of motion, making an action either impossible or inefficient, can be a significant contributory factor in the overuse scenario.

Short leg syndromes and other anatomical anomalies, either developmental or traumatic, will be covered in the section on biomechanical factors.

4.3.2 Muscular imbalance and weakness – implications, causes, assessment and treatment

(a) The causes of muscular imbalance and its implications

Natural development carries with it the tendency for one-sided dominance – most people are either right- or left-handed. In many cases the dominant side may be bigger, stronger and have superior control and coordination. This naturally leads to a tendency to hold a racquet in one hand, kick a football more confidently with one foot and adopt a certain stance when playing golf or cricket. This therefore leads to a naturally occurring muscular imbalance, altering the stresses on the system and thus contributing to the potential for an overuse injury.

Racquet sportspeople generally have an increased muscular development and strength on their dominant side at the expense of their range of movement. This restricted range of shoulder joint movement will also affect the movement of the neck, shoulder girdle and thoracic spine and, despite being small in magnitude, can significantly contribute to the potential for injury elsewhere.

As well as imbalances between the right and left sides of the body, there can be similar stressful relationships between the front and back. This is quite commonly seen in people who have had an injury to one muscle group which has not been fully rehabilitated following the injury. This can alter the normal balance between muscle groups and indirectly affect the timing of contraction/relaxation, thus contributing to the potential for injury by placing additional stresses upon certain body parts.

This front–back imbalance can also occur without the presence of related injury (Figure 4.3).

For example, in those sportspeople who have a naturally occurring lordosis (increased arch in the lower back) there is often an imbalance between the spinal and abdominal musculature, which leads to altered postures, muscle-fibre firing patterns and therefore altered movement patterns. Similarly, in

those people who have a thoracic kyphosis (rounded shoulders), where the head of the humerus can drop forwards and downwards, altered muscle tensions and firing patterns between the controlling muscles can produce abnormal movement, leading to repetitive microtrauma and eventual overuse injury (section 4.3.2(a)).

Weakness of one muscle group or another in relative terms will always be part of imbalance. This is obviously different from any specific weakness that exists as a result of injury, inactivity, illness or neural dysfunction, such as a prolapsed disc with nerve compression. When assessing a person who appears to be suffering from an overuse injury it is vital to consider the influence of all of the above, which sometimes makes it easier to understand the development of the problem.

(b) Isokinetic evaluation – a measurement of muscular performance.

This form of evaluation can be very valuable in many cases, as it can:

- provide an objective measurement, thereby allowing a more specific rehabilitation programme to be planned;
- objectively gauge progress or otherwise;
- be used along with other more functional tests to decide when to return to activity.

In the late 1960s the concept of isokinetic exercise was developed by James Perrine. Instead of traditional exercises which involve using a constant weight or resistance with the movement being performed at variable speeds, Perrine developed the concept of **isokinetics**, which involves performing the movement at a preset fixed speed, against a resistance that is totally accommodating throughout the range of motion (ROM). This therefore ensures that the muscles are worked throughout the entire range of movement. Sophisticated isokinetic machines working on these principles can assess any weakness in a range of movement at a particular speed

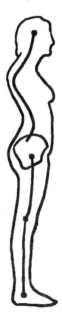

Figure 4.3 Lordosis and thoracic kyphosis.

and the exact phase of the movement during which the weakness occurs. By comparing the values for different muscle groups and opposing limbs the experienced practitioner can use this information to assess the individual for weaknesses and imbalances. However this does take a considerable amount of experience and skill and is an area of assessment that is still developing.

(c) The different types of muscular rehabilitation/strengthening exercise available

There are various forms of musculoskeletal exercise available for the practitioner to select from when rehabilitating a patient. The four types of exercise commonly used are isometrics, isotonics, isokinetics and closed chain/functional exercises.

Isometrics

Isometrics work against a fixed resistance and therefore there is no movement involved. The muscles contract statically.

Advantages of isometric exercises:

- They can be used early in rehabilitation without causing further joint irritation as there is no joint motion.
- They will increase static muscular strength.
- They help to retard atrophy.
- They assist in the reduction of swelling.
- They can be performed anywhere.
- No special equipment is needed.
- They can be performed in short periods of time.

Disadvantages of isometric exercises:

- Muscular strength gains are fairly specific to the joint angle at which they are performed, i.e. within 20°.
- They are subject to psychological influences.
- It is difficult to provide patient motivation.
- They do not contribute to muscular endurance.

- No eccentric work is provided.
- They may cause a large increase in blood pressure due to the Valsalva manoeuvre.

Isotonic exercises

These are performed against a set resistance through a particular range of movement. The speed may be variable and they are likely to include both concentric and eccentric work. During the concentric phase the muscle fibres will be activated and cause an overall shortening in the length of the muscle, while in the eccentric phase the muscle fibres will be activated but there will be an overall lengthening of the muscle as it lengthens under tension. A simple example of this would be the action of biceps brachii during controlled raising (concentric action) and lowering (eccentric action) of a weight. In general, more force can be developed using eccentric contractions, as fewer muscle fibres are activated during the contraction. This development of greater tension can lead to greater strength gains, but often at the cost of residual muscle soreness, probably due to microtrauma of the connective tissue, which can contribute to pain inhibition.

Advantages of isotonic exercises:

- Some can be relatively inexpensive.
- They are readily available.
- They provide motivation by achievement.
- Incremental progression can be easily incorporated.
- Work takes place through the range of movement.
- Work occurs at speeds greater than $0°s^{-1}$.
- They have a concentric and eccentric component.
- They can improve muscular endurance.
- They can be objectively documented.
- Variation is possible using different components, e.g. altering the weight or the number of repetitions and sets.
- They increase muscular strength in a few repetitions.

Disadvantages of isotonic exercises:

- They load a muscle at its weakest point in the range of movement.
- They are not safe in the presence of pain (supporting a weight).
- There is a danger of using them incorrectly and thereby causing trauma.
- There is a momentum factor once the weight starts moving.
- They do not develop accuracy at functional speeds.
- It is difficult to exercise at fast functional speeds.
- They are not usually performed in a diagonal or functional plane.
- It is impossible to spread the workload evenly over the entire range of movement.
- Machines work only one muscle group.
- It is impossible to vary resistance within a movement as the skeletal leverage changes occur.
- Isotonics do not accommodate to pain.
- Fatigue causes a decrease in the range of movement.
- Velocity, work and power are not controlled or measured and cannot be reproduced.

Isokinetic exercise

Isokinetic exercises occur at a fixed and predetermined speed from $1–450°s^{-1}$ against an accommodating resistance. Isokinetics have a fixed speed with a variable resistance that is totally accommodating to the individual throughout the range of movement (ROM). Therefore the resistance varies to exactly match the force applied at every point in the ROM. By controlling the velocity of the exercise, maximum resistance throughout the full ROM is achieved. This variable resistance, which matches the force applied at any one point, matches the changes in the amount of torque that can be produced as the length–tension ratio changes in the muscle group

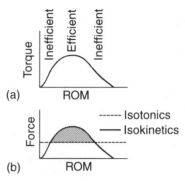

Figure 4.4   Diagram of length–tension relationship versus torque.

with biomechanical skeletal leverage changes (Figure 4.4).

The unique advantages of isokinetics are as follows.

- **Safety** – as the resistance is equal to the force applied.
- **Efficiency** – maximal loading at all points through range.
- **Accommodating resistance** – allows for safety and efficiency.
- **Decreased joint compressive forces at higher speeds** – i.e. the faster the movement of a surface over a fluid, the less the surface pressure.
- **Joint nourishment** – submaximal short arc isokinetics produce positive compressional forces, which stimulate synovial fluid production.
- **Physiological overflow** – various studies have shown an overflow phenomenon where training at one speed may have a positive beneficial effect at other speeds. This certainly occurs at slower speeds and perhaps at faster speeds. However, most gains are made very close to the training speed, thus isokinetics often allows training and rehabilitation to be carried out at closer to functional speeds.
- **Velocity spectrum training** – functional and sporting activities occur at varying velocities. Specificity of training means that it is important to be able to train at various functional velocities.

Further general advantages of isokinetics:

- Accommodating resistance – maximal loading throughout ROM
- Inherent safety factor with minimal risk to patient
- Reliability of equipment
- Reproducibility of testing
- Objective record of performance
- Exercise through velocity spectrum
- Use of concentric/eccentric muscular contractions
- Helps force development of quickness
- Develops force control accuracy
- Decreases reciprocal innervation time of agonist/antagonist contractions
- Accommodation to pain
- Accommodation to fatigue
- Joint nourishment
- Decreased joint compressive forces at high speeds
- Physiological overflow
- Provides feedback to patient.

Disadvantages of isokinetics:

- Cost of equipment
- Availability of equipment
- Lack of practitioner knowledge in use of equipment
- Difficulty of positioning and repositioning, to isolate movement to one joint
- The sensitivity of the equipment and recording devices in testing large muscle masses, e.g. the hip
- inconvenience and time factor involved with switching attachments for various joints and setups.

Assessments using isokinetic machines. This can be a useful adjunct to other clinical assessments and diagnostic investigations. The comparative peak torques achieved between a muscle or group of muscles of one limb to the other can be very useful, as is the percentage relationship between agonist and antagonist. In conducting this form of analysis the relative performance at different speeds and through specific ranges of motion need

to be measured, recorded and analysed. Isokinetic machines enable the 'work done' in different parts of the ROM to be measured as well as the 'fatigue rate', which is important when considering the endurance capacity of a muscle or group of muscles. This information can then be used to assess the potential contribution of muscular performance to overuse or repetitive injury, as well as being a 'benchmark' for the planning and progressing of a rehabilitation programme following injury. Alternatively, it may be used to evaluate the individual's vulnerability to injury and hence have a preventative function. Certain studies, and many clinicians, claim that isokinetic test information and associated curve analysis can be used diagnostically. This may be possible, although the practitioner needs to have a vast experience of clinical usage to be able to use its diagnostic potential.

Closed chain/functional exercises

There is no machine or exercise station that is yet capable of exactly reproducing a functional or sporting movement. It is therefore vital that in any rehabilitation programme the practitioner uses practices that are similar to the actual functional activity. This will help to ensure the re-education of a 'mature motor pattern', i.e. to establish a naturally occurring, coordinated, efficient and controlled action. This is why closed chain/functional exercises are important – they involve the contraction of associated muscle groups, with loading of the joint above and below. They also require the coordinated relaxation and/or static contraction of related muscles which function as fixators, regulators and neutralizers during the normal production of the action. Examples of closed chain/functional exercises include small range squats, step-downs or single leg squats.

The principle of coactivation plays a major role in functional movements. In using these exercises practitioners must analyse the type of muscle work involved in the required action – concentric, eccentric, isometric or synergistic – and then try to 'train' or rehabilitate that muscle using repetitions of the primary contraction type. Coactivation involves the fine controlled agonist/antagonist relationships to produce precise, controlled movements in functional positions at functional speeds. An example is the coactivation of quadriceps and hamstrings primarily, as well as calf and buttock muscles, to control a squat or knee bend just after heel contact when walking or running. Often functional movements involving naturally occurring coactivation are less stressful and therefore potentially less damaging.

(d) Muscular imbalance related to 'normal movement': hypertonicity and hypotonicity

To appreciate the factors involved with normal movement the practitioner has to be aware that certain muscles have a tendency to **hypertonicity** (shortening), while others have a tendency to **hypotonicity** (lengthening.) Given below is a list of the muscular tendencies; this information can be used to analyse movement at the pelvic and shoulder levels in particular.

Muscles with a tendency to hypertonicity/ shorten – mainly muscles with a postural function:

- Sternocleidomastoid
- Pectoralis major (clavicular and sternal)
- Trapezius (upper part)
- Levator scapulae
- Flexors of the upper extremity.
- Quadratus lumborum
- Back extensors:
  - Erector spinae
  - Longissimus thoracis
  - Rotatores
  - Multifidus
- Hip flexors:
  - Iliopsoas
  - Tensor fascia lata
  - Rectus femoris

- Lateral rotators of hip:
  - Piriformis
- Medial rotators of hip:
  - Pectineus
  - Adductor longus
  - Adductor brevis
  - Adductor magnus
- Hamstrings:
  - Biceps femoris
  - Semitendinosus
  - Semimembranosus
- Plantar flexors:
  - Gastrocnemius
  - Soleus
  - Tibialis posterior.

Muscles with a tendency to hypotonicity/ weaken – mainly muscles with a dynamic function:

- Scaleni
- Pectoralis major (abdominal part)
- Subscapularis
- Extensors of the upper extremity
- Trapezius (lower part)
- Rhomboids
- Serratus anterior
- Rectus abdominis
- Oblique abdominals
- Gluteus maximus, medius and minimus
- Vastus medialis and lateralis
- Tibialis anterior
- Peronei.

(e) The crossed pelvis syndrome

If the spinal extensors, quadratus lumborum and the hip flexors are hypertonic while the abdominal and gluteal muscles are hypotonic, then there will be abnormal compressional and shear forces on the spine, pelvis and hips leading to abnormal movement patterns (Figure 4.5).

Testing for muscle imbalance

The hip extension pattern (Figure 4.6)   Lie the patient comfortably in the prone position

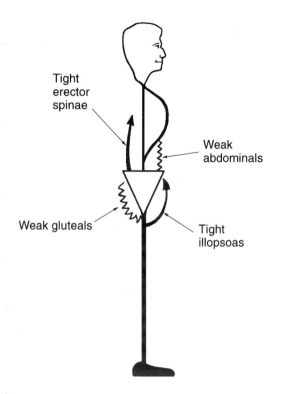

Figure 4.5   Crossed pelvic syndrome.

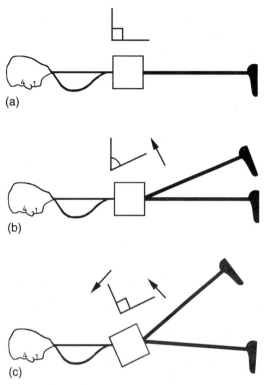

Figure 4.6   Hip extension. **(a)** Resting position: neutral position of pelvis. **(b)** Correct extension: pelvis remains neutral; angle between femur and pelvis reduces. **(c)** False extension: pelvis tilts anteriorly, increasing lumbar lordosis; femur remains at 90° to pelvis.

(on the front). Hip extension should then be initiated by the gluteus maximus, followed by a contraction of the hamstring on the same side and the spinal extensor muscles on the opposite side. Common anomalies are as follows.

- The gluteus maximus comes in too late.
- The gluteus maximus works minimally or does not work at all.
- There is overworking of the same-side spinal extensors.
- The lumbar spine extends and/or rotates, as a result of hypermobility or a hypertonic quadratus lumborum.

The hip abduction pattern (Figure 4.7) When lying comfortably on the side and well supported in that position, hip abduction (lifting the leg away from the mid-line) should be initiated by gluteus medius and minimus, followed by a stabilizing, gentle contraction of

quadratus lumborum on the same side. Common anomalies are:

- reduced gluteal contraction;
- overactive quadratus lumborum;
- abduction initiated by quadratus lumborum (producing a hitch);
- overactive tensor fascia lata, producing flexion and internal rotation instead of abduction;
- overactive piriformis, producing lateral rotation as well as abduction.

Although these testing positions are non-functional it is not unreasonable to assume that a correct pattern in lying has more chance of transferring into functional positions and *vice versa*.

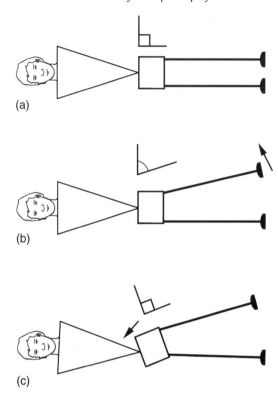

(a)

(b)

(c)

Figure 4.7 Hip abduction. **(a)** Starting position: neutral position of pelvis, legs resting. **(b)** True abduction: pelvis remains neutral; angle between femur and pelvis reduces. **(c)** False abduction: pelvis tilts laterally; angle between femur and pelvis is unchanged.

Treatment of crossed pelvis syndrome

Although always dangerous to generalize, with this type of presentation the treatment approach is one of (1) stretching out the hypertonic muscles, followed by (2) stimulating the hypotonic muscles. The aim is to restore a correct movement pattern, which can easily be reassessed at any stage. It could take anywhere from days to months to restore a correct pattern, and occasionally this cannot be achieved because of some other contributory problem, such as an instability or a severe degenerative joint problem.

(f) The shoulder and scapulothoracic area

In this area the patterns of movement and muscular control of them are more difficult to assess. This is primarily a result of the vast range of motion available at the shoulder and the very subtle interrelationships between the cervical, thoracic, ribs, shoulder joint and girdle.

In practical terms therefore, it is suggested that the practitioner becomes familiar with the muscular tendencies of hypertonia and hypotonia and incorporates this into basic assessment procedures. The treatment procedure is then as outlined above – stretch out the hypertonic and then stimulate the hypotonic muscle groups.

Once again factors such as pain, inflammation, hypermobility and loss of movement, and other factors that have the potential to change patterns of movement, will need to be taken into consideration.

4.3.3 Biomechanical factors, including gait and gait analysis

If the practitioner is going to analyse posture and gait in a way that is going to help him/her to understand the factors contributing to overuse, then a very clear understanding of the theoretical norms is required, followed by an ability to analyse the anomalies that occur during sporting activities and therefore to decide where and when any 'interference' is necessary. Factors to consider include:

- natural posture;
- muscular imbalance;
- the proprioceptive response;
- hyper or hypotonicity of relevant muscle groups;
- flexibility of relevant muscle groups;
- range of movement available at relevant joints;
- limb length discrepancies;
- limb alignment discrepancies;
- foot anomalies in the subtalar neutral position;

- functional anomalies in relaxed mid-stance;
- functional anomalies during training or competition.

Often, practitioners are able to observe pronation (lower-arched appearance) or supination (higher arched appearance) without analysing the factors that contribute to these presentations. In-toeing or out-toeing gait is easy to observe, but to work out the cause can be much more difficult. The same can apply to valgus (knock-knee) or varus (bow-leg) anomalies and to limb length discrepancy, which can be apparent or real, with many contributory factors. To be able to perform this analysis the practitioner must at the very least be able to identify the subtalar neutral position and relate this to theoretical normal motion.

The subtalar neutral position (Figure 4.8(a)).

The subtalar neutral position is the position whereby the subtalar joint is neither pronated nor supinated and the head of the talus does not protrude from behind the navicular on the medial or the lateral side. From this position of the joint, maximal function can occur in any permissible direction.

Pronation (Figure 4.8(b)).

This is a triplane axial motion occurring at the subtalar joint combining:

- abduction of the forefoot;
- dorsiflexion of the ankle;
- eversion of the heel.

Supination (Figure 4.8(c)).

This is a triplane axial motion occurring at the subtalar joint, combining:

- adduction of the forefoot;
- plantarflexion of the ankle;
- inversion of the heel.

(a) Theoretical normal motion (Figure 4.9)

1. The heel should strike the ground at the posterolateral aspect, in approximately 5–7° of relative supination (Figure 4.9).
2. As the weight is transferred forwards into the midfoot, pronation should occur at the subtalar and midtarsal (talonavicular and calcaneocuboid) joints, until subtalar neutral or just past neutral is achieved. The talus moves downwards and inwards during this pronatory movement, taking the tibia into internal rotation. In turn, the femur will follow the tibia, producing

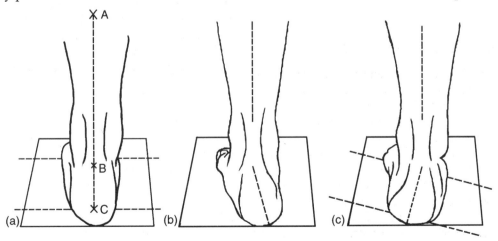

Figure 4.8 **(a)** Subtalar neutral position. **(b)** Pronation. **(c)** Supination.

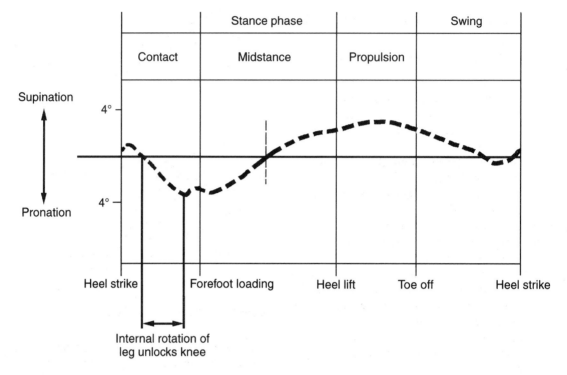

Figure 4.9   Theoretical normal motion.

internal rotation. This naturally occurring pronation is the body's own inherent mechanism, designed to absorb shock and to allow adaptation to uneven surfaces, by becoming more mobile. The foot is now in **mid-stance**.

3. As the bodyweight moves further forward from midfoot to forefoot, re-supination occurs, causing external rotation of both tibia and femur. This re-supination locks the calcaneocuboid joint, making the foot into a rigid lever, allowing the peroneus longus tendon to hold the first metatarsal firmly on the ground so that the first metatarsophalangeal joint can act as a pivot to allow effective forward motion.

4. This rigid lever is maintained as the heel lifts off the ground, requiring extension of the first metatarsophalangeal joint to make use of the **'windlass effect'**, which is the tensioning of the plantar aponeur-

osis, assisting with maintenance of re-supination and support of the longitudinal arch.

Any deviation from this theoretical normal motion can lead to alterations in gait, which could be totally responsible for or a contributory factor to the development of an overuse injury.

(b) Gait anomalies

Gait anomalies tend to fit into one of the following categories:

- excessive pronation from heel strike to midstance
  - with associated tibial internal rotation only
  - with associated tibial and femoral internal rotation also;
- failure to re-supinate during middle to late mid-stance.

- late pronatory motion, i.e. occurring during the push-off phase.

Possible causes of excessive pronation are:

- functional hallux rigidus – a limitation of movement of the big toe into extension;
- foot anomalies in subtalar neutral;
- ligamentous laxity, leading to increased joint movement;
- distal tibial varum above 3–4° (bowing of the lower limb);
- genu varum (bow legs) or genu valgum (knock knees);
- genu recurvatum (hyperextended knees);
- leg-length discrepancy with increased pronation of the longer limb;
- hypertonicity or loss of elasticity of the soft-tissue structures, particularly around the pelvic region or the calf muscles (especially the gastrocnemius);
- external tibial torsion (an outward rotation of the lower leg in relation to the upper leg);
- femoral anteversion (an alignment of the femur giving on appearance of internal rotation).

Functional hallux rigidus (FHR)

The hinge action of the toe joints is essential during the re-supinatory and heel-off phases of gait. This action requires dorsiflexion (extension) of the metatarsophalangeal joints, especially of the great toe. This continued hinge action provides four essential functions.

- The toes stay in contact with the ground to act as an anchor.
- It provides a fulcrum point for the weight-bearing limb's lever action against the support surface.
- It allows the windlass effect to occur, creating osseous stability (Figure 4.10).
- It allows the body to pass directly over the joint, efficiently advancing forward with each step.

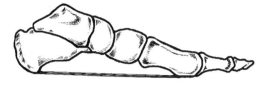

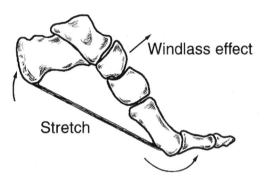

Figure 4.10   The windlass effect.

To allow this hinge action to occur, 65° of dorsiflexion (extension) is required at the first metatarsophalangeal joint. Only 20–30° of this movement is true dorsiflexion of the phalanges, the rest of the movement coming from plantarflexion of the first metatarsal (Figure 4.11).

In functional hallux rigidus there is reduction in the range of dorsiflexion available, causing a malfunction of the naturally occurring pivotal mechanism. This leads to:

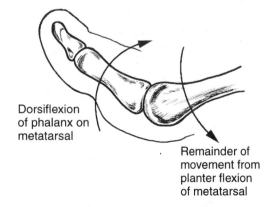

Figure 4.11   Plantarflexion of the metatarsals.

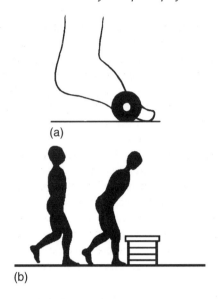

(a)

(b)

Figure 4.12   Postural changes.

- pronation late in the heel-off phase and consequent rolling off the forefoot, with potential deformation of the great toe towards the second toe (**hallux valgus**);
- postural changes (Figure 4.12) as a result of increased forward lean, which reduces the range of naturally occurring hip extension, preventing 'elastic recoil' of the hip flexors. Iliopsoas is therefore brought into action in an attempt to initiate hip flexion but, because the femur is locked beneath the pelvis, iliopsoas acts in reverse, causing lumbar spine and sacral rotation towards the fixed site rather than away from it in accordance with pelvic rotation. As this occurs with every step, lumbosacral and sacroiliac joint dysfunctions are common, as well as the muscular imbalances discussed above.

Clinical testing for functional hallux rigidus   The patient is seated in a non-weight-bearing position. The first metatarsal is stabilized and the hallux is dorsiflexed and plantarflexed to assess non-loaded range of motion. Loading of the plantar surface of the

first metatarsal is now performed by maximally dorsiflexing it. Hallux dorsiflexion is attempted once again. Minor resistance to 20–30% of dorsiflexion is the norm; considerable resistance or complete locking are definite signs of FHR. It must be remembered that the force used to dorsiflex the metatarsal is to equate the body's load against the floor, and therefore must be adequate to ensure correct findings. Although hallux rigidus is a functional disorder and this is a clinical test, if performed correctly it will give a very strong indication as to whether the condition does exist.

Treatment of FHR
- Orthotic prescription with the first ray cut out, allowing the first metatarsal head to 'drop' over the edge of the orthotic, thus artificially increasing the range of dorsiflexion.
- Compression mobilizations of the first metatarsophalangeal joint with the first metatarsal maximally dorsiflexed.
- Manual stretching and release techniques for the plantar aponeurosis.
- Stretching and release techniques for iliopsoas.
- Re-education of movement patterns around the pelvis and hips.
- Postural and proprioceptive re-education.

Foot anomalies in subtalar neutral

To be able to assess anomalies of any sort the practitioner must have a clear understanding as to the 'normal' rearfoot-to-forefoot relationship in subtalar neutral (Figure 4.13).

In the subtalar neutral position, the line bisecting the lower leg (A–B in Figure 4.13) and the line bisecting the calcaneum (B–C) should be continuous with each other. The plane of the forefoot, represented in the figure by metatarsal heads 2–4, should be at a right angle to A–B–C. (Metatarsal heads 2–4 are used because 1 and 5 tend to be mobile and have a tendency to deformation.)

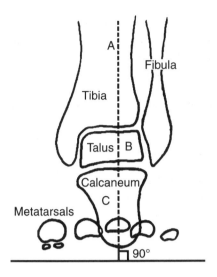

Figure 4.13 Normal rearfoot-to-forefoot relationship in subtalar neutral.

Many foot pathologies can exist in subtalar neutral although only the five most common are described here. The practitioner involved with gait analysis related to overuse injuries must have a basic knowledge of the five foot types discussed below and be able to understand how they can contribute to an abnormal gait pattern. However they must never be considered in isolation: other structural and functional anomalies must be taken into account simultaneously. When considering the movements occurring at the foot it is important to also observe the lower limb as a whole, looking for rotations, valgus (knock-knee) or varus (bowed) reactions and to consider what muscles could counteract or control the unwanted movements. When considering muscular control the practitioner must also be aware of the type of muscle activity being performed, i.e. concentric, eccentric, fixator or other.

With regard to the treatment of foot anomalies it must be remembered that the introduction of modified insoles or orthotics is a very skilled area and should be left to those who have the required knowledge and skills. Practitioners who do not feel confident in this area should attempt to develop a close professional relationship with those who do.

Rearfoot varus This is a structural anomaly which causes the calcaneum to be inverted to the ground when the subtalar joint is in the neutral position (Figure 4.14(a)). The cause of rearfoot varus is usually the failure of the posterior of the calcaneum to completely de-rotate from its infantile position. Anywhere from 3–5° of rearfoot varus is quite common.

Compensation for rearfoot varus anomaly will usually be via pronation until the medial border of the calcaneum and the forefoot reach the ground (Figure 4.14(b)). In such cases it is important to remember that very rarely is only one anomaly in existence, and other contributory factors leading to more

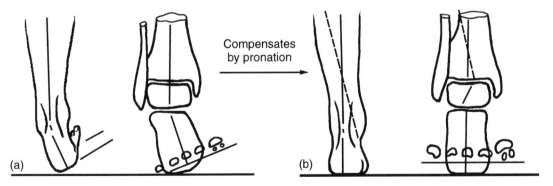

Figure 4.14 Rearfoot varus. **(a)** Neutral position. **(b)** Compensation.

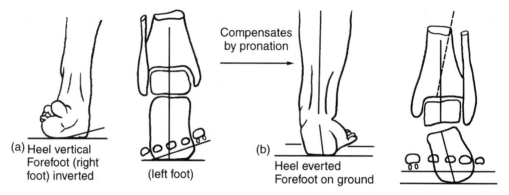

Figure 4.15 Forefoot varus. **(a)** Neutral position. **(b)** Compensation.

pronation than would be expected are also likely to be present.

Forefoot varus   This is a structural anomaly where the plane of the forefoot (represented by metatarsal heads 2–4) is inverted to the rearfoot when the subtalar joint is in the neutral position and the mid-tarsal joint is fully pronated (Figure 4.15(a)). The cause of forefoot varus is usually the failure of the head and neck of the talus to completely de-rotate from its infantile position.

Compensation will usually be via pronation, causing the calcaneum to evert in order to bring the forefoot on to the ground. A true forefoot varus will always lead to considerably more pronation than a rearfoot varus (Figure 4.15(b)).

Forefoot supinatus   This is an acquired inversion contracture of the forefoot around the longitudinal axis of the midtarsal (talonavicular) joint. This condition is often mistaken for a forefoot varus deformity as they appear very similar. The difference is that a forefoot supinatus is a compensatory situation that develops as a result of prolonged pronation at the subtalar joint; thus the forefoot is pushed via ground reaction force into a relatively supinated position. If this position is maintained for long enough then a soft-tissue contracture will develop around the talonavicular joint. A forefoot supinatus can be reduced while maintaining the subtalar joint

in its neutral position, whereas any attempt to reduce a forefoot varus would cause pronation at the subtalar joint. Compensation for forefoot supinatus will be similar to a forefoot varus, i.e. via pronation, although the treatment may differ somewhat.

Equinus   This refers to any condition, either structural or functional, that restricts ankle joint dorsiflexion to less than 10° when the subtalar joint is in neutral and the midtarsal joint is fully pronated (Figure 4.16).

Differentiation must be made between an osseous block and a soft-tissue limitation. This is achieved by examining the range of ankle dorsiflexion in the knee-straight compared to the knee-bent position. When the knee is straight the gastrocnemius (superficial calf muscle) is the most likely limiting factor, whereas when the knee is bent (releasing gastrocnemius tension) any limitation is likely to be osseous. It should be remembered that the soleus (the deeper calf muscle) could also limit movement when the knee is bent.

Compensation for an equinus condition can be:

- full compensation – the person excessively pronates as this actually creates more ankle joint dorsiflexion;
- partial compensation – the person walks with a premature heel lift, thus avoiding the restricted range;

Functional restriction
(knee extended)

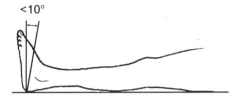

<10°

Structional restriction
(knee flexed)

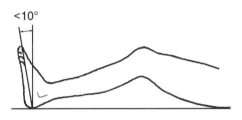

<10°

Figure 4.16 Equinus. **(a)** Functional restriction (knee extended). **(b)** Structural restriction (knee flexed).

• uncompensated – the person walks and runs on his/her toes, the heels being unable to reach the ground.

All these gait variations will lead to abnormal stresses somewhere within the chain and could be partly or totally responsible for the development of an overuse injury.

Plantarflexed first ray This is a structural abnormality where the first ray (i.e. the medial cuneiform, first metatarsal and its phalanges) has more plantarflexion than dorsiflexion available to it in relation to the plane of the metatarsals 2–5. Often the first ray is abnormally pulled down into plantarflexion (Figure 4.17(a)). The cause of this anomaly is often congenital, although it can be compensatory, as a result of an uncompensated rearfoot varus where no pronation occurs at the subtalar joint and the peroneus longus tendon (inserting into the plantar aspect of the first metatarsal) pulls down on the first ray to get it on to the ground, thus allowing the pivotal mechanism to occur.

Compensation for plantarflexed first ray depends on whether it is mobile or not. For example, if the first ray is rigidly fixed into plantarflexion then the compensation will be one of supination, where the weight is pushed back onto the lateral aspect of the foot (Figure 4.17(b)), whereas if the plantarflexion is mobile then it will only minimally influence the movement of the foot and other existing anomalies (if any) will be more significant.

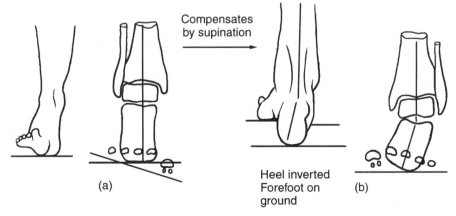

Compensates by supination

Heel inverted
Forefoot on ground

(a)   (b)

Figure 4.17 **(a)** Plantarflexed first ray pulled down. **(b)** Compensation.

(c)   Gait anomalies – factors affecting running gait

Ligamentous laxity leading to increased joint movement

The practitioner will find that certain individuals are hypermobile in some areas. This can be related to functional or sporting activities: for example gymnasts who work relentlessly on their mobility can become hypermobile.

However, it is also possible for some people simply to have a slightly greater than average amount of elastin in their ligamentous makeup. Occasionally this can be noted in all their joints, although it often seems to relate to only certain areas such as the ankle or shoulder. If this increased elasticity of the ligaments coincides with joint surfaces that are shaped to allow more movement than 'the norm', the person may be 'at risk' through excessive movement being available at that joint.

In gait analysis terms, if a sports performer has an excessive range of movement in the foot and ankle areas because of the shape of the joint surfaces, and also has increased amounts of ligamentous elastin, even a minor foot anomaly in subtalar neutral may lead to considerable pronatory movement. In the same circumstances a heavier person who spends all day on his/her feet will also be more 'at risk'.

Distal tibial varum

Tibial varum is the relationship between the transverse plane of the ground and the varus (bowing) angle of the distal (lower) one-third of the leg. The bisection of the lower one-third of the leg can be marked, the sportsperson stands with his/her subtalar joint in the neutral position, and the angle is measured (Figure 4.18).

Normal is 3–40. The greater the angle of tibial varum, the more pronatory move-

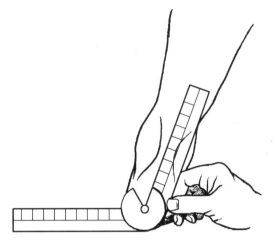

Figure 4.18   Measurement of tibial varum.

ment one would expect to see at the subtalar joint, except in those presentations where the gait anomaly is one of remaining in supination.

Genu varum (bow legs)

In cases of severe genu varum, the sports performer will often have relatively rigid, high-arched feet in association with his/her bowed legs leading to a supinated foot maintained through the gait cycle. Those people with minor to moderate genu varum often fit into the same category as those with an increased distal tibial varum, i.e. there is an increase in pronation at the subtalar joint.

Genu valgum (knock knees)

Genu valgum usually occurs in association with femoral anteversion internal rotation and can have many different causes (Figure 4.19):

- weakness of the external hip rotators;
- tightness of the hip adductors and internal rotators;
- wide pelvis – this occurs in women far more commonly than in men;
- tight hamstrings and calf muscles;

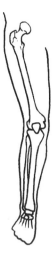

Figure 4.19 Genu valgum.

- a knock-on effect from excessive pronation at the subtalar joint.

Generally speaking, genu valgum will be a cause of or a reaction to pronation at the subtalar joint.

Genu recurvatum (hyperextended knees)

This can be a sign of an excessive range of joint motion with or without ligamentous laxity. It can also be a reaction to an equinus condition, where the sports performer locks the knees out abnormally in an attempt to avoid the restricted range of ankle dorsiflexion. Generally, genu recurvatum leads to increased stress on the knees, altered gait pattern, a muscular imbalance and often an increase in pronation at the subtalar joint.

Limb-length discrepancy

Where a true leg-length discrepancy does exist it is likely that the longer leg will have increased pronation at the subtalar joint. Pronation will reduce the length of the limb through associated internal rotation of the leg, often causing a valgus and flexed knee at the same time.

Common methods used to examine leg-length difference include:

- simultaneous palpation of both iliac crests in a standing position;
- the 'block method' – placing narrow blocks under the observed shorter leg until the iliac crests are level;
- simultaneous palpation of both anterior superior iliac spines in a standing position;
- the tape measure method – measuring between the anterior superior iliac spine and the inferior margin of the medial malleolus;
- radiographic measurements.

Of the above methods only the radiographic method has been shown to be inter-tester-reliable: all the other techniques show intertester difficulties. However, because of monetary costs radiographic measurements are often impractical. Therefore the practitioner has to choose the method that best suits his/her circumstances and use it when appropriate.

Hypertonicity of soft-tissue structures around the pelvic region

Short or hypertonic muscles, such as iliopsoas, hamstrings, tensor fascia lata and the iliotibial band, that rotate the femur or tibia either medially or laterally may be a cause of functional pronation (Figure 4.20).

The iliopsoas is a hip flexor and lateral rotator. Shortness of this muscle can be detected by the **Thomas test**, in which the supine patient brings the knee to the chest. If the opposite hip flexes, the iliopsoas on that side may be short. Tight iliopsoas may produce a lateral rotation of the limb, which will be compensated for by pronation in order to walk in a straight line.

Either medial or lateral hamstrings may be tight, causing the leg to rotate to its tight side. To test for medial hamstring tightness, flex a supine patient's hip to 90° and extend

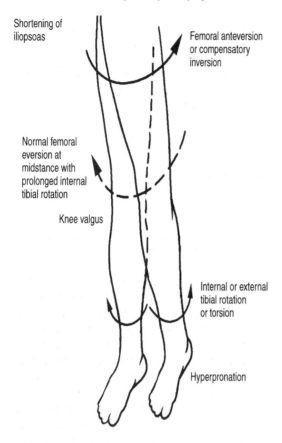

Shortening of iliopsoas

Femoral anteversion or compensatory inversion

Normal femoral eversion at midstance with prolonged internal tibial rotation

Knee valgus

Internal or external tibial rotation or torsion

Hyperpronation

Figure 4.20   Causes of functional pronation.

mine tightness in TFL and ITB. The patient should be on his/her side with the bottom knee flexed and the leg to be tested on top. The practitioner should then hold the ilium in a position perpendicular to the table as s/he raises the flexed upper thigh and leg into abduction and extension. In doing so s/he should allow the upper leg to drop in a controlled manner. If the thigh and leg stay abducted and if the leg does not fall below or at the level of the table, then TFL and ITB may be tight. This test may also be indicative of tight gluteus medius.

External tibial torsion

This may be congenital or acquired, as shown in Figure 4.21. If the tibia is externally rotated

the knee in the frontal plane until tension occurs (usually about 20–30° from extension). At this point, if the medial hamstrings are tight the leg will rotate inwards. This test does not take into account neural tension possibilities but can give an indication of hamstring tension as a possible contributory factor to pronation. If the medial hamstrings are tight this may cause toeing in, which is often compensated for by external rotation of the tibia in an attempt to walk in a straight line.

The tensor fascia lata (TFL) and iliotibial band (ITB) are hip flexors and internal rotators. Tightness can again contribute to pronation via external tibial torsion, in an attempt to straighten the limb from its internally rotated position. The **Ober test** will deter-

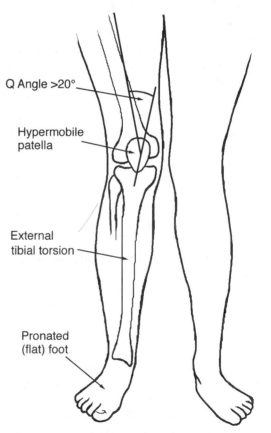

Q Angle >20°

Hypermobile patella

External tibial torsion

Pronated (flat) foot

Figure 4.21   External tibial torsion.

it is likely that this will lead to compensatory hyperpronation, or it may be that the external tibial torsion is a compensation for tight medial hamstrings or TFL, which are turning the leg internally.

Femoral anteversion

During the normal movement of the foot during the running action it is necessary for pronation to occur from heel-strike to early mid-stance. During this movement the talus moves medially, taking with it the tibia and the femur. Internal rotation is therefore a naturally occurring movement. For every 2° of pronation at the subtalar joint there will be 1° of internal rotation of the hip joint on that side.

Excessive femoral anteversion can be:

- congenital;
- trauma- or 'disease'-related – e.g. as a result of Perthes' disease or a slipped upper femoral epiphysis in children and adolescents;
- a result of tight tensor fascia lata, medial hamstrings and/or adductor muscle groups;
- a result of weakness in the muscles that externally rotate the leg, especially the gluteals;
- a result of hyperpronation at the subtalar and midtarsal joints.

As the patella sits on the femur, the practitioner can use the patella position to determine whether femoral anteversion is present. If the patella is parallel to the frontal plane then no femoral rotation exists. If the patella rotates internally or externally then a rotation is occurring.

The same criteria can be used to determine whether toeing in or toeing out is occurring above or below the knee. When there is toeing in or out and the patella is parallel to the frontal plane, then the pathology is below the patella (lower leg, foot or both). If the patella rotates then the pathology is probably related to the hip or femur.

In the standing relaxed mid-stance position the sports performer should have minimal turnout of the feet, be in the subtalar neutral position (with reasonable medial arch formation) and have the patella parallel to the frontal plane.

4.3.4 Neuromuscular–skeletal imbalance

(a) Introduction

Under this heading the practitioner must consider the relationships between the nervous system and the musculoskeletal system. In recent years this concept, of injury to the nervous system influencing the relationship between it and the musculoskeletal tissues it supplies, has come to be known as **adverse neural tension**. The concept of examining and treating neural tissue is not new, it has simply been explored from a neuroanatomical and neurophysiological viewpoint in greater depth, and its contribution to injury and the pain associated with it, be it acute or chronic, is therefore beginning to be better understood. The potential contribution of adverse neural tension to overuse injuries in sportspeople is very high.

The definition of adverse neurological tension is: 'abnormal physiological and mechanical responses produced from nervous system structures when their normal range of movement and stretch capabilities are tested' (Butler, 1991). In simplistic terms the concept hinges on injury to the nervous system that may or may not have been apparent (it is possible to have 'subclinical' injury that only becomes clinical at a later date when another injury or trauma occurs), which causes disturbance of the normal neurophysiological functions at that site, thus influencing the function of tissues elsewhere. Examples could be altered blood supply, muscle strength, muscle tone, nutrition of the tissues and electrical impulse conduction.

Sites of injury within the nervous system are:

- **soft tissue, bony or fibro-osseus tunnels** – the spinal nerve in the intervertebral foramen or the median nerve in the carpal tunnel are classic sites; there is always potential for friction of the nervous tissue structures within a tunnel;
- **where the nervous system is relatively fixed** – e.g. the radial nerve to the head of the radius or the common peroneal nerve to the head of the fibula;
- **where the nervous system branches** – e.g. the union of the lateral and medial plantar nerves to form the common plantar digital nerve to the web space between the third and fourth toes; a neuroma may develop if traumatized;
- **where it passes close to or over unyielding structures** the nervous system may be susceptible to trauma – e.g. the brachial plexus over the first rib and any nerves passing through the plantar fascia;
- **naturally occurring tension points** – e.g. the tibial nerve posterior to the knee and the sixth thoracic vertebral level.

Prior injury, such as an old fracture, can trigger off 'subclinical' injury, which lies apparently dormant (sometimes for years) until a further injury occurs that activates symptoms from the old injury site. Car accidents produce 'whiplash' injury, which traumatizes the nerve roots in the intervertebral foramen and perhaps the brachial plexus over the first rib and commonly lies dormant until another injury comes along and contributes to the development of severe tennis-elbow-type symptoms. The new injury does not have to be severe. Repetitive actions (as in overuse), sustained stressful body postures (as in racing car drivers) and biomechanically stressful movements (such as tumble turns or throwing the javelin) can be enough to trigger a response. Even trauma at relatively non-vulnerable sites can have repercussions at other more vulnerable areas. For example, ankle

inversion sprains can damage the common peroneal nerve, especially at its attachment to the fibula, even though there is no trauma to the fibula itself.

All of these possibilities mean that the practitioner must be aware that injury to the nervous system, past or present, chronic or acute, can be a potential contributory factor in overuse or repetitive injury.

(b) *Tension testing*

Tension testing is one of the investigative procedures used when dealing with overuse or repetitive injuries. It contributes to the assessment and examination proceedings and helps the practitioner to get as clear a picture of the presentation as possible. Treatment techniques based on tension testing findings will be discussed in some detail in the sections referring to specific injuries.

The scope of this text only allows a basic description of some of the testing positions (for more detail see Butler, 1991). The following basic tension tests will be outlined with an explanation of 'normal responses' and the information to be gathered:

- passive neck flexion (PNF);
- straight leg raise (SLR);
- prone knee bend (PKB);
- slump test;
- upper limb tension test 1 (ULTT1);
- upper limb tension test 2 (ULTT2);
  - with median nerve bias
  - with radial nerve bias.
- upper limb tension test 3 (ULTT3).

Passive neck flexion (PNF)

The person lies supine (on the back), preferably without a pillow. The practitioner then passively flexes the neck in a 'chin on chest' direction. Any reproduction of the person's symptoms, the range of motion achieved and the resistance encountered should be recorded and analysed (Figure 4.22). PNF is indicated for all possible spinal disorders and where arm or leg pain could be of spinal origin.

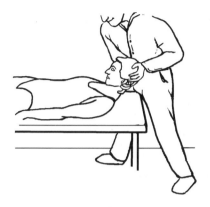

Figure 4.22 Passive neck flexion.

The normal response is painlessness, other than a minor pulling at the junction of the lower neck and upper back.

Straight leg raise (SLR)

The person lies supine at the side of the couch nearer to the practitioner. The hips and trunk should be in neutral and there should be no pillow under the neck unless absolutely necessary. One hand is placed under the Achilles tendon and the other just above the knee. The leg is then lifted keeping the knee straight (Figure 4.23).

Again, symptom response, range of movement and resistance are all noted and compared with the other limb, as well as normal responses to the test procedure. SLR is indicated for all spinal and leg symptoms and can be made more sensitive and therefore informative by adding other components, for example:

- ankle dorsiflexion;
- ankle plantarflexion/inversion;
- hip adduction;
- hip medial rotation;
- passive neck flexion.

The range of SLR can vary in normal healthy individuals from 50–120°, commonly producing symptoms of 'stretch' or 'irritability' in the posterior thigh, posterior knee and posterior calf into the foot. The practitioner is always trying to interpret the resistance and symptomatology compared to the contralateral limb.

Prone knee bend (PKB)

The PKB is recommended for any sports performer who presents with hip, anterior thigh, knee and upper lumbar problems. The person

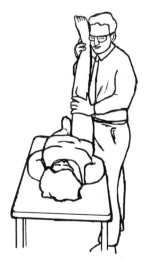

Figure 4.23 Straight leg raise.

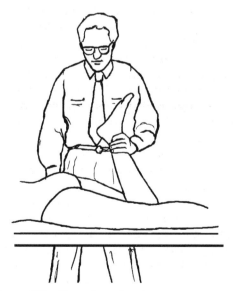

Figure 4.24 Prone knee bend.

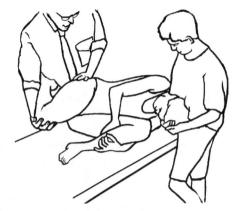

Figure 4.25   The slump test and prone knee bend.

lies prone (on the front) at the side of the couch nearest to the practitioner, with the head turned towards that side. The lower leg is then grasped and the knee flexed, bringing the heel towards the buttock (Figure 4.24). Symptoms, range of movement and resistance are all compared to the other side.

The test can be made more sensitive by adding hip extension, especially combined with adduction, or by adding the slump test to PKB (Figure 4.25), which can be a way of differentiating between nervous-system and non-nervous-system structures.

The normal response is a pulling or pain in the front of the thigh muscle as the heel approaches the buttock.

The slump test (Figure 4.26)

1. The person sits well back on the end of a plinth with thighs well supported and knees together. The person is asked to link the hands together behind his/her back and the practitioner stands to the side but close (Figure 4.26(a)). Any resting symptoms are noted, as are any changes with each addition that follows.

2. The person is asked to 'sag' in the middle – to lower the back while keeping the neck in neutral (Figure 4.26(b)). Overpressure is now applied to the thoracic and lumbar components through the arm resting over the shoulders. Any changes in symptomatology are noted.

3. The spinal flexion position is maintained and the person is asked to bend his/her neck, 'chin on chest' and then overpressure is applied (Figure 4.26(c)). Any change in symptoms after neck flexion and after overpressure is applied are noted.

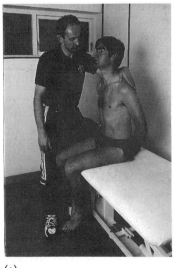

(a)

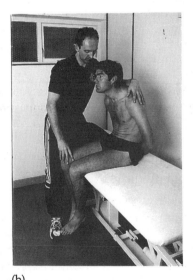

(b)

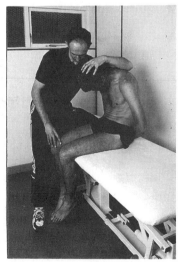

(c)

Figure 4.26   The slump test.

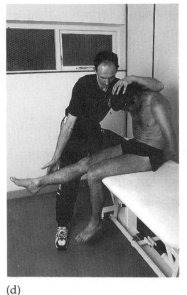

(d)

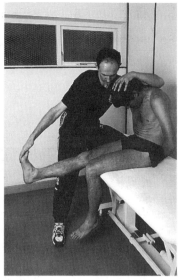

(e)

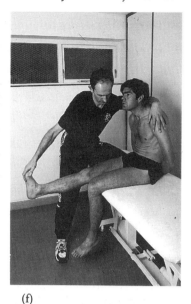

(f)

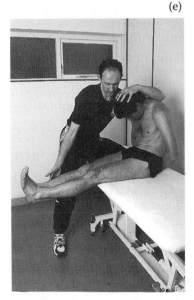

(g)

Figure 4.26 (cont.) The slump test.

4. The person is then asked to straighten the knee actively, range of movement, resistance and symptoms being noted. If there is a pain-dominant side then the non-painful leg should be extended first so as to get a better idea about what to expect from the painful side (Figure 4.26(d)).

5. The person is now asked to dorsiflex the ankle or 'pull his/her toes up' (Figure 4.26(e)). Any changes in symptoms are noted.

6. Neck flexion is now slowly released and the response is carefully assessed (Figure 4.26(f)).

7. The same procedure is now repeated for the other leg and any differences are noted.

8. In the slump position, both knees are extended and the effect of release of neck flexion is noted (Figure 4.26(g)).

The slump test is a powerful test of many structures, so care must be taken to accurately assess and interpret the findings. It is not always necessary to perform the whole test, particularly if the person's symptoms are reproduced when, for instance, overpressure is applied or as the knee is actively extended. Considerable care must be taken if there is any suspicion of a discogenic disorder. In this case the test should be either not performed or performed short of the onset of symptoms. The neural tissues can still be examined in discogenic disorders by the use of the passive neck flexion and straight leg raise tests.

The normal responses noted are as follows:

- **slump/neck flexion** – pain in the mid–lower thoracic area;
- **slump/neck flexion/knee extension** – pain in the hamstring and behind the knee, with some restriction of knee extension;
- **slump/neck flexion/knee extension/dorsiflexion** – some restriction of ankle dorsiflexion and a minor increase in symptoms in all areas;
- **on release of neck flexion** – a decrease in symptoms in all areas and an increase in range of knee extension and ankle dorsiflexion.

When necessary, sensitizing additions such as increasing hip flexion, hip adduction or medial rotation, plantarflexion/inversion of the ankle and even side flexion of the trunk to the opposite side can be used.

Upper limb tension test 1

The test for the left arm is described (Figure 4.27).

1. The patient is positioned in the neutral supine position, towards the left-hand side of the couch. The practitioner faces the patient in stride standing, his/her right hand holding the left hand of the patient. The upper arm rests on the practitioner's left thigh (Figure 4.27(a)).
2. Constant depression of the shoulder girdle is maintained by the practitioner's left hand, thus preventing elevation of the shoulder girdle during abduction. The patient's arm is then abducted to approximately 110° using the practitioner's left thigh (Figure 4.27(b)).
3. With this position maintained, the forearm is then supinated and the wrist and fingers are extended (Figure 4.27(c)).
4. The shoulder is then laterally rotated (Figure 4.27(d)).
5. The elbow is then extended while maintaining the previous components (Figure 4.27(e)).

6. With this position held, cervical lateral flexion to the right is added and then released (Figure 4.27(f)).

Symptoms and symptom changes must be identified and interpreted after each step. The normal responses are:

- deep stretch or ache in the front of the elbow extending down the front/outside of the forearm to the first three fingers;
- a definite tingling sensation in the first three fingers;
- stretch in the anterior shoulder area;
- cervical lateral flexion away from the tested side increases the above responses;
- cervical lateral flexion towards the tested side reduces the test response.

ULTT1 is recommended for all patients with symptoms anywhere in the arm head, neck and thoracic spine.

Upper limb tension test 2

As with ULTT1, ULTT2 should be performed in all cervical, thoracic and upper limb disorders. The bias of the test will be determined by the patient's symptoms: for example, a 'tennis-elbow'-type presentation with symptoms in the radial nerve distribution will require priority examination using ULTT2 with a radial nerve bias, whereas a carpal-tunnel-type syndrome may be initially investigated with a median nerve bias and perhaps examined further using sensitizing additions for the ulnar nerve, or even a different test altogether.

With median nerve bias The test is described for the left arm (Figure 4.28).

1. The patient lies slightly diagonally across the couch with his/her head towards the left-hand side and the scapula free of the bed. The practitioner's right thigh rests against the patient's left shoulder. The practitioner's right hand holds the patient's elbow and the left hand holds the wrist (Figure 4.28(a)).

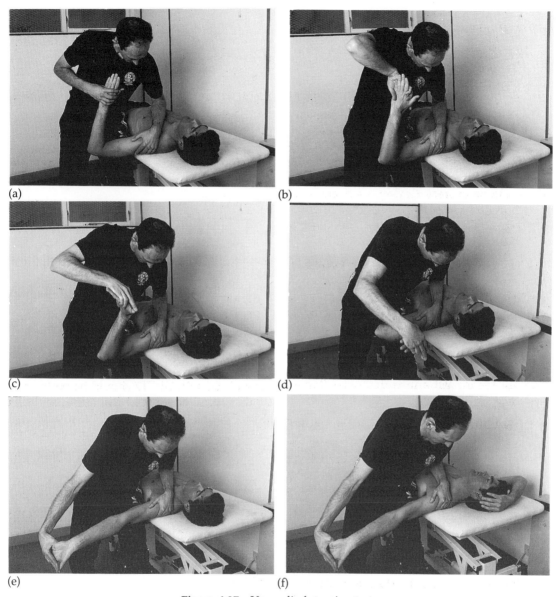

(a)

(b)

(c)

(d)

(e)

(f)

Figure 4.27 Upper limb tension test.

2. The shoulder girdle is depressed carefully using the practitioner's thigh (Figure 4.28(b))

3. Shoulder depression is maintained while the elbow is extended with the shoulder approximately 10° abducted, so that the arm is clear and parallel to the couch (Figure 4.28(c)).

4. The shoulder girdle depression/elbow extension pattern is maintained while the practitioner laterally rotates the whole arm (Figure 4.28(d)).

5. While this position is maintained the practitioner slides his/her left hand down to the patient's hand, slipping the thumb into the web space between the

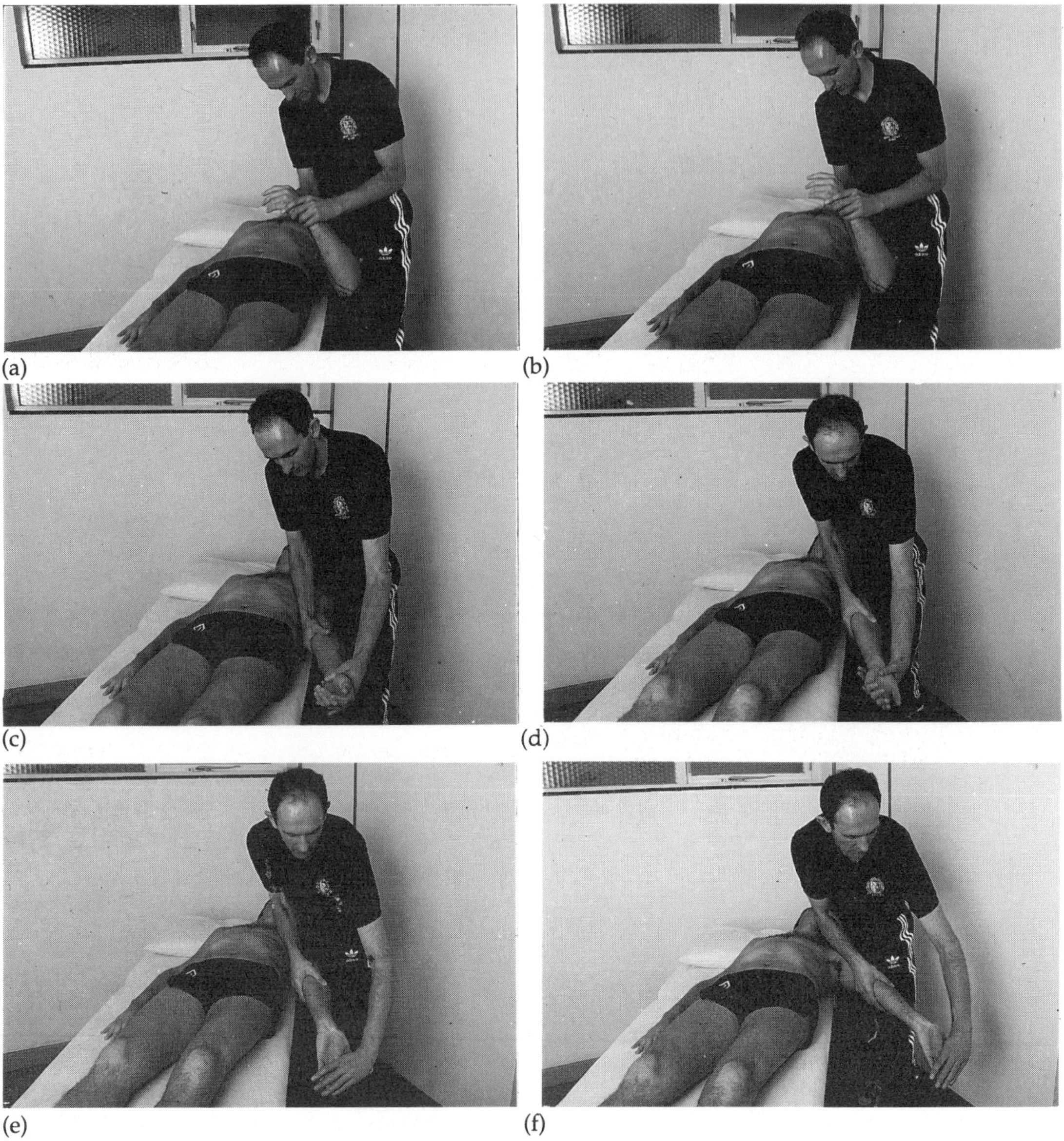

Figure 4.28 Upper limb tension test with median nerve bias.

thumb and index finger and then extending the patient's wrist, fingers and thumb (Figure 4.28(e)).

6. Abduction can be added as a sensitizing movement (Figure 4.28(f)).

With radial nerve bias The test is described for the left arm (Figure 4.29).

1. The starting position, shoulder girdle movements and elbow extension are the same as for the test with the median nerve bias.

2. With this position maintained, the shoulder is then medially rotated. The practitioner must reach under the patient's arm as far as possible with his/her left

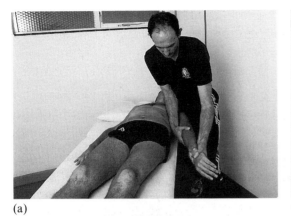

(a)

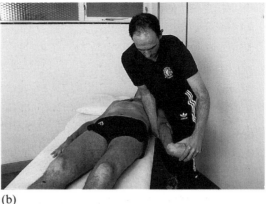

(b)

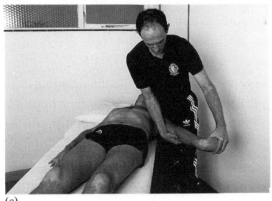

(c)

Figure 4.29   Upper limb tension test with radial nerve bias.

arm and grasp the patient's wrist (Figure 4.29(a)).
3. The patient's wrist is then flexed passively using the practitioner's left hand (Figure 4.29(b)), or the patient can be asked to perform an active movement into flexion.
4. Abduction can be added as a sensitizing movement (Figure 4.29(c)).

Very few studies have been published indicating normal responses to ULTT2, so comparisons are generally made with the other arm. However, it does appear to be normal to feel some symptoms along the innervation fields of either radial or median nerves, depending on the bias of the tension test performed.

Upper limb tension test 3

This test differs from ULTT1 and 2 insofar as it uses elbow flexion to tension the nervous system, thereby targeting the ulnar nerve. This test is described for the left arm (Figure 4.30).

1. The patient and the examiner take the same starting position as described for ULTT1. The patient's elbow is supported just below the examiner's anterior iliac spine (Figure 4.30(a)).
2. With the wrist held in extension and the forearm in supination, the elbow is flexed (Figure 4.30(b)).
3. The examiner maintains depression of the shoulder girdle by pressing into the couch with a clenched fist, immediately proximal to the shoulder (Figure 4.30(c)).
4. While maintaining the above components of the test movement, the shoulder is rotated laterally (Figure 4.30(d))
5. Shoulder abduction is then added by a movement of the examiner's body, which pivots around the arm which is in contract with the couch, to maintain shoulder depression (Figure 4.30(e)).
6. As with the other ULTT this one can be performed with the neck in neutral or in positions of lateral flexion (Figure 4.30(f)).

Symptom responses should be ascertained after each step of the test. In symptomatic individuals there may be tingling or stretch

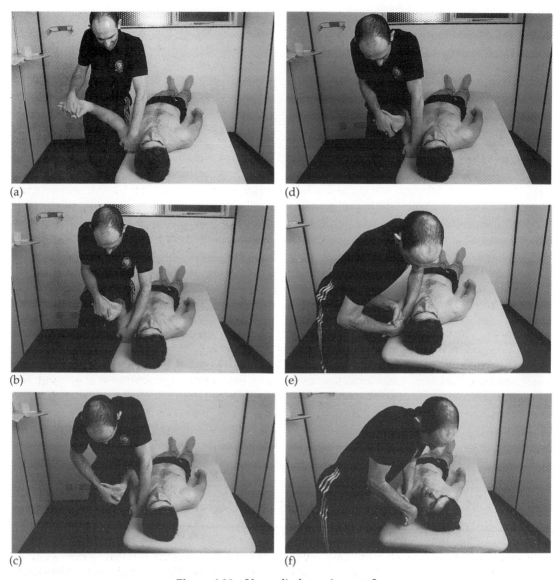

Figure 4.30   Upper limb tension test 3.

discomfort at the medial aspect of the elbow or in the ulnar aspect of the hand.

4.3.5   Prior injury

(a)   Introduction

The effects prior injury can have on the potential to develop an overuse or repetitive injury are based on:

- changes within the makeup of that structure, e.g. loss of tensile strength, altered fibre alignment, loss of tissue extensibility or elasticity and altered nerve and blood supply to the tissues;
- muscular imbalance as a result of the above changes
  - within that muscle group
  - in relation to other muscle groups;

- altered movement patterns as a result of the changes above.

(b) Changes within the makeup of the structure

Irrespective of which soft-tissue structure is damaged, it is generally accepted that injury will lead to loss of tensile strength. The type and severity of injury will to a certain extent determine the degree of lost strength. All tissues generally go through the same healing processes of acute inflammation, proliferation and remodelling. Reported time scales for healing and strength gain vary considerably between authors, but it is generally accepted that maximum loss of strength occurs between 2 and 7 days but return to near normal strength can take anywhere between 2 and 4 months, with some authors suggesting it can take up to 1 year or more.

The time scales are less clear when repetitive or overuse injuries are considered because the repetitive microtrauma initiates then maintains an ongoing inflammatory response until the adaptive ability of the tissue is exceeded.

Tensile strength will be further reduced by invasive therapies such as corticosteroid injections. Immobilization, other than that necessary to settle the original acute inflammation, is also a weakening factor.

Taking these factors into consideration will often make it easier to understand the development and maintenance of many repetitive injuries. To illustrate this point a couple of fairly typical scenarios are described below.

Example 1: the swimmer

The swimmer, who originally complained of soreness over the point of the shoulder after long swim sessions (but it was never bad enough to require rest), presents 2 months later with severe pain in the front of the shoulder into the upper biceps area. A true long head of biceps tendinitis develops, requiring rest and treatment, but because the national championships are only 2 weeks away, training begins after only 5 days of rest and no specific strengthening exercises are introduced. Poor performances at the championships are explained away in terms of interruption of preparation, not the pain, weakness and altered stroke action that has developed as a result of the ongoing microtrauma. Eventually, 4 months after the original complaint, a full-blown subacromial impingement syndrome develops, which requires another 2 months of treatment and rehabilitation before any swim training can recommence. Is this swimmer now at risk?

Example 2: the middle-distance runner

The middle-distance athlete partially tore her calf muscle in a 1500 m race in the early part of the season. There was a history of two less severe but similar incidents in the last 18 months. Stretching technique was good but no specific strengthening had been done as both times the pain was gone after 3 weeks and the muscle had just felt a little tight for another month or so.

On this occasion the athlete understands the necessity to perform strengthening exercises but loses interest 1 month later when she can no longer feel any pain. In an attempt to capture as much of the season as possible she increases her training quite quickly and begins to run quite well, as cardiovascular fitness had been maintained by running in water. In her second 3000 m race a soreness develops in the Achilles tendon of the same leg, which ends the season and takes 2 months to settle. Where did it all go wrong ?

(c) Muscular imbalance and altered movement patterns

This is always a possibility following a previous injury and can often result from the performer trying to compensate for the injured structures. This can place unfamiliar stresses upon other structures as a well as the injured part. For further consideration see section 4.3.2.

(d)   *Overloading due to repetition of specific action*

As previously mentioned in this chapter all bodily tissues have an adaptive ability or tolerance level. The tolerance level of one tissue type to another will vary, as will the tolerance from one person to another. With increasing years the same person's ability to tolerate load may also vary. Some or all of the factors listed at the beginning of this chapter under the causes of overuse injuries will determine the sportsperson's tolerance level at any one time.

Simplistically the bodily tissues are more able to cope with variable stress rather than repetition of the same action time after time.

What must be considered is the cumulative stress of repetitions performed on a daily, weekly, and monthly basis – hitting 500 golf balls in one day may be okay, but hitting 500 balls every day for a month may cause an overuse injury.

Rest, adequate nutrition for recovery, appropriate preparation and working on quality rather than quantity wherever possible are very effective ways of minimizing the potential for overuse.

4.4   REFERENCE

Butler, D. (1991) Mobilization of the nervous system. Churchill Livingstone, Edinburgh.

5. Examination, assessment and treatment of injuries

5.1 EXAMINATION AND ASSESSMENT OF INJURIES

5.1.1 Introduction

To simply list and describe a selection of injuries and conditions without first making reference to some of the principles that should underpin their examination, assessment and treatment could foster a naive approach to the management of sporting injuries. Many of the injuries sustained by sportspeople that will be described and discussed later frequently overlap with other conditions and may well be related to predisposing physical factors. To successfully treat the injured athlete who presents with a complex set of inter-related signs, symptoms, pathoanatomy and possible predisposing physical factors, requires a thorough and methodical approach to all aspects of examination. This examination procedure should be guided by sound clinical reasoning processes and should be based upon a comprehensive knowledge base. While it is beyond the scope of this text to cover these important issues in any depth, they will be discussed briefly in an attempt to stress their importance, particularly in the treatment and management of the more complex sports injury presentations.

5.1.2 Clinical reasoning

This term relates to the thought processes that are used by the clinician in terms of examining, assessing, treating and managing patient problems. It does not relate to specific examination or treatment actions or to particular clinical decisions. The term 'clinical reasoning' has been used by medical educationalists for some time, but it has only been in recent years that its relevance and application to physiotherapy has been stressed. Higgs (1992) in a review of the subject noted that the clinical reasoning processes that are used by experienced therapists are similar to those used by their medical counterparts but that therapists tended to place greater emphasis on treatment and subsequent evaluation, while members of the medical profession tended to emphasize diagnosis formulation. The examination process can be described as a hypothetico-deductive process. This involves the therapist making hypotheses about numerous aspects of the patient's presenting problem, e.g. diagnosis, contraindications to treatment, type of treatment to be undertaken, likely prognosis and factors predisposing to the presenting problem. By a process of subjective and objective evaluation these hypotheses are then tested. How effective this process is depends to a large degree on how comprehensive the clinician's knowledge base is and how effectively this is organized. According to Jones and Butler (1991) one of the fundamental differences between the 'expert' and the 'novice' is the content and the structure of this knowledge base. Jones and Butler noted that inexperienced therapists had relatively few clinical patterns stored in their memories and that many of these patterns, which were learned through texts, were too rigid. This can result in a line of examination questioning being closed before sufficient information has been

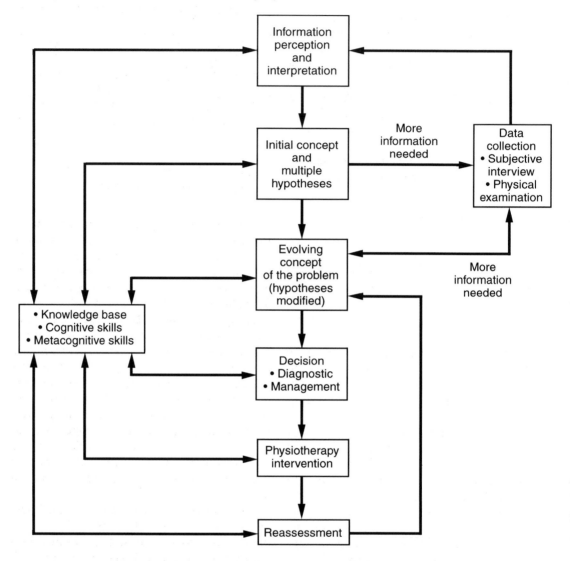

Figure 5.1   The clinical reasoning process, based on the hypothetico-deductive reasoning model. (Source: reproduced from Higgs, 1992, with permission.)

gleaned or in indiscriminate action being taken on every clinical detail. In contrast, the experienced clinician tends to structure the examination process in response to the information that is elicited from the patient. In other words, there is immediate synthesis and interpretation of the information into hypotheses, which are then tested with further examination and treatment. Conver-sely, the novice tends to adhere to a set examination process that has been learnt by rote and instead of interpreting patient information in terms of clinical patterns and hypotheses, tends merely to record specific examination findings. Jones and Butler (1991) advocated the adoption of a clinical-reasoning-based examination and treatment approach as a way of efficiently developing a well-structured knowledge base. The desired relationship between a hypothetico-deductive clinical reasoning strategy and a clinician's knowledge base is depicted in Figure 5.1.

It is hoped that this text will help to enhance and increase the clinician's knowledge base by providing information in a manner that will help clinician's to endorse some of the clinical patterns they have already encountered and to recognize new ones.

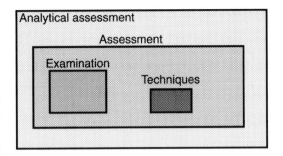

Figure 5.2 The relative importance of treatment technique, examination and assessment.

5.1.3 Principles of examination and assessment

There are many texts which comprehensively cover important aspects of musculoskeletal examination procedure (Grant, Jones and Maitland, 1988; Jones and Butler, 1991; Maitland, 1986, 1991). As far as orthopaedic physiotherapy is concerned, it has been the clinicians who have worked in the fields of manipulative therapy who have recognized that examination and assessment have greater importance than specific treatment modalities alone. The reason for this emphasis is that individual treatment modalities can only have an optimum effect if they are delivered appropriately and this can only be achieved if an efficient and logical examination and assessment strategy is implemented. Maitland (1988) graphically represented the relative importance of treatment techniques, examination and assessment (Figure 5.2) as part of his description of a manipulative physiotherapy model. It is this concept of examination and assessment that is advocated for the management of the sports injuries that will be presented in this text.

This model of physiotherapy is one which primarily uses the presenting signs and symptoms of the patient to dictate the type of treatment and management that is appropriate. This approach is fundamentally different from treatment systems that are based primarily on the formulation of a diagnosis, which itself then dictates which treatment and management should be implemented. A 'signs and symptoms' approach advocated by Maitland does not diminish the importance of the 'diagnostic' approach and indeed pays very close attention to the formulation of a diagnosis where this is possible. By adopting a 'signs and symptoms' approach to the management of the injured athlete, the therapist will be encouraged to employ clinical reasoning skills and this in turn will foster a holistic approach to the management of the condition. This is of particular importance when dealing with more complex sports injuries, which may be multifactorial in origin and pathology and which require more than just 'local' treatment to ensure complete recovery without unnecessary relapse.

The approach proposed by Maitland (1988) stipulates that the treatment techniques selected be closely analysed so that their efficacy can be determined. While this approach has been used widely by therapists in relation to manual therapy techniques, it has not generally been applied to other treatment modalities such as exercise and electrotherapy. The successful treatment and rehabilitation of the majority of sports injuries involves multiple treatment modality usage and if such regimens are to be of optimum efficacy, each modality must be applied in a logical manner and evaluated, where possible, along the same lines as individual manipulative therapy techniques.

Some of the basic principles of the type of examination, assessment and treatment procedures that are advocated will now be described. This is done only to act as an *aide memoire* or as a brief overview. The texts by Maitland (1986, 1991) and Jones and Butler (1991) are recommended for further information.

5.1.4　Subjective examination

It is vital to find out the exact nature of the patient's problem in terms of his/her chief complaint and how it affects his/her function. Areas of symptoms must be precisely ascertained and the behaviour of the symptoms, especially as regards functional activities, must be studied. This basic information often gives very strong clues as to the anatomical source of the symptoms and helps the clinician to determine the severity and irritability of the condition. This information will help to dictate the type of objective examination testing that will be required and will help when making a prognosis. When interviewing the patient and later when performing tests and treatments the clinician should always try to 'make features fit' (Maitland, 1986). For example, the presenting complaint should be accompanied by a history and a set of signs and symptoms that accounts fully for the condition in question. One frequently encountered scenario which illustrates this is the runner who complains of a long-standing 'hamstring strain' but on questioning has no history of a specific sudden onset of symptoms, which is always the case when a muscle has actually been 'strained'. Instead the patient recounts an insidious onset that corresponded with the onset of hill running. Another incongruity in this case is the area of symptoms, which the patient usually experiences in the mid-posterior thigh but which on occasions spread to affect the calf. In this case the mode of onset and the symptomatic areas are not suggestive of a primary hamstring muscle problem and the

clinician at this early stage of the examination would probably be hypothesizing that vertebral and neuromeningeal structures might be implicated. Further questioning and objective examination would test this hypothesis.

5.1.5　Objective examination

This part of the examination process should be a direct extension of the subjective examination and seek to test anatomical structures to either implicate or clear them. In addition to performing standard musculoskeletal clinical tests, it is often useful to perform functional tests. Where appropriate these could consist of activities that actually reproduce the patient's symptoms or could involve the movements that were involved in the injury's onset. The point of this is twofold. Firstly, functional tests, which are invariably combined and sometimes complex movements, frequently provide information regarding the anatomical structures that are at fault, when testing those same structures in isolation does not. Secondly, this type of testing can sometimes be used to differentiate between the involvement of different structures in the presenting condition.

5.1.6　Assessment

This is not the same as 'examination'. There are three types of assessment (Maitland, 1991). The first is the type of assessment that the clinician should make during the initial examination; this could involve, among other things, relating the examination findings to the behaviour of the patient's symptoms and to the diagnosis. The second type is an assessment/reassessment process, which is crucial to the testing of examination hypotheses and the identification of clinical patterns. This process involves monitoring the patient's signs and symptoms prior to and following the application of a specific treatment, to see if it is effective. The third type of assessment is analytical assessment, which should be undertaken during and at the completion of the treatment programme. This type of assessment retrospectively evaluates the effect of the treatment programme and is used to formulate a prognosis.

5.2 TREATMENT MODALITIES

5.2.1 Introduction and overview

This section will give an overview of some commonly used modalities that are employed to treat and rehabilitate injured athletes. This overview will hopefully put into context some of the specific treatment recommendations and guidelines that appear in the sections dealing with individual sports injuries.

It is probably true to say that each therapist has a particular bias towards one type of therapy, such as manual therapy, exercise therapy or electrotherapy. The reasons for such a bias could include an emphasis of one particular therapy in the practitioner's training or to clinical experiences that result in him/her empirically selecting a certain treatment approach in response to certain clinical presentations. Many of the treatment modalities currently in everyday physiotherapy practice have not been subjected to sufficient scientific scrutiny to enable a definitive conclusion to be reached as to their actual physiological effects or efficacy. This is particularly true of many electrotherapy treatments. The reason for this is that it is extremely difficult, and in some instances impossible, to perform scientifically validated tests on many of the physiotherapy treatments currently employed that would give definitive answers to the basic questions of 'how does it work?' and 'how effective is it?'. This state of affairs should not, however, prevent the clinician from employing specific treatment modalities in an evaluative manner and where possible basing his/her treatment selection on the scientific data available. In so doing therapists will avoid the pitfall of selecting treatments simply out of habit and will ensure that their treatments are of optimum effect.

The treatment modalities that will be described and discussed here come under the headings of electrotherapy, exercise, taping and manual therapy. It is hoped that this section will give those who are unfamiliar with the treatment aspects of physiotherapy practice a basic understanding of the subject. For those clinicians who are relatively inexperienced, it is hoped that the following discussion on treatment strategies and the specific treatment recommendations that are made regarding specific injuries and conditions, will provide tried and tested approaches to injury management. This may serve as a starting point for individual professional development. For the experienced practitioner, the text will either confirm his/her own preferred treatment strategies and/or stimulate thought and discussion.

5.2.2 Electrotherapy

There are a multitude of electrotherapy machines, which therapists of many persuasions use to treat and in some instances 'diagnose' various physical ailments. Some of these treatments have over the years become accepted as conventional methods of treatment and some therapists rely heavily on electrotherapy as a mainstay of their clinical practice. Many of the claimed effects of most electrotherapies are scientifically unsubstantiated. This does not, however, deter the electrotherapy manufacturers from devising ever more ingenious, microprocessor-controlled, high-tech devices and launching them on to the multi-million-pound electromedical equipment market. These machines are frequently accompanied by pseudoscientific marketing literature which very often baffles therapists, let alone the intended recipients – the patients. Nevertheless, the clinical experiences of countless therapists have, over the years, indicated that some of the electrotherapies have a positive effect on a wide range of sports injuries and it would be foolish to dismiss these clinical observations just because of shortfalls in orthodox scientific testing.

Most experienced therapists use various electrotherapy modalities but do so in as evaluative a manner as possible and look upon electrotherapy as an adjunct to more direct forms of physical treatment, such as manual and exercise therapies. Some of the more commonly used electrotherapies will now be discussed. These have been selected because of their current popularity.

(a) Ultrasound (US)

Ultrasound is probably the most widely used electrotherapy and is employed in the treatment of acute and chronic soft-tissue injuries. The technology involved is relatively simple and involves the application of an electrical current to a piezoelectric crystal, which is encased in a metal treatment probe. This generates a sound wave between 0.75 MHz and 3 MHz, which is applied to the patient's skin via some form of liquid or gel coupling medium (Figure 5.3).

The ultrasound energy output is controlled by three parameters: time, power output (measured in watts) and pulsing of the output. If the output is of sufficient power and duration, thermal effects will be experienced. However, many if not all of the therapeutic effects of ultrasound are thought to be produced by non-thermal mechanisms. In the early stages following injury, ultrasound is used with the intention of modulating the inflammatory response. It is also claimed to be effective in producing analgesia and in reducing the post-traumatic exudate that is responsible for soft-tissue swelling. Some therapists use ultrasound in the treatment of chronic conditions and one frequently cited effect is an increase in scar tissue plasticity, although there is no firm scientific evidence to support this.

Ultrasound is probably the most widely researched of all the electrotherapies. Despite this there is still uncertainty as to its actual effects on the cellular repair mechanisms that occur following injury (Maxwell, 1992). This makes it impossible for the therapist to base dosage and treatment frequency entirely on scientific data. However the fact remains that ultrasound has been used therapeutically for over half a century and has been clinically proved to be safe (in the hands of qualified therapists) and to have observed clinical effects in optimizing recovery following soft-tissue injuries.

(b) Laser therapy

Laser therapy has been a popular treatment for acute and chronic soft-tissue injuries since the mid 1980s. Its proponents claim

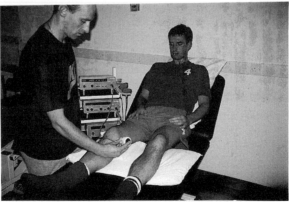

Figure 5.3 The application of ultrasound.

that it produces analgesia and promotes healing. Therapeutic lasers are sometimes termed 'soft lasers' and produce beams with wavelengths of between 660 nm and 904 nm. The clinical effects of laser therapy and the exact physiological responses have not been conclusively proved.

(c)   Pulsed electromagnetic energy

Pulsed electromagnetic energy (PEME) is a modality that is commonly used to treat a wide range of chronic and acute musculoskeletal conditions. It is derived from the established use of electromagnetic energy to produce a heating effect on body tissues, which dates back many years and uses radio waves of 27.12 MHz . This form of treatment using electromagnetic energy is commonly referred to as short wave diathermy (SWD) and has been used by therapists to produce a 'deep ' heating of muscles, joints and body cavities in order to increase circulation and produce analgesia. Whether or not SWD is truly effective in producing physiological effects that optimize healing or reduce pain has never been conclusively proved (Kitchen and Partridge, 1992). Developments in technology and treatment modalities have produced refinements in this mode of treatment and since the 1950s PEME has been used to treat the same range of conditions as SWD. This treatment uses the same type of waveform as SWD but it is pulsed in such a way that at low frequencies and pulse widths (both of which can be altered by the therapist) there is no appreciable thermal effect. Some of the claimed effects of PEME are a decrease in post-traumatic swelling, the reabsorption of haematoma, an increase in fibrin and collagen formation and the acceleration of nerve growth and repair. Such observations have not, however, been universally observed (Kitchen and Partridge, 1992). More research is required if these claims are to be substantiated and if optimum treatment parameters are to be established.

(d)   Electrical stimulation

Electrical stimulation (ES) is used in physical therapy to produce muscular contractions and to produce analgesia. Another claimed effect is the stimulation of circulation, which it is claimed can optimize tissue healing and aid in the reduction of traumatic soft-tissue and joint effusions. ES is available in many different wave-forms and frequencies and these are altered in order to produce different physiological effects. For instance, a waveform with a high amplitude and low pulse width could be used to produce involuntary muscular contractions. The machines that produce these therapeutic currents are many and varied and are marketed under a bewildering array of names. The original machines used to produce muscular contractions emit a 'faradic' current which has a pulse width of 1 ms and is delivered at a frequency of 50 Hz. While effective, such currents produce significant cutaneous discomfort and modern machines use wave-forms and frequencies that are more easily tolerated.

ES is frequently used to elicit muscular contractions when they cannot be performed actively by the patient, as a result of inhibition and/or weakness. In these situations they can be used to re-educate the desired muscular activity. Muscular stimulation can also sometimes be of value when treating chronic muscle tears that have resulted in deep scarring and as a result are symptomatic during activity – for example the athlete may experience a localized pulling or tight sensation, usually during ballistic movements. In such cases the ES can be given across the symptomatic site while the affected limb is positioned so that the affected muscle is at full stretch and no joint movement is possible. The strong isometric contraction obtained by the application of the ES can be augmented by an active contraction and this produces a localized increase in muscular tension, which may result in greater scar tissue plasticity.

Some therapists and athletic trainers have endorsed the use of ES as a means of producing strength gains and there was considerable interest in the so called 'Russian' currents during the 1970s. However, simple logic would suggest that, if such currents were superior to voluntary muscular contractions in producing strength gains, then they would have to produce greater muscular tension than voluntary contractions. This has not been consistently demonstrated to be the case and it is doubtful that, in practice, ES offers any real advantages over orthodox strengthening exercise programmes.

ES is probably of most value in treating pain and for most therapists this is its main application. Some of the commonly used methods of modulating pain perception are transcutaneous nerve stimulators (TNS), interferential currents and high-voltage galvanic stimulators. While the use of ES to produce analgesia is an accepted and common part of physiotherapy practice it should rarely if ever be the sole treatment modality used for musculoskeletal disorders. For optimum results it should complement more direct means of treatment such as manual and exercise therapies.

(e) Electromyographic biofeedback

Electromyographic biofeedback (EMGBF) involves measuring the electrical activity of working muscles with surface electrodes and amplifying the resultant electrical impulses. These are then relayed to the therapist and patient, either audibly or visually. As there is a proportional increase in electrical activity with an increase in muscular effort, the patient is made aware of this by an increase in the volume of the EMGBF and/or an increase in the number of lights that are illuminated on the EMGBF display. Electromyography has been used in 'physical medicine' as a diagnostic tool for decades. however, its use in everyday clinical settings has been a relatively recent development. This has been due entirely to advances in electronics technology which have enabled the equipment to be miniaturized and vastly improved in terms of reliability and performance. Modern EMGBF machines fit into the palm of a hand and the surface electrodes are reusable and require no special skin preparation. They can be used in everyday settings and they provide an invaluable analysis of functional muscular activity, which can be used to aid muscular re-education and strengthening exercise programmes.

5.2.3   Exercise therapy

The prescription of exercise has been an integral part of physiotherapy practice for generations (Figure 5.4).

Over the past two decades there have been considerable advances in the disciplines of

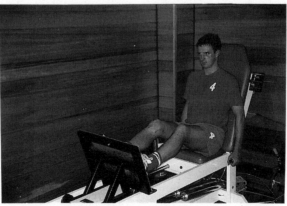

Figure 5.4 Exercise therapy.

kinesiology and biomechanics and some of this knowledge has been applied to everyday clinical practice, particularly in the field of lower limb rehabilitation following anterior cruciate reconstruction (Palmitier *et al.*, 1991). Consequently, exercise therapy has been re-evaluated by many contemporary therapists and its central role in the management of the majority of sports injuries has been recognized.

Exercise therapy serves two purposes following injury. Firstly, it can help rectify the physical problems that are a direct consequence of the injury, and secondly, it can be used to maintain general and sport-specific skills and fitness.

This second use of exercise is often termed **substitute training**. Substitute training involves omitting or swapping certain preferred training activities for those that will not unduly stress the injured area, so that appropriate treatment and the passage of time can rectify the problem. The appropriate type of substitute training depends upon the type and severity of the injury and on the sport of the athlete in question. For example, a javelin thrower who presents with an early-stage shoulder tendinitis may only need to temporarily reduce the number of throws carried out in training or the number of throwing sessions and perhaps modify strength training exercises to avoid positions of full shoulder abduction. For a more serious and long-term problem such as a completely ruptured Achilles tendon in a football player, there would have to be major changes to the preferred training programme. Instead of running to maintain cardiovascular fitness, the footballer would perhaps cycle or row so that the injury was not overloaded. In the early stages of the injury it would also be inappropriate to undertake any skills training. In such a case the substitute training programme would have to be radically different from the one employed when fully fit. Substitute training has the practical benefits of maintaining various aspects of fitness during

periods of injury and it also helps to keep the athlete in a positive frame of mind. This in turn helps to keep him/her motivated and compliant with any physical restrictions that have to be imposed and the rehabilitation programme that has been implemented.

It was mentioned earlier that exercises are used in injury rehabilitation to rectify some of the physical problems that have resulted either from injury or from subsequent surgery or immobilization. Exercise can be used to improve:

- Muscle function
- Joint function
- Movement patterns
- Coordination
- Proprioception
- Flexibility
- Bone and soft-tissue 'strength'.

Muscle weakness is a common problem following many different types of injury. Improving strength with suitable exercise is often a goal of the rehabilitation process but, in practice, this should not be an isolated objective. For instance a restriction of muscular flexibility and/or a restriction of joint mobility will result in a 'weakness' of the associated muscles and attempts to strengthen the affected muscle groups without rectifying the associated joint and muscular stiffness will not give optimum results. It is rarely if ever the case that the rehabilitation programme strives to achieve only one of the above objectives. For example, if the main clinical problem seems to be of joint stiffness, then strengthening work should be given in addition to mobilizing exercises so that muscular strength improves through the newly acquired ranges of motion.

When a specific muscle group is targeted for strengthening, it is important to ensure that imbalances do not occur. An appropriate balance should be made between agonists and antagonists and between opposite limbs. This will ensure that optimum function is restored and re-injury is prevented (Atha, 1981).

It is also important to ensure that the muscles that are being strengthened are also re-educated so that they and their associated muscle groups are able to produce coordinated patterns of movements that are functionally relevant to the sport in question. In practice this coordination training is intimately related to the exercises that are given to improve proprioception. For the exercise programme to fulfil all these inter-related aims, it is vital that emphasis is placed on functional and sport-specific exercises. In addition to being able to achieve multiple rehabilitation goals, functional and sport-specific exercises adhere to the accepted convention of 'specificity of training' (Harris, 1984). This relates to the fact that gains in muscular performance are specific to the actual exercises and activities practised and will not necessarily transfer to different activities (Harris, 1984). For example, a basketball player who has a weak quadriceps following a knee injury may have a functional complaint of 'weakness' when jumping. Improved quadriceps strength obtained from performing weight-resisted seated knee extension exercises would not necessarily result in an improved ability to jump or drive off from the affected limb. If improvements in muscular performance are to be of functional use to the athlete, the exercises that are used must be related to the function and/or sporting activity in question (Rutherford, 1988). The seated knee extension exercise is a non-functional exercise for the quadriceps muscles, which are worked in isolation, while a step up would be a functional activity.

In addition to some important biomechanical differences (which are explained in the section on anterior cruciate ligament injuries), one of the most obvious differences between the seated knee extension and the step exercise is that the latter involves multiple muscle work. Another is that the step exercise involves lower-limb weightbearing forces. These two factors are prerequisites if optimum improvements are to be made in

lower-limb proprioception and if correct movement patterns are to be re-established in addition to the basic goal of 'strengthening'. Although the example of functional exercise was related to lower-limb muscle groups, the same principles apply to the upper limb. It is important that functional exercise be progressed in such a way that incorrect movement patterns are not adopted and this is best achieved by stressing quality of movement rather than quantity and by progressing to quicker movements only after they have been mastered at slow speeds (Palmitier *et al.*, 1991).

The final point to consider is the effect that exercise can have on non-contractile tissues such as bone, articular cartilage, tendons and ligaments. It has been demonstrated that periods of rest and immobility result in a weakening of these structures and that there are positive changes in response to physiological stresses (Booth and Gould, 1975; Reid, 1992). Conversely, if these tissues are overstressed – and this can easily be done following injury – structural damage can result. For these reasons, it is desirable for postinjury and postsurgery periods of rest, protection and/or immobilization to be kept to an absolute minimum and for a closely monitored and carefully progressed exercise programme to be instituted. In this way the injured athlete will be sidelined for the minimum amount of time and his/her functional outcome will be optimized.

5.2.4 Taping

The terms 'taping' and 'strapping' are interchangeable and relate to the application of adhesive fabric, either elasticated or rigid, so that it supports joints or soft tissues. Strapping can be of use immediately following injury, during rehabilitation or as a prophylactic measure. As a first-aid treatment its main use is to control the bleeding and soft-tissue swelling that can occur immediately following injury. It also supports the injured tissues in such a way that the likelihood of further damage is reduced. During the rehabilitation phase, taping can be used to facilitate and improve movement, by supporting injured tissues in such a way that discomfort is alleviated and any resultant pain inhibition is reduced and proprioception enhanced (Millar, 1973). The use of functional taping in the rehabilitation of certain injuries, fits well with the current sports medicine philosophies of limiting postinjury and postsurgical immobilization to a minimum and of encouraging active management (MacDonald, 1994).

Another important use of taping is to correct abnormal joint positions and to alter the alignment of soft tissues such as tendons in such a way that improvements in function are facilitated. The most common application for this type of taping is in the management of patellofemoral problems. This was described by McConnell (1986) and involves the identification of abnormal patella positions, which are then corrected with tape so that function is improved and rehabilitation of any associated muscular dysfunction and inhibition is optimized. This approach to taping, which is based upon a thorough clinical and functional assessment followed by a careful re-evaluation process, should serve as the basis for the application of all taping.

The prophylactic use of taping is common practice among many athletes across many different sports, for both training and competition. The areas of the body that are routinely taped in an attempt to prevent or limit the extent of an injury depend to a high degree on the sport in question. For example, boxers will routinely use hand taping to protect their metacarpophalangeal joints, while some rugby players and American footballers (particularly defensive and offensive linemen) use a modified boxer's handwrap to provide support. It is thought that injury-preventative taping has its effects partly by physically restricting potentially injurious ranges of movement and partly by stimulating skin sensory afferent nerve pathways which, via spinal pathways, facilitate active control mechanisms (Millar, 1973). While most body parts can be taped it is undoubtedly the ankle which is most commonly taped for prophylactic reasons. Studies have demonstrated the decreased incidence of sprains with the use of such taping (Garrick and Roqua, 1975), but devices such as laced ankle stabilizers have been shown to be more effective (Miller and Hergenroeder, 1990). Given the fact that they are re-usable and easier to apply, the use of such devices seems to be preferable, though individual choice on the part of the athlete should be the deciding factor.

Taping can be of value in preventing and in treating a wide range of sports injuries (Figure 5.5).

However, it will only be of benefit if the injury is properly assessed. Inappropriate tap-

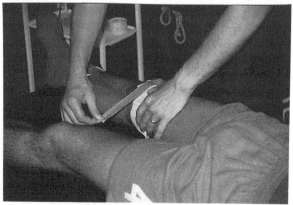

Figure 5.5 The application of taping.

ing can not only be ineffective but can increase the severity of the injury in question and cause damage to other areas.

5.2.5 Manual therapy

In the following discussion, the term 'manual therapy' will be used to cover all the therapies that involve the manipulation (i.e. movement rather than forceful high-velocity joint manipulation) of any anatomical structure. These are massage (in all its many guises) and joint mobilization/manipulation.

Manual therapy is invaluable in the effective management of the majority of sports injuries. Some of the indications and effects of manual therapy are discussed below.

(a) Mobilization and manipulation

'Mobilization' and 'manipulation' are terms that are frequently used to describe the techniques of passive movement used to treat a wide variety of vertebral and peripheral joint conditions together with associated pathologies of the nervous system. There are numerous schools of manipulative therapy, which have their own philosophies and methods of examination, assessment and treatment. The manual therapies recommended for the treatment of the conditions that have been selected for description and discussion do not relate to one specific concept of manipulative therapy.

However, for manipulative therapy to be truly effective, it must be applied in such a way that its effects are closely monitored both during and after each treatment. The concept of manipulative therapy, as described by Maitland (1986, 1991), is probably the most complete in this regard.

Passive movement can be used to:

- improve restrictions of motion;
- reduce protective muscle spasm;
- treat pain (of mechanical rather than of inflammatory origin).

The latter two effects of passive movement are frequently overlooked.

While the effective management of most sports injuries involves the use of many different types of treatment, such as exercise and electrotherapy treatments, it is probably true to say that passive movement therapy should play a central role in the management of the majority if the best results are to be achieved. Specific techniques and indications for their application will be described in relation to specific injuries and conditions.

(b) Massage

Massage is routinely used for pre- and post-sporting participation in order to prepare the athlete for competition and to help limit or prevent postexercise fatigue and stiffness. However these undoubtedly beneficial

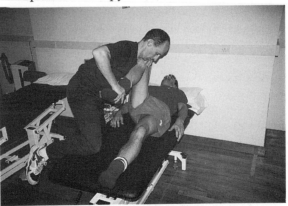

Figure 5.6 Passive mobilization of the knee.

applications of massage will not be discussed here. Instead, the application of massage techniques to soft-tissue injuries will be considered.

In the treatment of sports injuries, massage techniques have been routinely used to improve the flexibility of thickened tissues such as muscle, tendon and ligaments. Techniques such as transverse frictions, as described by Cyriax (1984), are of proven clinical value in the treatment of subacute and chronic injuries. Such techniques have no place in the treatment of acute injuries as they will probably cause further tissue damage. They can be effective in improving flexibility and in modulating pain but their efficacy is dependent upon the correct timing following injury and on the dose (i.e. the vigour with which they are applied), the duration of the treatment and the treatment frequency. Most clinicians apply friction-type massage with the intention of achieving the previously mentioned effects of improving tissue flexibility or mobility and of 'breaking down adhesions'. One often overlooked reason for applying these and similar techniques is to stimulate the healing process in such a way that the soft-tissue repair is as strong as possible. It has been demonstrated that injured soft-tissues that are subjected to controlled amounts of external stress respond in such a way that the ultimate strength of the repaired tissue is stronger than would be the case if the tissue had been 'rested' (Gomez *et al.*, 1991; Maxwell, 1992). Specific soft-tissue techniques can in theory be used to stimulate increases in soft-tissue tensile strength. If they are to be effective in achieving this, they must be applied at the appropriate time following injury and, to do this, the clinician must have a detailed knowledge and a thorough clinical understanding of the healing process – specifically with regard to the time scales that relate to the formation and maturation of collagen. Hunter (1994) described the application of what he termed 'soft-tissue mobilizations' with the intention of improv-ing soft-tissue tensile strength following injury, and he advocated the use of a grading system similar to that used by Maitland (1991) for joint mobilization techniques. This recommendation was made so that the clinician could subjectively quantify the load that is applied. It also helps with treatment progression and the delivery of optimum force. This evaluative approach to massage application, which is based on a sound understanding of soft-tissue pathophysiology is the ideal on which to base this most effective treatment modality.

5.3 REFERENCES

Atha, J.(1981) Strengthening muscle. *Exercise and Sports Science Review*, **9**, 1–73.

Booth, F.W. and Gould E.W. (1975) Effect of training and disuse on connective tissue, in *Exercise and Sports Sciences Review*, (eds Whitmore and Keough), Academic Press, London.

Cyriax, J. (1984) *Textbook of Orthopaedic Medicine*, vol. 2. Baillière Tindall, Eastbourne.

Garrick, J.G. and Requa, R.K. (1975) Role of external support in prevention of ankle sprains. *Medical Science of Sports*, **5**, 200–203

Gomez, M.A., Woo, S.L.Y., Amiel D. *et al.* (1991) The effects of increased tension on healing medial collateral ligaments. *American Journal of Sports Medicine*, **19**(4), 347–354.

Grant, R., Jones, M.A. and Maitland, G.D. (1988) Clinical decision making in upper quadrant dysfunction, in *Physical Therapy of the Cervical and Thoracic Spine*, (ed. R. Grant), Churchill Livingstone, New York.

Harris, F.A. (1984) Facilitation techniques and technology adjuncts in therapeutic exercise, in *Therapeutic Exercise*, 9th edn, (ed. J.V. Basmajin), Williams & Wilkins, Baltimore, MD.

Higgs, J. (1992) Developing clinical reasoning competencies. *Physiotherapy*, **78**(8), 575–581.

Hunter, G. (1984) Specific soft tissue mobilisation of soft tissue lesions. *Physiotherapy*, **80**(1), 15–21.

Jones, M.A. and Butler, D.S. (1991) Clinical reasoning, in *Mobilisation of the Nervous System*, Churchill Livingstone, Edinburgh.

Kitchen, S. and Partridge, C. (1992) Review of shortwave diathermy continuous and pulsed. *Physiotherapy*, **78**(4), 243–252.

McConnell, J. (1986) The management of CMP: a long term solution. *Australian Journal of Physiotherapy*, **23**, 220–221.

MacDonald, R. (ed.) (1994) *Taping Techniques. Principles and Practice.* Butterworth-Heinemann, Oxford.

Maitland, G.D. (1986) Vertebral manipulation, 5th edn, Butterworth, London.

Maitland, G.D. (1988) A manipulative physiotherapy model. IFOMPT Congress proceedings.

Maitland, G.D. (1991) Peripheral manipulation, 3rd edn, Butterworth Heinemann, Oxford.

Markku, J., Jarvinen X., Matti, V.K. *et al.* (1993) The effects of early mobilisation and immobilisation on the healing process following muscle injuries. *Sports Medicine*, **15**(2), 78–89.

Maxwell, L. (1992) Therapeutic ultrasound: its effects on the cellular and molecular mechanisms of inflammation and repair. *Physiotherapy*, **78**(6) 421–425.

Millar, J. (1973) Joint afferent fibres responding to muscle stretch, vibration and contraction. *Brain Research*, **63**, 380–838.

Miller, E.A. and Hergenroeder, A.C. (1990) Prophylactic ankle bracing. *Pediatric Clinics of North America*, **37**, 1175–1185.

Palmitier, R.A., An, K., Scott, S.G. *et al.* (1991) Kinetic chain exercise in knee rehabilitation. *Sports Medicine*, **11**(6), 402–413.

Reid, D.C. (1992) Sports injury assessment and rehabilitation, Churchill Livingstone, Edinburgh.

Rutherford, O.M. (1988) Muscular co-ordination and strength training: implications for injury rehabilitation. *Sports Medicine*, **5**, 196–202.

6. Selected injuries by body region

6.1 THE SHOULDER COMPLEX

6.1.1 Introduction

The shoulder complex is composed of the following functionally related synovial joints; the **glenohumeral joint**, the **acromioclavicular joint** and the **sternoclavicular joint** (Figure 6.1).

It also includes the **scapulothoracic 'joint'**. These articulations allow the arm to be moved through large and complex ranges of movement. However, the price for such mobility is a compromise in the stability of some of these joints, most notably the scapulothoracic and the glenohumeral articulations. The inherent mobility of the glenohumeral joint predisposes it to both traumatic and overuse injuries. Such injuries are common in contact sports and among 'overhead' athletes, i.e. throwers, racquet-sport competitors and swimmers.

6.1.2 Functional anatomy

(a) The sternoclavicular and acromioclavicular joints

The sternoclavicular (SC) and acromioclavicular (AC) joints provide the only ligamentous connections between the upper limb and the axial skeleton. As such their role is to transmit and dissipate the external forces that are applied to the upper limb (both compression and tension). In addition to force transmission, the SC and AC joints help to control both the ranges and amounts of movement that are available in the glenohumeral and scapulothoracic joints. The clavicular joints work as a functional unit, with the clavicle

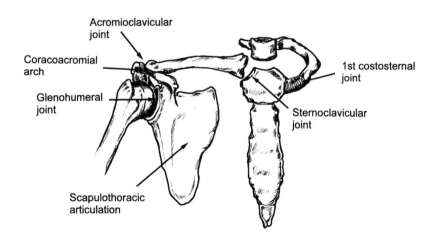

Figure 6.1 The shoulder complex.

transmitting forces and consequent ranges of motion, from one joint to the other. During full elevation of the arm the lateral portion of the clavicle moves through approximately 45–60° of movement (Schenkman and De Cartaya, 1987). The actual directions of movement that occur in the SC and AC joints are dependent upon the direction of movement in the corresponding upper limb, and *vice versa*. If movements of the SC and AC become limited by pain or stiffness, e.g. as a consequence of injury, there will usually be a significant reduction in glenohumeral and general shoulder complex function.

(b) The scapulothoracic 'joint'

The scapulothoracic (ST) 'joint' is the term used to describe the articulation of the scapula and the upper posterolateral aspect of the thorax. Scapular stability is dependent upon complex and coordinated muscular activity and its function is to provide a stable, yet mobile base upon which the upper limb can move. The scapula, by virtue of its mobility, permits significantly larger ranges of arm movement than would be the case if the glenohumeral joint operated in isolation. Normal ST and glenohumeral motion is dependent upon a finely controlled pattern of muscular activity and the interaction of these joints in producing arm movements is often referred to as **scapulohumeral rhythm** (Codman, 1934). During the first 30° or so of arm elevation, the scapula remains relatively immobile so as to provide a stable base on which the humerus can move. This has been termed the 'setting phase' (Doody, Freedman and Waterland, 1970). As arm elevation continues, the scapula protracts, i.e. it rotates laterally and slides anteriorly around the thorax. Between approximately 30 and 90° of arm elevation there is approximately 1° of scapular movement for every 2° of humeral movement. After the humerus passes the horizontal, the rate of scapular elevation matches that of the humerus (Codman, 1934).

ST movements may exhibit reductions in movement quality and quantity, when the scapular musculature (particularly trapezius, rhomboids, levator scapula and serratus anterior) become inhibited by pain-provoking conditions, e.g. injuries that affect the muscles directly or, more frequently the joints of the shoulder complex. Consequently, an alteration in the length–tension relationship of the glenohumeral joint soft tissues can result. This may then either cause or perpetuate a glenohumeral joint injury.

(c) The glenohumeral joint

The glenohumeral joint can be subdivided into the glenohumeral (GH) and the subacromial (SA) articulations. The glenohumeral articulation, in common with all synovial joints, relies upon capsular and ligamentous structures to provide passive stability. These structures are, however, relatively lax so as to allow large ranges of movement in multiple directions. The bony configuration of the relatively large humeral head and the relatively shallow glenoid cavity of the scapula also permit large excursions of movement (Warner *et al.*, 1992). Glenohumeral capsular laxity is most pronounced when the arm is by the side of the body and in this position the superior and inferior glenohumeral ligaments provide most of the passive support to the humeral head against inferior displacement. As the arm is abducted the inferior glenohumeral ligament contributes more (Neer, 1983). When the arm is simultaneously elevated and laterally rotated, the anterior glenohumeral ligament broadens and acts as a sling to prevent excessive anterior translation of the head of the humerus (O'Brien *et al.*, 1990). A failure of this passive stabilizing mechanism can result in anterior humeral head subluxation and consequent pain and poor function when the arm is in the overhead position.

The greater tuberosity of the humerus provides the infraspinatus and the supraspinatus with a prominent attachment which gives a mechanical advantage to their actions. When the arm is elevated, an accompanying lateral rotation of the humeral shaft takes place and this prevents the greater tuberosity from impacting against the superiorly placed acromion process and coracoacromial ligament. The underside of the acromion and the coracoacromial ligament form the coracoacromial arch, which has a synovial lining known as the subacromial bursa. This articulates with the superior part of the humeral head and has been termed the 'subacromial joint' (Corrigan and Maitland, 1994). The rotator cuff muscles lie in this relatively confined space and the subacromial bursa minimizes the forces that they are subjected to.

(d) The rotator cuff

The rotator cuff is the name given to the four muscles that pass from the scapula, spread around the humeral head and insert on to the upper portion of the humerus. These are the anteriorly placed **subscapularis**, the superiorly positioned **supraspinatus** and the posteriorly placed **infraspinatus** and **teres minor**. The glenohumeral articulation is unique in the way that its associated supporting musculature physically interacts with the joint capsule. These supporting muscles are immediately adjacent to and attached to the capsule. These physical connections enable the tension generated by the contraction of the rotator cuff muscles to be transmitted to the capsule. As a result the capsule then tightens and holds the humeral head centrally against the glenoid cavity (Kamkar, Irrgang and Whitney, 1993).

The subscapularis muscle produces internal humeral rotation and in throwing activities and forehand racquet strokes (particularly overhead) it functions with pectoralis major and latissimus dorsi in generating forward arm momentum. However its maximum effort occurs when it works eccentrically to limit the arm from excessively rotating laterally, e.g. in the preacceleration or 'cocking'

phase of throwing/stroke playing (Glousman, 1993).

Supraspinatus works with deltoid to abduct the arm, with its main contribution probably occurring in the first part of the range. It also works to stabilize the humeral head when the arm is fully abducted (Corrigan and Maitland, 1994).

The infraspinatus and teres minor muscles produce lateral humeral rotation. Their most important role is in countering excessive anterior displacement of the head of the humerus. Normal glenohumeral dynamic stability and quality of movement is dependent to a high degree on efficient infraspinatus function (Kamkar, Irrgang and Whitney, 1993).

While the rotator cuff muscles can produce specific glenohumeral movements, their main role is to stabilize the humeral head against the glenoid cavity, both at rest and when the upper limb is moved. They perform this work in combination with one another and with the deltoid and long head of the biceps. Excessive anterior and posterior glenohumeral stresses are countered by the actions of subscapularis and infraspinatus while vertically directed forces are countered by deltoid and the inferiorly placed rotator cuff muscles (Kamkar, Irrgang and Whitney, 1993).

6.1.3 Selected injuries of the shoulder complex

The following injuries and conditions will be considered:

- Musculotendinous
  - Rotator cuff lesions
    Supraspinatus tendinitis
    Subscapularis tendinitis
    Infraspinatus tendinitis
    Rotator cuff ruptures
    Impingement syndromes
  - Bicipital tendinitis (long head)
  - Long head of biceps subluxation
  - Biceps tendon rupture

- Joint
  - Glenohumeral instability
  - Clavicular joint injuries
- Other
  - Suprascapular nerve entrapment
  - Long thoracic nerve entrapment.

(a) Rotator cuff lesions

Lesions to the individual components of the rotator cuff will be described. However, as most of these conditions have an overuse component to their aetiology and pathology, and as the rotator cuff muscles function together rather than individually, it is not surprising to find that, in practice, injury is more likely to affect multiple structures. In the clinical setting it is frequently impossible to precisely implicate one particular anatomical structure when making a diagnosis, e.g. to differentiate between injury to the supraspinatus tendon and injury to the subacromial bursa. In the case of rotator cuff lesions the term 'impingement syndrome' has been used, rather than nominating specific anatomically titled lesions, which gives an oversimplified and rather too narrow view of the actual pathology involved. Impingement syndromes will be discussed later in reference to glenohumeral instability.

Supraspinatus tendinitis

Isolated supraspinatus tendinitis can be set in motion by a single episode of injury but is more commonly attributable to overuse forces; the tendon is injured along with other structures. These injuring forces usually involve repetitive overhead arm movements and could be linked to faulty throwing or racquet technique.

Signs and symptoms   Pain is the chief complaint; it is situated deep in the point of the shoulder and may refer into the proximal upper arm. In the most acute cases, the inflammatory response may cause constant discomfort, which disturbs sleep and is interspersed with episodes of severe catching pain, usually with movements of the arm into elevation. In the chronic stages, pain is experienced intermittently with resisted shoulder abduction or as an 'arc of pain' as the arm is elevated.

Examination   The tendon may be palpated to reveal tenderness and thickening. This is most easily done by palpating the tendon between the greater tuberosity and the examiner's finger while simultaneously distracting the arm and rotating it laterally and medially. Pain may be elicited by resisting shoulder abduction. Movement of the arm through abduction frequently produces an 'arc' of pain, which usually occurs between 60° and 110° of abduction, i.e. as the inflamed tendon is compressed beneath the coracoacromial arch. When this arc of pain is present on passive shoulder abduction, a confirmatory test of supraspinatus tendinitis can be performed by applying an inferiorly directed force to the humeral head while it is in the painful arc of movement. A reduction in the pain intensity confirms a supraspinatus lesion. It is important to differentiate a supraspinatus tendinitis and for that matter any rotator cuff lesion, that occurs independently of a glenohumeral instability from one that occurs as a result of an instability, as this will have a crucial bearing on the management (see section 6.1.3(c)).

Treatment   In the acute stage, modification of pain-provoking activities is mandatory. Non-steroidal medication, electrotherapy and cryotherapy can be used for pain relief and to modulate the inflammatory process. Passive accessory glenohumeral movements may also be employed for pain relief as described by Maitland (1991). When the condition is in the subacute and chronic phases, the use of passive glenohumeral mobilization techniques can be progressed from the pain-free range treatments for pain control, to pain-provoking glenohumeral accessory and phy- siological movements, which are designed to 'clear the joint' in relation to symptomatic ranges. One such range of movement, which is frequently symptom-provoking, is the posi- tion of shoulder elevation referred to as the 'quadrant position'; another is the 'locking position', which is a combined movement of the shoulder into abduction while the upper arm is maintained in slight horizontal exten- sion and in medial rotation (Maitland, 1991). End-range passive mobilization techniques directed to such painful/stiff restrictions are often effective treatments. Transverse friction massage to the supraspinatus tendon may also be used in the chronic phase. This type of treatment is contraindicated in the early or acute phases of the condition. Before sporting activities are resumed it is advisable to test for muscle imbalances in the shoulder complex and to correct any aberrations so as to avoid a recurrence. For the same reason it is import- ant to ensure that correct sporting technique, and in the case of racquet sports correct equipment, is used. The exercise protocol out- lined for glenohumeral instabilities is suitable for this condition.

Subscapularis tendinitis

This is most common in throwing sports, swimming and racquet sports. Subscapularis works eccentrically as the arm is elevated to prevent excessive lateral rotation and then concentrically to accelerate the upper limb into flexion and medial rotation. This type of eccentric–concentric coupling produces very high forces, which can result in microtrauma to the tendon substance when repetitive movements are performed. This is frequently the case when unaccustomed amounts of throwing, swimming or forehand racquet strokes are performed. In such cases there is a gradual onset of symptoms and accompany- ing stiffness, usually towards the end of the exercise session. Like all the rotator cuff tendinitis conditions, individual acute epi-

sodes of trauma are rarely the cause of the problem.

Examination   Local tenderness of the sub- scapularis tendon can be elicited on palpation medial to the lesser tuberosity of the humerus and this is most easily done with the shoulder in some lateral rotation. A painful arc of movement may be present when the arm is simultaneously abducted and laterally rotated.

Treatment   This is along the lines outlined for supraspinatus tendinitis. A graduated strengthening exercise programme should be followed prior to the re-commencement of sport. This should be progressed to include plyometric or stretch–shortening exercises that are of functional relevance to the sport in question. This will ensure that full strength and appropriate neuromotor control is regained, thus optimizing performance and limiting the chance of a recurrence.

Infraspinatus tendinitis

While infraspinatus, and the smaller teres minor, which lies immediately below it, are capable of laterally rotating the humerus, their prime functional role is to stabilize the humeral head against the glenoid cavity. In throwing, EMG studies have shown that infraspinatus works maximally to laterally rotate the arm as it is 'cocked', i.e. prior to the acceleration phase (Glousman, 1993). It also works hard during the acceleration phase to prevent the shoulder flexors and medial rotators (pectoralis major, subscapu- laris, anterior deltoid and latissimus dorsi), from anteriorly subluxing the humeral head and to decelerate the upper limb (Kamkar, Irr- gang and Whitney, 1993). These findings can be extrapolated to overarm racquet strokes and certain swimming strokes. As with the other rotator cuff muscles, excessive amounts of and overvigorous overarm movements are usually the cause of the injury. Any resultant pain will invariably lead to inhibition, which will result in reduced infraspinatus activity and reduced posterior glenohumeral stability.

Signs and symptoms   As the anatomy of the muscle would suggest, pain is usually experienced when the arm is laterally rotated, particularly when this is combined with elevation. In chronic cases, pain may not only be localized to the area of the infraspinatus tendon. In addition, generalized and particularly anterior shoulder pain may be a feature as the anterior glenohumeral capsular structures may be stressed by the anteriorly subluxing humeral head.

Examination   Observation of the scapula may reveal atrophy of infraspinatus. Tenderness can often be elicited by palpating the tendon at and near its insertion on the posterior portion of the greater tuberosity with the arm by the side. Stretching the muscle may also reproduce pain. This can be done by holding the upper arm in 90° of abduction and keeping the elbow at right angles. The humerus is then medially rotated to stretch the infraspinatus. From this fully rotated position the movement of lateral humeral rotation, i.e. back to the starting position, can be resisted, and this may also reproduce the patient's pain and implicate the infraspinatus. In chronic cases of infraspinatus tendinitis, the movements of medial humeral rotation and of horizontal flexion are usually limited by stiffness, which is probably due to posterior glenohumeral capsular contracture. In such long-standing cases, this capsular hypomobility is usually in contrast to hypermobility of the anterior glenohumeral capsule. This capsular pattern is frequently associated with anterior instability of the glenohumeral joint (see section 6.1.3(c)).

Treatment   The physical treatment modalities that have been described for the treatment of supraspinatus tendinitis also apply to the treatment of infraspinatus tendinitis.

Once the acute phase has passed, re-establishment of infraspinatus function should be a central theme in the successful rehabilitation of this injury. However, this will only be possible if full pain-free mobility is restored to the glenohumeral joint, particularly as regards stretching out the posterior capsular structures. EMG biofeedback is a valuable tool in helping the athlete to regain infraspinatus strength and control. EMG can be used from the early stages of regaining isometric infraspinatus control to the later stages when its function is stressed during the cocking phase of overarm throwing and racquet positioning through to stabilizing the humeral head as the shoulder flexors/internal rotators accelerate the arm forwards.

For this type of muscular re-education to be effective, the following points should be considered.

- Quality of movement must be stressed at all times.
- Submaximal loads should be used and muscle fatigue should be avoided.
- Muscular activity should be progressed from isometric to concentric to eccentric.
- Initial exercises should be at slow speeds. Increased speed should be used as a progression.
- Relevant ranges of movement must not be limited by pain or resistance – if they are, clear them with passive mobilizations.
- No pain should be provoked – it will cause inhibition and be counterproductive.

Rotator cuff ruptures

These can occur as a direct result of one traumatic incident, or more usually as a sequel to ongoing degenerative changes within the structure of the tendon. In the early stages of this pathology, such degenerative changes usually occur asymptomatically. This process is one of collagen breakdown, which occurs at a rate that outstrips the rate of collagen formation. These changes could be seen as an acceleration of the natural changes that occur in tendon structure with the passage of time, the physical demands that are placed upon the shoulder of the 'overhead' athlete being the factor that causes the acceleration. The pathological process is initially one of microscopic cellular damage within the tendon. Inflammation causes local oedema and this restricts the microcirculation of the tendon. As a consequence the healing process is disturbed. Because this process is usually asymptomatic, or only results in mild discomfort, the athlete invariably continues to exercise, so causing further damage to the tissues and compounding the problem. Inflammation and swelling of the cuff results in muscular inhibition and more stress is then applied to the glenohumeral passive stabilizing structures. The cellular microtrauma causes a reduction in the tensile strength of the tendon substance and continued athletic endeavours convert the microtrauma to macrotrauma. At this stage the athlete may present for treatment, with the condition well established and resistant to the first-line treatment of rest and modulation of the inflammatory response, which is usually effective in the early stages of the condition. Alternatively, the athlete may continue to work with and around the problem until a specific traumatic incident (which is often trivial in itself), partially or completely ruptures the pathological tendon.

Signs and symptoms Pain and an associated loss of function are the chief complaints. Resting pain and pain that disturbs sleep can be attributable to partial and complete ruptures (Kvitne and Jobe, 1995). A specific site of pain and tenderness is usually identifiable by the athlete, but more generalized shoulder pain usually accompanies this, which often refers to the upper arm and occasionally to the elbow and forearm. Any movements of the shoulder into elevation invariably provoke pain, which is inhibitory

in nature and greatly reduces the quality of shoulder movements. A specific injuring incident may be recalled by the athlete, but where this involves relatively trivial forces and where there is a history of ongoing chronic shoulder pain, the predisposing factor of tendinosis should be suspected. This is an important factor to identify as it will have a bearing on the amount of time that healing and rehabilitation will take, with or without surgical repair. Continued athletic activity by the overhead athlete may be possible but this will entail extra force being absorbed by the other components of the rotator cuff and the glenohumeral capsule, which may result in their failure.

Examination There are no specific tests for detecting partial or complete tears of the rotator cuff. The examination should include the passive movement tests and muscle contraction tests that were mentioned in reference to rotator cuff tendinitis. Complete tears would be suspected in the presence of gross weakness or altered movement patterns. In the case of supraspinatus rupture there is poor quality and weakness of the first part of the range of abduction. Even in the case of acute ruptures with no obvious background of degenerative tendon changes, atrophy of the affected muscle occurs within a few days. Because of the usual chronic soft-tissue degenerative background to these ruptures, it is important to examine for signs of glenohumeral instability. It is usually impossible to determine the exact pathology and its extent by clinical examination alone. Soft tissue scanning and arthroscopy are essential tools in this respect.

Treatment Where a definite diagnosis has been made and where the symptoms are functionally limiting, surgical repair is indicated. As rotator cuff tears are often associated with impingement pathology beneath the coracoacromial arch, acromioplasty and/or subacromial decompression may be performed simultaneously to prevent reinjury. Conservative management may be implemented as a first-line approach if the symptom severity, functional limitations and pathology are deemed not too severe. This should follow the same lines as the management of the post-repaired/decompressed shoulder. The mobilizing techniques and muscular re-education and strengthening protocols that are used for treating glenohumeral instabilities are appropriate for conservatively and operatively managed cases, the fundamental difference being the need to protect the repaired structures from potentially injurious passive and active forces in the immediate postoperative period. This does not mean, however, that lengthy periods of postoperative immobilization are required. Postoperative immobilization should be minimized because of the risk of rotator cuff atrophy, glenohumeral stiffness and poor neuromotor control. Modern methods of soft-tissue repair and fixation often allow immediate postoperative passive and active/assisted shoulder movements, together with rotator cuff stabilizing exercises. This approach will minimize the amount and severity of postimmobilization complications (Wilk and Arrigo, 1993).

Impingement syndromes

Impingement refers to the intermittent pressure that is exerted (usually in certain positions of shoulder elevation) upon the rotator cuff tendons where they lie beneath the coracoacromial arch. This can set in motion inflammatory and degenerative pathology and result in attrition of the tendon. Two types of glenohumeral impingement have been described, and in order to implement effective management it is important to differentiate between the two when making a diagnosis. This is not straightforward as the syndromes share signs and symptoms. However, different injury mechanisms are involved. The first type of impingement is termed 'primary' impingement and can be due to crowding of the subacromial space; for example, a traumatic incident or an overuse training scenario could cause tendon inflammation and thickening or a subacromial bursitis. Other causes could be glenohumeral capsular contracture or an imbalance between the strong deltoid and weaker (perhaps due to injury or poor conditioning) rotator cuff muscles, which results in the humeral head migrating upwards. The second type of impingement is termed 'secondary' and is a relative reduction in the subacromial space, caused by instability of the glenohumeral joint (see section 6.1.3(c)).

Primary impingement The pathological changes involved in this type of impingement have been classified into three stages, although, as with all injury classifications, there is considerable overlap of pathology in the clinical setting – Table 6.1 (Neer, 1983).

Table 6.1 Three stages of impingement (adapted from Neer, 1983)

Stage	Tendon pathology
One	Oedema and inflammation
Two	Fibrosis and tendinitis
Three	Tendinosis, rupture and bone spurs

Treatment and short-term rest, plus modification of aggravating activities, is usually effective for stage one primary impingements. Once stage two and three tissue changes have occurred, the pathology is not reversible and surgical management, followed by long-term rehabilitation or even permanent cessation of sport, may be required. Attempts to conservatively manage these cases should stress glenohumeral and scapulothoracic movement re-education as well as strengthening exercises, and these must not provoke any symptoms. The exercise protocols outlined for glenohumeral instability are appropriate.

Examination: A positive impingement sign, i.e. reproduction of pain, may be elicited by any glenohumeral movement that closes down the subacromial space. This may be done by performing passive glenohumeral abduction while stabilizing the shoulder girdle and preventing scapular protraction and upward rotation. Another method is to flex the shoulder to the horizontal position and then perform internal rotation. Both tests are positive for impingement if pain is reproduced.

Secondary impingement Secondary impingement occurs as a consequence of a functional decrease in the subacromial space brought about by glenohumeral instability and/or altered glenohumeral rhythm. The pathological soft-tissue changes are the same as for primary impingement. These changes are also caused by a 'pinching' of the rotator cuff between the greater tuberosity and the coracoacromial arch or by pressure from the posterosuperior glenoid rim against the underside of the infraspinatus and supraspinatus tendons.

A reduction in the amount of scapular protraction and the accompanying upward rotation of the glenoid cavity during movements of the arm into elevation can result in excessive subacromial compression between the coracoacromial arch and the greater tuberosity. Causes of such alterations in scapular movement patterns could be weakness and poorly coordinated scapular stabilizer, particularly serratus anterior (Glousman, 1993).

Glenohumeral laxity, usually in an anterior direction (see section 6.1.3(c)) can also predispose to secondary impingement. This type of instability results in an anterior and superior translation of the humeral head and the superiorly placed rotator cuff tendons are compressed in positions of shoulder elevation. The tendons of supraspinatus and infraspinatus may also be compressed against the posterosuperior glenoid rim (Kvitne and Jobe, 1995) as the humeral head translates forwards, as the arm is elevated. This mechanism of injury may account for the rupture of the undersides of these tendons.

Examination: The tests described for primary impingement can be used to elicit pain and confirm impingement in the 'secondary' group. However these must be accompanied by tests for glenohumeral instability (especially in an anterior direction). The assessment of serratus anterior weakness and/or reduced scapulothoracic stability relies mainly on the observation of abnormal scapular postures such as winging of the scapular and poor or altered quality of scapular movements when compared to the non-affected side, particularly when the arm is moved into elevated positions. It may also be possible to quantify the scapular muscle's ability to stabilize the scapula by taking measurements of the gap between the inferior angle of the scapula and its closest thoracic spinous process in three different positions of humeral abduction. This has been described by Kamkar, Irrgang and Whitney (1993) (after Kibler). The first measurement is taken with the arms by the side, the second with the hands resting on the iliac crests (thumbs pointing posteriorly) and the final measurement with the shoulders abducted to 90° with full internal rotation. Bilateral measurements are made and compared. In cases where serratus anterior, trapezius and the rhomboids do not effectively stabilize the scapula, there is an increase in the measurements obtained on the affected side.

Treatment: As the underlying cause of secondary impingement is anterior glenohumeral instability, the instability must be treated as a priority. Failure to do so, and merely treating the impingement syndrome symptoms, will predispose the overhead athlete to further tissue damage and possible rupture (Kamkar, Irrgang and Whitney, 1993).

(b) Long head of biceps tendon injuries

The long head of biceps attaches to the superior portion of the glenoid cavity, passes intracapsularly, where it is invested by a synovial sheath, and exits from the lower anterior portion of the glenohumeral capsule. The tendon lies between the tendons of supraspinatus and subscapularis in the sulcus between the greater and lesser tuberosities of the humerus.

The position of the tendon, as it runs in this sulcus, predisposes it to wear directly against the humerus as well as beneath the coracoacromial arch when the arm is used above the head. The tendon of the long head of biceps prevents excessive upward humeral head migration when the humerus is moved by the deltoid. In cases of anterior glenohumeral instability, a greater force is applied to the tendon, which over time can lead to attrition, inflammation and rupture.

Biceps tendinitis

The long head of biceps is commonly affected by inflammatory lesions. As with rotator cuff lesions, the mechanism of injury is more commonly overuse than acute trauma.

Signs and symptoms   Pain is the main complaint and is usually localized to the front of the shoulder, but may radiate distally. The shoulder movements that produce symptoms are usually combinations of elevation and lateral rotation.

Examination   Stretching the tendon and isometric biceps contractions can reproduce pain and confirm a diagnosis. Palpation of the tendon can be performed with the arm abducted to 90° or by the side and with the elbow flexed to a right angle. The humerus is passively rotated back and forth via the forearm. The tendon can then be felt to roll under the palpating fingers. Stretching the tendon is best achieved by the examiner standing behind the patient, to the side being tested, and placing the heel of one hand on the upper dorsal aspect of the shoulder to stabilize it. The fingers of the same hand palpate the tendon. With the other hand, the examiner extends the shoulder, maintaining elbow extension and forearm pronation. Static test-

ing can be carried out with the arm by the side, with the elbow flexed to 90° and with the forearm in the mid position. The examiner then resists simultaneous elbow flexion and supination. In all these tests, pain reproduction is a positive result.

Treatment   This follows the same lines as for that detailed for rotator cuff lesions (see supraspinatus tendinitis, above, and section 6.1.3(c)).

Long head of biceps subluxation

The transverse humeral ligament holds the tendon in the bicipital groove, augmented by the more superiorly placed coracohumeral ligament. Defects of these supporting ligaments, caused by either a specific traumatic incident or by repetitive activities such as throwing, may result in the subluxation of the biceps tendon. Another cause could be a relatively shallow bicipital groove.

Signs and symptoms   Pain is usually the main complaint; it is experienced at the front of the shoulder during forceful shoulder movements or throwing activities. Complaints of simultaneous 'snapping' or 'clicking' sensations are strongly suggestive of this lesion.

Examination   The tendon is usually tender and thickened when palpated and it may be possible to palpate a 'click' at the front of the glenohumeral joint as the upper arm is repeatedly taken from internal to external rotation. The patient's pain and accompanying tendon subluxation may be reproduced by lifting a small dumbbell (with the elbow straight) into elevation through abduction. The examiner should palpate the tendon as the arm is raised so as to feel the 'snap' of the tendon as it subluxes. This usually occurs after 90–100° of movement.

Treatment   If the cause is a single episode of trauma and the other glenohumeral passive and active stabilizers are not affected, it will be down to how functionally limiting the symptoms are, before surgical intervention is considered. This would involve fixation of the tendon to the floor of the groove. Where the cause is linked to an overuse scenario, it is vital that the shoulder complex is thoroughly examined so that other associated lesions to the glenohumeral passive and active stabilizers are identified. When such associated injury exists, surgery may be indicated to repair/reconstruct the damaged tissues as well as to decompress the subacromial structures. Appropriate postoperative rehabilitation will be vital for the optimization of athletic ability. Details of such a rehabilitation programme are given in section 6.1.3(c).

Biceps tendon rupture

Partial or complete ruptures may occur as isolated lesions following specific episodes of trauma but, as with similar injuries to the rotator cuff, such pathology is usually the sequel to long-standing degenerative tissue changes. These occur in tandem with and possibly as a result of subclinical glenohumeral instability, which itself is caused by excessive external forces from training and competition.

Signs and symptoms A distinct episode of trauma can usually be recalled by the athlete and a sensation of tearing or snapping is often described and localized to the anterior shoulder. As a result there is usually an immediate loss of function, pain and inhibition of all or most shoulder movements. In the case of degenerative pathology that predates the rupture, the forces involved in the injuring movement may be relatively trivial. There is usually a long-standing history of chronic recurrent shoulder symptoms.

Examination Careful questioning and observation are all that is usually required to make a diagnosis. Active elbow flexion reveals a 'Popeye'-contoured biceps, which is caused by a distal contraction of the ruptured long head.

Treatment Surgical repair gives the best chance of regaining adequate function for the overhead athlete. Postoperative rehabilitation must address all aspects of shoulder complex mobility, strength, stability and neuromotor control (section 6.1.3(c)).

(c) Glenohumeral instability

Repetitive and forceful movements that are performed in positions of elevation and external rotation can cause a passive stretching of the glenohumeral capsule and ligaments, particularly the anterior structures. A gradual process of soft-tissue attenuation and breakdown usually occurs over long periods of time and as the initial symptom severity is usually not enough for the athlete to curtail training, the rate of tissue deterioration eventually exceeds the rate of repair. Initially the joint hypermobility is controlled by the restraining effect of the rotator cuff. Fatigue of these muscles over time may limit the effectiveness of this active control mechanism (Kvitne and Jobe, 1995) and the presence of soft-tissue oedema and pain can also inhibit this active control mechanism. A muscular imbalance then occurs and the humeral head is displaced anterosuperiorly. This places the infraspinatus and supraspinatus tendons into positions where they may become impinged and it also places extra stress upon the long head of biceps. This type of impingement is therefore termed 'secondary' impingement, i.e. secondary to a pre-existing glenohumeral instability.

Signs and symptoms Episodes of severe, disabling pain, which has a sudden onset, is usually the chief complaint. Pain is usually linked to a specific range of overarm motion such as the wind-up phase or acceleration phase of throwing. In chronic cases (and many are by the time the athlete presents for the first consultation), there will often be multiple pathology such as tendinitis, partial rotator cuff ruptures and capsulolabral tears. Glenohumeral instability (and its associated pathology) can be career-threatening and early recognition and implementation of the correct management is therefore vital.

Examination   Overhead athletes frequently exhibit hypermobility into positions of elevation and lateral rotation. This is due to stretching of the anterior shoulder soft tissues and is sometimes in contrast to posterior capsular tightness, which limits internal rotation and horizontal flexion. Gross glenohumeral instability, which is usually in an anterior direction, is relatively easy to determine through questioning the patient and by performing simple passive testing of the anterior glenohumeral capsular structures. There are, however, a large number of overhead athletes who exhibit very subtle signs and symptoms suggestive of mild glenohumeral instability. As there is usually multiple pathology associated with instability problems, the examination must cover all components of the shoulder complex. The specific tests described for lesions to the rotator cuff and long head of biceps should form part of the examination, as should an evaluation of scapulothoracic function.

Active and passive movement tests that cause deep-seated crepitus or 'clunks' could indicate glenoid labrum tears or the presence of loose bodies. Reduced range of movement in the absence of acute trauma could be linked with rotator cuff tendinitis or tears, or to chronic subacromial bursitis. Specific areas of tenderness and thickening in relation to any of these structures would help confirm this. Observation of muscular wasting (particularly of the scapular muscles) and muscle testing can be indicative of weakness and poor control. This is particularly the case for infraspinatus. Functional testing of this muscle is facilitated by the use of EMG biofeedback equipment.

Stability tests for the glenohumeral joint are of most significance but in many cases the findings are subtle and need careful interpretation and crossreferencing with the information gained from subjective examination. Testing the amount and the end feel of anterior humeral head translation and comparing this with the non-affected side can give important information on joint stability. In the anteriorly unstable joint there is often a degree of anterior humeral head laxity, with a loose end feel. The tests described by Kvitne and Jobe (1995), which are modifications of the apprehension test for recurrent glenohumeral dislocation, are particularly helpful both in diagnosing cases of anterior instability and in differentiating between primary and secondary impingements. The tests are performed with the patient in supine lying and involve passive movement into the 'apprehension test' position of 90° abduction and 90° of lateral rotation. In this position a gentle anteriorly directed pressure is applied to the head of the humerus. If the patient experiences marked apprehension with or without pain, then this is indicative of gross glenohumeral instability, as in the case of recurrent dislocations. Pain without apprehension could indicate either a primary impingement or mild anterior instability with secondary impingement.

Differentiation between anterior instability with secondary impingement from primary impingement is possible by performing the 'relocation test'. This simply entails positioning the patient in the above apprehension testing position and then placing a posteriorly directed force to the humeral head. Patients with primary impingement experience no change in their pain level, while those with anterior instability and secondary impingement experience a lessening of their pain. This results from the posteriorly moving humeral head relieving the impinging pressure on the underside of the rotator cuff against the posterosuperior glenoid rim.

Treatment Surgical treatment may be required in cases of gross instability or in cases of mild to moderate instability that have not been helped by physiotherapy. Surgical management could involve the repair of rotator cuff tears, the repair of glenoid labral lesions or the tightening of a lax anterior capsule. The rehabilitation protocols for both conservatively and surgically managed cases are identical. With surgically managed cases, the surgical procedures that have been undertaken will dictate the timing and the dosage of physiotherapy treatments. The treatment and rehabilitation of conservatively and surgically managed instabilities can be considered under the headings of mobility, strength, stability and neuromotor control.

(d) Additional factors to consider with rotator cuff lesions

Mobility

The restoration of normal joint and associated muscular function is dependent to a high degree on the presence of full pain-free joint mobility. The use of active and particularly passive joint mobilizing procedures is invaluable in controlling pain and in overcoming joint stiffness. Pain treatments could in the early postoperative stages or in cases of severe, irritable pain, involve the application of gentle glenohumeral accessory movements. For non-irritable pain, which is often experienced at end of range elevation, strong oscillatory end-range mobilizing techniques are effective treatments. The control of pain and the restoration of optimum range of movement by passive mobilization, greatly improves the functioning of the shoulder complex musculature by reducing inhibition.

Strength

All joints work most effectively if their associated musculature is of optimum strength.

Whatever method is chosen to bring about strength gains, the amount and duration of the exercises must not compromise the tissues, which will probably be weakened by either degenerative pathology, disuse or the effects of surgery. The standard progression of muscle work from isometric to isotonic (emphasizing concentric before eccentric), and finally using plyometrics is a logical approach and prevents injury through overload. Such a carefully progressed exercise 'dosage' optimizes gains in non-contractile soft-tissue strength as well as improving muscular strength.

It is important for the exercises not to be pain-provoking as this will cause muscle inhibition and be counterproductive. Exercises to strengthen the deltoid that involve abduction with internal rotation risk causing subacromial impingement and should be avoided. Exercises to improve the strength of the shoulder rotators, particularly the lateral rotators, which in many overhead athletes become relatively weak, should be used throughout the rehabilitation process. Selecting exercises that are functional in respect to the muscles that need to be strengthened and the particular sport of the athlete will ensure that strength gains are of direct relevance to the athlete.

Stability

The important role of the rotator cuff muscles as glenohumeral stabilizers should be borne in mind when rehabilitating shoulder function. The same applies to the scapulothoracic muscles. Before progressing to quick, forceful movements, slower submaximal work should be performed to enhance the stabilizing role of the rotator cuff. Specific weaknesses should be targeted and it is particularly important to ensure that infraspinatus function is fully rehabilitated. PNF techniques are valuable in improving this type of control and they should also be used to improve scapulothoracic control.

Neuromotor control

Coordinated and efficient overhead athletic arm function is dependent upon adequate neuromotor control. Damage to mechanoreceptors in the periarticular structures of the shoulder, and pain stimuli, adversely affect this mechanism and it can only be re-established by stressing quality of movement and correcting any faulty or abnormal movement patterns that may occur in the exercise programme. Before sporting activities are recommenced, the sporting shoulder movements that will be required must be practised submaximally. In the case of complex patterns of movement, these should be broken down into subcomponents and practised before being amalgamated.

6.1.4   Clavicular joint injuries

The acromioclavicular joint (ACJ) is more frequently injured than the sternoclavicular joint (SCJ) and, while both can succumb to degenerative pathology, most sport-related injuries to these joints are caused by single episodes of trauma. Injury to the ACJ usually produces localized pain. Shoulder movements are usually pain-provoking, particularly horizontal flexion. The SCJ is usually injured by very strong forces such as a direct blow or medially directed shoulder girdle movements.

The ACJ is usually damaged by falls on to the outstretched arm or the point of the shoulder. Disruption to the acromioclavicular ligaments and to the coracoacromial ligaments can occur and can result in a deformity of the joint. This is sometimes referred to as a 'separated shoulder' and an observable step can be identified, where the lateral end of the clavicle sits higher than the acromion, which is depressed by the weight of the upper limb. These deformities can be quite gross, but athletic ability is rarely affected. In many cases the damaging forces are transmitted through the glenohumeral joint and this may also be a cause of pain.

SCJ dislocation can result from violent episodes of trauma and usually involves the medial end of the clavicle being displaced forwards and up. Rarer cases of posterior displacement must be treated as medical emergencies because of the chance of injury to the upper mediastinal contents (Corrigan and Maitland, 1994). Reduction may be achieved by positioning the patient in the supine position with a pillow under the shoulder blades, which places the shoulder girdles into some retraction. In this position the arm of the affected side is held in an abducted and slightly extended position while traction is applied along the axis of the arm (Reid, 1992). Successful anterior reduction of the medial clavicle may be accompanied by a 'pop' and reduction of pain.

Treatment   In the early stages following ACJ and SCJ sprain, pain control can be gained by the use of gentle accessory movements and the application of electrotherapy. Discomfort may also be reduced by the use of a supportive strapping which can also improve shoulder function. General shoulder mobilizing and strengthening exercises are introduced and progressed as pain allows.

6.1.5   Nerve entrapment

The majority of nerve injuries that result from sporting accidents involve neuropraxia and therefore cause transient disability. Injuries to the suprascapular and long thoracic nerves will be discussed briefly.

(a) The suprascapular nerve

The suprascapular nerve is derived from C5 and C6 and supplies supraspinatus and infraspinatus. It also supplies sensory innervation to the acromioclavicular joint and to the posterior glenohumeral capsule. It sits in the suprascapular notch and runs in the supraspinous fossa. The nerve is relatively immobile in the suprascapular notch and may be damaged by repeated traction forces that are applied to the upper limb. It is also tensioned by movements of the shoulder into horizontal flexion.

Signs and symptoms Poorly localized pain may be experienced in the posterior shoulder region. Feelings of shoulder weakness in positions of abduction may also be reported. The resulting muscular imbalance could lead to an impingement syndrome.

Examination Prolonged entrapment may result in wasting of supraspinatus and infraspinatus. Weakness and altered quality of movement of the first part of abduction can be caused by supraspinatus weakness and weak lateral shoulder rotation by infraspinatus weakness. Pain may be reproduced by sustaining a position of full horizontal shoulder flexion or by applying direct pressure to the nerve at the suprascapular notch.

(b) The long thoracic nerve

The long thoracic nerve is derived from C5, C6 and C7 and innervates serratus anterior. It descends dorsally to the brachial plexus and is at most risk of injury at the root of the neck. A blow to this area or prolonged forceful traction, e.g. by a rucksack, could result in its injury.

Signs and symptoms Diffuse pain in the neck and shoulder girdle may be experienced, together with a feeling of weakness and awkwardness when elevating the arm. This weakness is due to a partial or complete paralysis of serratus anterior and the subsequent reduction in scapulothoracic coordination and strength.

Examination Elevation of the medial border of the scapula away from the posterior chest wall (winging), may be obvious in standing and more obvious when the arm is abducted. Testing the strength of shoulder protraction reveals obvious weakness.

Treatment The majority of these injuries are neuropraxias and resolve partially or completely with time. In cases of partial recovery, suitable strengthening programmes may be able to produce compensatory hypertrophy. Strengthening and re-education exercises are made more effective by the use of EMG biofeedback.

6.2 THE ELBOW

6.2.1 Introduction

The elbow is a common site for both traumatic and overuse injuries in many different sports. Acute injuries can occur in contact sports or in sports that may involve a risk of accidental high-impact loading to the joint. Overuse elbow injuries are common across many sports, the commonest diagnosis probably being epicondylitis, i.e. tennis elbow and golfer's elbow. The treatment of choice for these common overuse conditions is a matter of contention among clinicians and the methods used to treat problems of elbow hypomobility (the invariable sequel to serious acute injury), often provoke controversial debate. Some clinicians feel that passive elbow movements are completely contraindicated because they have allegedly been linked with incidences of heterotopic bone formation in the surrounding soft tissues. There is little if any evidence to support this, and as long as passive movements are not applied vigorously to acute elbow injuries or to conditions where there is marked protective muscle spasm, there will be no greater chance of precipitating such adverse tissue responses at the elbow than at any other joint. Omission of passive movements from the treatment of a wide variety of elbow conditions greatly reduces the therapeutic possibilities available to the clinician.

This discussion will stress the need for careful differential diagnosis and will encourage treatment selection based upon the presenting signs and symptoms rather than on diagnostic titles. This approach, if accompanied by an ongoing process of treatment evaluation, should ensure that treatments are of optimum efficacy.

6.2.2　Functional anatomy

The elbow functions with the shoulder complex to move and position the hand. Limitations of movement in the elbow, which may be brought about by injury, can to a degree be compensated for by extra or altered shoulder complex and trunk movements. This compensatory mechanism may explain why many overuse injuries that result in subacute pain during sport are played with for some considerable time before the athlete eventually presents for treatment.

The elbow joint is composed of three separate joints (Figure 6.2), which share the same synovial capsule.

The humeroulnar and humeroradial joints allow flexion and extension movements, while the humeroradial and superior radioulnar joints permit the rotary forearm movements of supination and pronation. Because of this shared capsule and synovial membrane and because of the overlap in function between the three joints, injury and associated pathology to one can lead to problems in the other two.

6.2.3　Selected elbow injuries

The majority of sports-related elbow pains are due to local musculoskeletal pathology. However, problems of the ipsilateral shoulder and of the cervical spine can cause referred symptoms in the elbow region, as can neural tissues. It is therefore mandatory to test these structures, actively and passively, in all presenting 'elbow' problems. Such 'excluding tests' help to identify specific elbow joint pathology, when associated with active and passive elbow movement tests. Special attention should be given to these passive 'joint' tests, as limitations in the range and end feel

of accessory and physiological elbow movements is encountered in a wide range of elbow soft-tissue conditions.

The exact site of the symptoms should be precisely defined, as this will often give a clue as to the origin of the symptoms. Poorly defined, diffuse symptoms, which may not be directly provoked by elbow movements, should raise the suspicion of a lesion in a more proximally placed structure, particularly when they are aggravated by shoulder or neck movements. Where symptom areas run in lines, or are described as 'bands' of discomfort, the problem could be one of adverse neural tension and the appropriate upper limb tension tests should be performed.

Elbow injuries will be discussed under the headings:

- Musculotendinous disorders
- Ligamentous disorders
- Joint disorders
- Nerve entrapments.

(a) Musculotendinous disorders

Epicondylitis

This term refers to inflammatory conditions that affect the lateral and medial humeral epicondyles, to which the common extensor and common flexor tendons, respectively, attach. The term 'tennis elbow' has been historically used to describe lateral epicondylitis and 'golfer's elbow' to describe medial epicondylitis. However these terms have, over many years, been used by lay and medical people alike to describe a wide range of painful elbow conditions and consequently their use as diagnostic titles has been undermined. The exact pathology involved in these lesions is uncertain, but it is often the case that longstanding cases of epicondylitis have signs and symptoms that emanate from more than one structure. For example, there may be elbow joint signs and indications of adverse neural tension in addition to the signs that

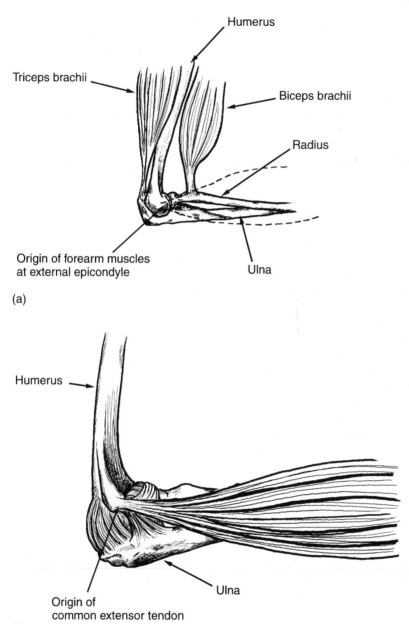

Humerus

Triceps brachii

Biceps brachii

Radius

Origin of forearm muscles
at external epicondyle

Ulna

(a)

Humerus

Ulna

Origin of
common extensor tendon

(b)

Figure 6.2   The elbow.

indicate specific epicondylar and tendon pathology.

Aetiology and pathology   The condition has traditionally been attributed to a chronic inflammation of the tendon and its insertion. Work by Regan *et al.* (1992) has, however, disputed this inflammatory cause. Studies of pathological tissue obtained from cases of recalcitrant lateral epicondylitis cases undergoing surgery, when compared to cadaveric specimens, showed degenerative rather than inflammatory changes within the tendon and bone interface tissues. The presence of primarily degenerative rather than inflammatory pathology may explain why some cases are resistant to inflammation-modulating treatments.

The cause of the condition is thought to be a repetitive contraction or stretching of the tendon, which produces local trauma. If injurious activities are continued the amount of cellular damage can exceed the rate of tissue repair. Overuse and/or poor technique among racquet sports players has been associated with lateral epicondylitis, while medial epicondylitis has been linked to throwing activities that impart valgus elbow stresses or excessive amounts of driving a golf ball (Reid, 1992). Such mechanical causes of degenerative and inflammatory tendo-osseous tissues may be only a part of the pathological picture. Chronic anomalies in the nervous system have also been implicated, with trophic changes in the soft tissues that they innervate. Alterations in axoplasmic flow may over a period of time cause a devitalization of these 'target tissues' and predispose them to injury (Butler, 1991). Irritation of the posterior interosseous nerve at the interface of supinator and extensor carpi radialis brevis may also cause lateral elbow symptoms, as may scarring of the small sensory nerves that innervate the lateral epicondylar soft tissues (Butler, 1991).

Signs and symptoms The main complaint is of intermittent lateral elbow pain. There is often a focal point of pain at the epicondyle and/or in the adjacent musculotendinous structures. This pain may refer distally along the forearm muscles, but associated areas of proximal arm pain are atypical of a local soft-tissue lesion and may be due to pathology of proximal structures. Pain is usually provoked by any activity that either stretches the affected tendon/bone or causes stress to

the same area by muscular contraction. Areas of acute tenderness are common, either directly on the epicondyle or on the adjacent tendon and tender 'trigger spots' may be located within the forearm muscles. Constant aching after activity is indicative of an inflammatory condition. This may be in response to mechanical tissue disruption or to degenerative tissue changes.

Examination This should consist of active and passive movement tests and static resisted contractions (SRCs) of the local joint and musculotendinous structures. Additionally, active and passive cervical spine movements should be examined, together with the full range of upper limb tension tests. ULTT2 is often positive in cases of lateral epicondylitis, especially when performed with a radial nerve bias. These 'nerve tests' and the examination of the cervical spine should be mandatory in all presentations of epicondylitis. Butler states that adverse neural tension signs need to be treated in three quarters of 'tennis elbow' presentations (Butler, 1991). In the case of lateral epicondylitis, SRCs applied to the forearm extensors via the middle finger place a contractile force upon extensor carpi radialis brevis (ECRB). Pain reproduction with this test could implicate a posterior interosseous nerve irritation where it interfaces with ECRB.

Restrictions of elbow mobility into terminal extension are frequently encountered and are often especially symptom-provoking when the extension movement is combined with the accessory movements of adduction or abduction.

Treatment The treatment of clearly defined cervical spinal joint signs and of adverse neural tension signs should be performed first in isolation from one another and from treatment directly to the elbow. This will help in deciding if, and by how much, these 'remote' structures are contributing to the problem. Passive mobilizations should be given to clear limited, pain-provoking ranges of elbow movements and this can be done in isolation from other structures or in positions of upper limb neural tension. This approach may elicit joint signs that are more relevant (e.g. more precisely located or more comparable) to the condition than is the case when the elbow is examined 'out of tension'.

Other manual therapies that regularly achieve symptomatic and functional improvement include transverse friction massage. How they affect beneficial change is open to debate, but this should not detract from their efficacy. Other frequently used modalities include ultrasound, laser and interferential therapy. While these treatments may improve symptoms, they do not address the movement anomalies mentioned earlier. Electrotherapy should therefore only be used as an adjunct to more direct methods of treatment.

The use of systemic and topical non-steroidal anti-inflammatory medication is widespread, as is the use of steroid injections into the offending tendon and soft tissues. However, the overall efficacy of these treatments in the management of these conditions is unclear.

When normal and asymptomatic ranges of joint and neural tissues have been regained and when the pain response has been cleared or reduced, it is important to institute a graduated programme of strengthening and stretching work for the elbow and forearm and to ensure that proper sporting technique is used (Tables 6.2, 6.3). Correct racquet stroke technique is vital if recurrences are to be avoided (Lifield, 1992). The patient should therefore be referred to an appropriate coach.

The use of epicondylitis clasps to control pain during functional activities has increased markedly over recent years. These devices come in many shapes and sizes and probably achieve their effect by compressing the forearm musculature just distal to the elbow. In this way a 'false' origin for the muscle is provided and consequently a reduced force

Table 6.2 Racquet sports: technical factors that may cause or perpetuate epicondylitis – directing unnecessary force through the elbow by excessively stretching the forearm muscles or by generating excess intramusculotendinous tension

Backhand

Common fault: Elbow/wrist extension used excessively to power the shot.

Solution: Adopt correct side-on body position with forward weight distribution and allow trunk and shoulder to power the shot. Double-handed backhand emphasizes trunk power over elbow/wrist power.

Forehand

Common fault: High stroke speed.

Solution: Emphasize style and timing to achieve power and speed.

Common fault: Wrist flexion and forearm supination used to impart topspin.

Solution: Emphasize body momentum and shoulder power. Lean into the shot, impacting the ball low and following through and over the ball to topspin it.

passes through the pathological and painful 'true' muscle origin.

Triceps and biceps tendon ruptures

These are uncommon sporting injuries but can occur when large external forces are exerted upon the tendon while it is in tension, particularly if these injuring forces are at speed. Significant tears must be identified as early as possible so that suitable treatment can be implemented.

Signs and symptoms There will be an incident of specific trauma, immediately followed by a loss of function in terms of strength and control. There may be significant bruising some hours after the injury.

Examination An observable and palpable gap may be obvious and there will be little

Table 6.3   Racquet sports: equipment faults that may cause or perpetuate epicondylitis

Grip size
Fault: Too small or too large, resulting in overstretching or overcontraction of the forearm muscles.
Solution: The correct grip diameter is equal to the distance from the tip of the ring finger to the distal palmar crease. Alternatively, there should be space to fit one index finger width between the thenar eminence and the fingertips when the racquet is gripped.

String tension
Fault: Too high.
Solution: Lower-tension strings permit more impact dissipation through the strings rather than through the arm.

Racquet weight and balance
Fault: Heavy racquet with most weight in head.
Solution: Graphite-framed racquets reduce overall weight and reduce arm forces. Lighter racquets also allow more precise shot selection. A neutral balanced racquet or one with a light head may reduce lateral elbow forces by reducing extensor radialis brevis loads.

Balls
Fault: Wet
Solution: Avoid playing on wet surfaces where the balls pick up water and become heavy, resulting in greater impact forces.

Court surface
Fault: Hard versus soft
Solution: Soft surfaces give lower bounces and may encourage increased wrist and elbow movements when reaching to retrieve shots.

or no resistance to attempted static resisted contraction of the muscle concerned.

Treatment   Surgical repair probably gives the best chance of regaining athletic ability. A period of postoperative immobilization is usually necessary and this should be followed by a progressive active and passive elbow mobilization programme and a progressive strengthening exercise regime.

(b) Ligamentous disorders

Acute episodes of injury to the elbow such as are caused by valgus and varus forces can result in collateral ligament damage, but these are relatively rare occurrences. The medial collateral ligament (MCL) is more prone to such injuries than the lateral collateral ligament. However the more common type of ligamentous elbow injury is a chronic overuse injury to the MCL.

Chronic medial collateral ligament injury

This is frequently encountered in throwing sports where the acceleration phase of throwing whips the forearm into a valgus direction. This places tension on to the medial joint structures, particularly to the anterior oblique band of the MCL, which is the main restraint to this force (Conway *et al.*, 1992). Over time the MCL may become attenuated and damage to the articular surfaces of the elbow joint may also occur. This is especially true for the humeroradial joint which is subjected to compressional forces as the elbow is repetitively forced into a valgus position.

Signs and symptoms   Chronic inflammation of the medial elbow soft tissues with occasional episodes of superimposed acute inflammation gives the patient a background of medial elbow discomfort with episodes of acute pain during throwing activities. Because of the overuse nature of the injury and the fact that associated joint structures may be pathological, there will often be postexercise pain. Pain at the commencement of exercise, which in the early stages of the condition may ease once the joint has been 'warmed up', is also a feature.

Examination   There may be medial joint line thickening and tenderness, and tenderness over the radial head and adjacent joint line. Stress testing of the collateral ligaments should be performed in approximately 15° of flexion (Norwood, Shook and Andrews, 1981) and this may reveal laxity and/or a loose end feel to overpressure.

Treatment   This condition can be very disabling and prevent any forceful throwing activities. Conservative treatment would consist of the usual electrotherapy modalities to modulate pain and inflammation, followed by mobilizing and strengthening work to address specific strength and range of movement anomalies. A very gradual return to throwing-related activities is essential and the strengthening exercises should, in the later stages of the rehabilitation process, be specific to the actions of the sport in question. At this stage and on returning to training, emphasis on good technique is vitally important and occurrences of the elbow being quickly snapped into terminal extension should be avoided. The use of joint taping to reduce terminal elbow extension forces may be helpful at this stage.

In cases that are resistant to conservative management, operative repair or reconstruction of the MCL may give the only chance of a return to throwing (Conway *et al.*, 1992).

(c) Joint disorders

Repetitive weightbearing elbow forces or repetitive throwing forces may cause injury to the joint surfaces, or, in the skeletally immature, epiphyseal trauma.

Epiphyseal trauma

Single episodes of excessive forearm flexor muscle work can result in medial humeral epiphyseal injury. Acute local tenderness and pain on resisted wrist flexion or passive wrist extension could indicate such a lesion in an adolescent. X-ray investigation would confirm this.

This age group can also sustain medial humeral epiphyseal problems following overuse. In the USA the term 'Little Leaguer's elbow' has been used to describe the problem of medial humeral epiphyseal injury in children involved in high-repetition throwing sports such as baseball pitching, although the condition could equally be provoked by other 'upper limb sports' such as gymnastics. Repetitive trauma can (through compressive medial elbow forces) result in fragmentation of the epiphysis. Rest and modification of throwing activities should resolve the presenting complaint, which is usually exercise-related elbow pain and limited terminal elbow extension. Failure to implement relative rest in these cases can lead to elbow deformity, arthritic changes and loose body formation.

Loose body formation

This may accompany many of the overuse injury scenarios that affect both adolescents and adults. The condition should be suspected when there are complaints of intermittent 'catching' pain, swelling and episodes of the joint locking, i.e. there being a mechanical block to extension. In such cases it may be possible to gently mobilize the elbow into the restricted range by oscillating an adduction/abduction movement at the end of the available range of extension. This manoeuvre should not be vigorously forced nor should it provoke pain. Freeing of the loose body should permit full extension. In these cases X-ray investigation and possible arthroscopic inspection and loose body removal is indicated.

(d) Nerve entrapments

Peripheral nerve lesions at the elbow can result in distal sensory and motor changes, the severity of which will be in direct proportion to the magnitude of the actual nerve injury. This section will concentrate on the entrapment syndromes that may be confused with symptoms arising from other elbow soft tissues.

Ulnar nerve

The ulnar nerve passes the elbow joint posteromedially and lies in a groove between the medial epicondyle of the humerus and the olecranon process. The nerve may be prone to direct trauma in this osseous groove and may also be prone to compression just distally to this point, where it lies beneath the medial epicondylar attachment of the flexor carpi ulnaris. Such compressive forces could be caused by a contraction of the muscle during strong wrist and elbow flexion movements. Positions of elbow flexion place tension on the nerve along its entire tract (Butler, 1991), especially at the elbow, where it interfaces with osseous and fibrous and muscular tissues.

Signs and symptoms If sufficient pressure is exerted upon the nerve, sensory changes in the medial forearm, wrist, hand and medial one and a half digits will be evident. There may also be motor changes with weakness and atrophy of the interosseous muscles and of the hypothenar eminence. Irritation of the nerves soft-tissue investments may result in medial elbow pain with little or no symptomatology attributable to disturbed nerve conduction.

Examination A full assessment of forearm and hand sensation and motor function should be performed. Subtle signs attributable to mild or intermittent compression may be elicited by sustaining a position of elbow flex-ion for a few minutes. A positive Tinel sign may also be present – the reproduction of forearm and hand paraesthesia by tapping the nerve behind the medial humeral epicondyle. ULTT3 should also be performed as this places large tension forces upon the ulnar nerve. By adding and removing some of this test's 'sensitizing' movements, it may be possible to differentiate between nerve and other soft tissues as to the cause of symptoms.

Treatment Cases of intermittent medial elbow pain that are thought to be attributable to ulnar nerve irritation and cases where there are only mild signs of forearm and hand sensory disturbances may benefit from nerve mobilization. This would be performed using positions of elbow flexion, with ULTT3 being the base technique of choice. Where there are obvious and significant motor changes, nerve conduction studies and soft-tissue scanning would probably be indicated prior to surgical decompression.

Radial nerve

At the elbow the radial nerve splits to form a superficial sensory branch and a deeper motor branch which is known as the posterior interosseous nerve. Irritation of this nerve may give rise to lateral elbow symptoms and it is most at risk of such mechanical irritation against the adjacent extensor carpi radialis brevis and the supinator muscles. This latter interface is termed the **arcade of Frohse** and is the point where the posterior interosseous nerve passes between the two heads of supinator. Athletes who participate in throwing sports are susceptible to entrapment at this site (Stroyan and Wilk, 1993).

Signs and symptoms Entrapment of the superficial sensory branch may cause pain or altered sensation over the lateral aspect of the wrist and of the thumb. The pain associated with posterior interosseous nerve entrapment can mimic that produced by inflamed lateral epicondylar soft tissues and may be mistaken for a 'lateral epicondylitis'.

Examination Pain may be reproduced by resisted forearm supination and resisted middle finger extension (Watrous and Ho, 1988). These tests may cause pain due either to a muscle–nerve interface problem or to a local non-neural soft-tissue lesion. Differentiation between these structures may be possible by performing these static resisted contraction (SRC) tests in positions of neural tension and comparing the results with the SRC tests performed out of tension. The use of neural tension tests such as ULTT2 (with radial nerve bias) can also be used as a differentiation test.

Treatment Radial nerve mobilizing procedures such as ULTT2 can be very effective at alleviating symptoms. Where a muscle interface problem is suspected, a stretching programme for the supinator and extensor carpi radialis brevis muscles may help to reduce local nerve tension. In cases resistant to conservative treatment, operative decompression may be indicated.

6.3 PELVIC AND GROIN INJURIES

6.3.1 Introduction

Pain in the pelvic and groin region is a common occurrence among athletes from many different sports and accounts for between 2% and 5% of all sports injuries (Karlsson *et al.*, 1994). The symptoms can be very limiting as regards sporting performance, persist for protracted periods of time and be resistant to treatment. Pain in these areas can come from many different structures and involve diverse pathology (Figure 6.3; Tables 6.4, 6.5) but the majority of sporting injuries in this region involve muscles and tendons.

Table 6.4 Musculoskeletal conditions and the nerves that can mimic/contribute to their symptomatology

Condition	Nerve
Adductor strain	Obturator nerve
Osteitis pubis	Obturator nerve
Psoas bursitis	Ilioinguinal/iliohypogastric nerves
Inguinal disruption	Ilioinguinal/iliohypogastric/genitofemoral nerves
Trochanteric bursitis	Lateral cutaneous nerve of the thigh

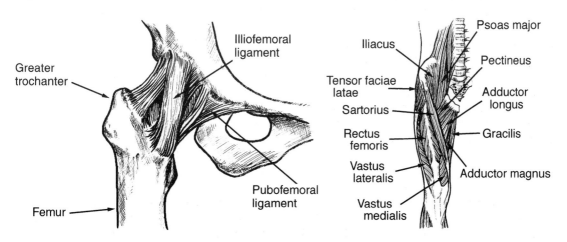

Figure 6.3 Anatomy of the pelvic and groin region.

Table 6.5 Nonmusculoskeletal pathologies that can be a cause of groin pain

- Prostatitis
- Urinary infections
- Pelvic abscess
- Gynaecological disorders
- Pelvic inflammation
- Hernias (femoral and inguinal)
- Tumours, e.g. osteosarcoma, chondrosarcoma
- Rheumatoid arthritis
- Reiter's syndrome

This is particularly true for the majority of acute injuries which often affect single structures. However, when the symptoms are chronic, it is invariably the case that multiple pathology exists, such as hip and vertebral joint hypomobility, muscle weakness, inhibition and imbalance as well as inflammatory and degenerative joint and soft-tissue changes. In such cases it is usually inappropriate and of little practical help to come up with a single diagnostic title. Instead, a systematic approach to the examination and evaluation of the patient's problem should be adopted and used to identify and prioritize the physical limitations that present. This will enable the clinician to classify the problem primarily in terms of dysfunction rather than pathology. It will then be possible to formulate a course of action to rectify the presenting dysfunction. It is not suggested that the clinician turn a blind eye to the actual pathology that is causing the symptoms and dysfunction. Indeed the discussion that follows will be based on individual pathological conditions and syndromes. This is done so as to act as a point of reference and to cover those welcome if uncommon eventualities when the athlete presents with single pathology. However, in practice it is usually necessary to treat and to rehabilitate the athlete in relation to the presenting signs and symptoms which arise from multiple, inter-related pathologies.

General considerations regarding acute and chronic muscle and tendon problems will be covered first. Following this, inguinal disruption, hip joint disorders, pubic symphysis instability, osteitis pubis and nerve pathology will be considered.

It is beyond the scope of this text to cover the subjects of vertebral and sacroiliac joint disorders. However it is mandatory in the presentation of all conditions that involve the pelvic and groin regions to undertake a musculoskeletal examination of the spine and sacroiliac joints, as these structures frequently refer symptoms to all parts of the abdomen, pelvis and groin.

6.3.2   Muscle and tendon injuries

The most commonly injured structures in this region are adductor longus, rectus femoris, rectus abdominis, and iliopsoas (Renstrom, 1992). These muscles and their tendons may be subject to acute or chronic pathology, or to a combination of the two. The following discussion will first deal with the general principles concerning the treatment and management of these conditions, which can be applied to the treatment and rehabilitation of all muscle and tendon injuries in this region. This is followed by more specific information regarding individual muscles.

6.3.3   Acute injuries

Acute injuries always date to a specific episode of trauma, whether this be direct, such as a kick, or indirect, such as an overstretch of the muscle/tendon. They are relatively easy to diagnose, as the signs and symptoms are linked directly to a specific injuring incident, the functional mechanics of which can be used to determine which structures have been damaged. This information, together with the clinical and functional signs, make it a relatively easy task to ascertain the degree of injury and to make a prognosis regarding the type of treatment that will be required and the time it will take for full sporting function to be restored.

These signs are the usual soft-tissue findings of localized tenderness, and pain in the same area when the muscle is stretched or made to contract. Swelling and bruising may also be evident, especially in superficial muscles and tendons such as adductor longus, which is the most commonly injured muscle in this region. In some cases of grade two strains, a gap may be palpable or observable, especially when the muscle is isometrically contracted. Injury to deeply placed structures such as iliopsoas or pectineus are less easily identified by observation or palpation.

Treatment of acute injuries consists of the usual RICE (rest, ice, compression and elevation). The use of crutches until the acute pain has subsided can prevent unnecessary and potentially aggravating forces from being applied to the damaged tissues. Many athletes prefer not to use walking aids but this should be discouraged and it should be explained that their use can, in the long term, save recuperation time by avoiding unnecessary secondary soft-tissue damage. Once the initial inflammatory response has settled, a programme of flexibility work should be undertaken to restore full pain-free extensibility of the injured area. These activities should not jeopardize the healing tissues and therefore should initially be pain-free. Primarily, non-weightbearing stretches are the techniques of choice and can be used with proprioceptive neuromuscular facilitation (PNF) techniques to overcome protective spasm and improve the range and quality of the stretches. These can later be progressed to more forceful weightbearing stretches and be incorporated into sport-specific activities. A carefully progressed stretching programme will stimulate the healing process, prevent scar tissue contracture and optimize function. This process will be enhanced by instituting a programme of graduated strengthening exercises.

As with the initial flexibility exercises, the strengthening exercises should initially be pain-free. For this reason, relatively low stress exercises such as isometric work are used initially and progressed to more forceful isotonic exercise, with this type of muscle work initially favouring the less demanding concentric components. Eccentric training can then be emphasized, with the final exercise progression for most sporting activities being eccentric–concentric coupling work. With these types of activity, progression should be made from slow to fast work.

The application of high loads in the form of non-weightbearing resistance such as weights to the hip musculature is not functional for most sporting activities. The muscle's role as a fixator and synergist as well as a prime mover, should be borne in mind when formulating suitable exercises and efforts should be made to rehabilitate the balance of strength and control between opposing groups and between more distal and proximal muscles.

6.3.4 Chronic injuries

Care should be taken when local muscle and tendon symptoms are not linked to a specific injuring incident. A gradual onset of symptoms in this region can be due to overuse and a resultant breakdown of muscle and tendon tissue. In these instances, the athlete may recount one particular incident that was associated with the onset of the symptoms, but where this is a relatively trivial injury, there could be a background of ongoing degenerative pathology which has predisposed the tissues to injury. It is important to classify such injuries as 'chronic' rather than to treat them as acute problems, as they invariably take longer to rehabilitate and it is often necessary to treat associated and possibly contributory or causative anomalies. These commonly include hypomobility syndromes of the vertebral, pelvic and hip joints. These hypomobility conditions may result in muscular shortening due to a combination of reflex hypertonicity and joint stiffness. Problems of this nature must be treated with a programme of passive and active joint mobilization if the exercise regime to restore muscular extensibility, strength, control and balance is to be of optimum benefit.

6.3.5 Injuries to specific soft tissues of the pelvis and groin

(a) Adductor longus

The adductor longus is the most superficial of the adductor longus, brevis and magnus trio and its action of adducting the hip is shared with gracilis and pectinius. In addition to being prime movers, these muscles have an important stabilizing and synergic role in relation to hip and pelvic motion. The adductor longus is the most frequently injured muscle in the pelvic and groin area and the proximity of its pubic attachment to that of rectus abdominis means that chronic inflammatory changes may affect both structures (Renstrom and Peterson, 1980). The frequency of acute injury is relatively high in the 16–25 years age group, especially among rugby and soccer players (Gordon, 1995). In these instances the mechanism of injury often consists of overstretching the muscle, as in lunging for a ball or sidestepping an opponent. Injury may also be caused by a sudden resistance to a strong adduction force, such as an opponent blocking forceful hip adduction in a block tackle. Chronic tendon and muscle pathology is also encountered in these sports, and in sports that entail repetitive hip abduction and adduction such as skating and cross-country skiing (Renstrom, 1992).

Signs and symptoms Pain in the region of the hip adductor muscle group is a common occurrence but in itself is not conclusive evidence that the cause is a local muscular injury. The adductor region is a common area for pain referral from vertebral structures, from the pelvic and hip joints and from associated peripheral nerves. Symptoms from remote joint structures tend to be diffuse, as does any tenderness elicited upon palpation. Adductor pain that is due to a local muscular

or tendon strain is usually localized to a relatively small area and in such cases the patient usually identifies the area specifically with one finger. Due to the superficial position of the muscle, swelling and bruising may be clearly evident and these signs are conclusive proof of a local strain. In such cases any activities that place the muscle under tension or involve its contraction will be pain-provoking. Significant grade two strains may result in an observable or palpable gap in the muscle and this may be most evident if the muscle is contracted isometrically.

Examination Stretching or contracting the muscle reproduces pain. In the case of adductor longus, this may be performed by abducting the hip with the knee flexed or extended. These two testing positions may be used to differentiate between adductor longus strains and strains to the gracilis, as this muscle inserts below the knee and is therefore stretched to a greater extent when hip abduction is performed with the knee extended. Tenderness, soft-tissue swelling and defects within the muscle are easily palpated in the superficially placed adductor longus and this is best achieved with the hip in a relaxed position of combined abduction, lateral rotation and extension.

Treatment The treatment for acute strains has been outlined earlier. Depending upon the severity and extent of the tissue damage, gentle stretching work can be instituted a few days following the actual injury. These must be initially performed in a pain-free range and this is best done in non-weightbearing, the movement of combined hip abduction and extension being performed in a position of approximately 60° of hip flexion. In this position, gravity imposes a stretch to the muscle and it may be necessary to initially support the limb with a pillow under the lateral aspect of the knee at the limit of the available pain-free range. In this way a sustained pain-free range stretch can be achieved. As range is restored and the pain response diminishes, gentle overpressure can be applied to the muscle in this same position, either manually or with the use of a weight bag placed over the knee. All these stretching activities can be performed by the athlete but, where possible, passive stretching should also be applied by a physiotherapist, as this is arguably the most efficient way of improving range of movement and can easily be integrated with PNF techniques to enhance the process.

Following this initial mobilizing work, weightbearing and functional activities must be used to impose sport-relevant stretch forces to the muscle so that full sporting function is restored. These should initially be performed slowly and only when a pain-free non-weightbearing stretch has been achieved.

The exercises that are appropriate for this stage of rehabilitation depend upon the sport of the athlete in question. For example, a footballer would need to practise non-weightbearing activities such as kicking movements with the instep, where the adductors work as prime movers. This exercise can be performed with elastic bandage resistance, which gives a submaximal loading. In this example, the adductors are made to work eccentrically and are then prestretched prior to working concentrically to produce the hip adduction component of the kick. For a throwing athlete such as a javelin thrower, the adductors would need to be rehabilitated as regards their prime moving role but in this case the movement in question is of the pelvis on the fixed foot. This could be achieved by planting the foot of the affected side on to the ground with the hip of the affected side in an abducted position. The athlete would then sidestep on to the affected leg, using the adductors of the weightbearing limb to adduct the pelvis upon the femur. The use of an elasticated harness to provide resistance to this movement is a simple and effective progression. In this example the final progression would be to sideways lunging and running drills.

(b) Rectus femoris

This muscle, which is the most anteriorly placed component of the quadriceps, has its proximal attachment at the anterior inferior iliac spine (the 'straight' head), with a 'reflected' head just below at a point just above the acetabulum. It therefore has a flexing action at the hip as well as contributing to the movement of extension at the knee. Because of the anatomical and biochemical properties of this muscle it has been classified as being a 'movement synergist' (Richardson, 1992). This type of muscle has the characteristics of fast twitch muscle fibres (type II) and is suited to the production of high-speed movement. The iliopsoas (which acts with the rectus femoris to flex the hip) and the vastus medialis (which acts with the rectus femoris to extend the knee) are classed as 'stability synergists' (Richardson, 1992), and as such have properties associated with slow twitch muscle fibres (type I). This includes the ability of the muscle to control low forces over long periods of time. If, therefore, fast hip flexion or knee extension movements are performed, as is the case during many different running and kicking sports, rectus femoris will be preferentially recruited to perform these movements ahead of the iliopsoas and vastus medialis muscles. This fact may go some way to explain why rectus femoris injuries are associated with speed activities such as sprinting and kicking. Another reason is that the muscle spans two joints and is at times subjected to opposing forces simultaneously. For example, when sprinting, the rectus femoris of the leading lower limb simultaneously contracts to flex the hip, while being stretched from below by the flexed knee. This imposes high force values on the muscle, particularly with high-speed movements, and requires a high degree of neuromotor control. If this control system fails to operate smoothly, due to poor coordination or fatigue, then a poorly timed contraction could occur and result in a strain. Strains to the upper musculotendinous portion of the rectus femoris may be caused by a specific episode of acute trauma or by overuse, such as prolonged and intensive shooting practice in soccer.

Signs and symptoms With acute injuries, there will be localized tenderness and possibly swelling, bruising and a palpable gap. Any contraction or stretching of the muscle produces pain and initially, following injury, this may be provoked simply by walking, as the affected hip is flexed to swing the non-weightbearing lower limb forwards and again as the affected limb is extended at the hip during 'push-off'. Less irritable symptoms, as frequently occur in many chronic conditions, may only be provoked with quicker movements such as running at speed, when the pain is usually experienced as the knee of the affected side is flexed quickly. Forceful movements such as kicking are also usually pain-provoking.

Examination Static testing of the muscle should include isometric testing of the rectus femoris as a hip flexor and as a knee extensor. Stretching the muscle by performing combined knee flexion and hip extension usually demonstrates a restriction, i.e. by stiffness and pain. It is often useful to perform this stretch in two ways. The first is by applying the hip component before the knee component and the second a reverse of this process. Each method may reproduce subtly different stretch and pain responses, as may the addition of rotation at the hip. The response that is most comparable to the patient's symptoms would be used in treatment. Adopting different testing positions to evaluate the muscle's contractile ability is also useful, as this can influence the site and degree of symptom response. For example, a test of knee extension with the hip flexed, as occurs in the sitting position, may give a different pain/range response from resisted knee extension performed with the hip extended, e.g. with

the patient lying supine with the knees flexed over the end of the treatment bench. The position that most closely replicates the patient's symptoms presumably stresses the muscle/tendon in the damaged area and could be used as a position in which to perform strengthening exercises.

Treatment Active exercise and passive stretching should commence after the initial inflammatory response has subsided. The specific stretches that should be used should be the ones that most closely replicate the patient's symptoms, as these will presumably stress the muscle/tendon in the appropriate region. For the same reason, the actual exercises used to strengthen the muscle should be progressed (as the severity of the pain response diminishes) to include those movements and positions that similarly reproduce relevant signs and symptoms. Initially, the usual progression from pain-free isometric exercise through to the various types of isotonic muscle work should be made. Because of the high force production that occurs in rectus femoris during high-speed movements, it is important to progress the speed of the strengthening exercises to those that are relevant to the sport in question.

(c) Iliopsoas

As the main flexor of the hip, iliopsoas is of prime functional importance in a wide range of running and power sports. It is prone to acute injury when a strong or quick contraction meets a forceful resistance, or to a chronic inflammatory injury following overuse scenarios, such as a large amount of unaccustomed uphill or sprint running.

Signs and symptoms Pain is the chief complaint and is usually located deep into the anterior aspect of the hip. The pain may result in protective spasm and this, together with a desire by the athlete to avoid the pain, can result in the affected hip being held in combined flexion, adduction and lateral rotation.

Examination Passive correction of the above antalgic hip deformity usually reproduces pain. Cases of subtle hip flexion deformities can be detected with a Thomas test. The presence of iliacus spasm can sometimes be determined by pressure being applied to Baer's point (located approximately two to three fingerbreadths medially from the anterior superior iliac spine), in which case marked tenderness is elicited. Static contraction of the affected hip flexors will also produce pain, as will digital pressure applied to the iliopsoas tendon.

Treatment After the acute phase has passed, passive and active stretches of the affected hip into extension should be performed to achieve full iliopsoas extensibility. PNF techniques are useful adjuncts to passive stretching and can be done in the supine lying Thomas test position of contralateral hip flexion and affected hip extension. This position helps to stabilize the pelvis and keep the lumbar spine in a neutral position. Strengthening exercises must be progressed in the final phases to include high-speed, full-range resisted hip flexion, from end-range hip extension. This is important as, in high-speed running, iliopsoas must be able to flex the hip quickly after being fully stretched. An elastic resistance bandage is a useful tool in such exercises. It provides a relatively low load and, in standing positions, can be aligned so as to assist the attainment of full hip extension prior to resisting hip flexion.

(d) Rectus abdominis

The two rectus abdominis muscles work as prime movers of the trunk into positions of flexion. They have been classified as being movement synergists (Richardson, 1992), i.e. they have a relatively high fast twitch fibre content and, during fast movements, are pre-ferentially recruited ahead of the transverse and oblique abdominal muscles, which have the functional attributes of slow twitch muscle fibres and are classified as stability synergists (Norris, 1995). Athletes who are most prone to strains of rectus abdominis are those whose sports impose forceful and quick trunk flexion movements, particularly involving outer range muscle work. Examples are tennis players serving or playing overhead shots (Balduini, 1988).

Signs and symptoms Pain is localized to the region of injury which is usually below the level of the umbilicus, usually affecting the musculotendinous portion or the muscle's insertion onto the superior pubic ramus. Any resisted trunk movements into flexion will be pain-provoking as will extremes of trunk extension which will place a tensional stress upon the muscle.

Examination Acute cases of injury may present with observable swelling and bruising. Static rectus abdominis work in supine, as occurs in raising the head and shoulders, may reproduce pain and be associated with a pain/inhibition tremor. Stretching the muscle is also usually symptom-provoking and can be best tested by the patient performing a half press-up in the prone lying position, i.e. using the arms to lift the shoulders clear of the treatment couch while keeping the pelvis on the couch, thus extending the trunk.

Treatment As with other muscle conditions characterized by pain, it is important to achieve some measure of pain control before instituting a programme of stretching and strengthening exercises, if these are to be of optimum benefit. In the case of acute injuries this may be achieved by a suitable period of rest and the application of treatment modalities such as ice and electrotherapy. When the pain response to active and passive movement has subsided, or in cases of relatively mild pain, as occurs with some chronic injuries, a progressive exercise programme should be instituted. It is important to regain full pain-free muscle extensibility, and exercises that can be used include the above-mentioned half press-up manoeuvre. An effective sustained stretch can also be obtained by positioning the patient in the supine position with his/her pelvis over the hinged head section of an adjustable-back treatment couch. The head portion of the couch can then be elevated to the desired position, placing the recti abdominis under tension. Once full pain-free muscle extensibility has been restored, strength and function must be fully rehabilitated before sporting activities are resumed. The exercise programme described for the postoperative rehabilitation of inguinal disruption repair is suitable for the rehabilitation of rectus abdominis tears.

(e) Inguinal disruption

This term will be used to describe the abdominal soft-tissue pathology which is known among other things as 'sports hernia' (Hackney, 1993), 'incipient inguinal hernia' (Lovell, Malycha and Pieterse, 1990) or 'Gilmore's groin' (Gilmore, 1993). 'Inguinal disruption' is the term used here because it is a more accurate description of this lesion than 'hernia'. It describes a pattern of soft-tissue disruption that affects the inguinal region of the abdomen without there being a true herniation of the abdominal contents. This latter type of pathology is a well-recognized clinical entity, with clear signs and symptoms. In contrast, inguinal disruption is a more difficult condition to conclusively diagnose.

The pathology, as described by Gilmore (1993), consists of:

- a torn external oblique aponeurosis, resulting in dilation of the superficial inguinal ring;
- a torn conjoined tendon;
- a dehiscence between the inguinal ligament and the conjoined tendon.

Associated pathological findings include a deficiency in the transversalis fascia with a bulging of the posterior wall of the inguinal canal (Hackney, 1993). It has been proposed that this weakening of the transversalis fascia results in pain when sporting activity produces an increase in intra-abdominal pressure (Polglase, Frydman and Farmer, 1991).

In the vast majority of cases, no one specific traumatic incident can be identified by the athlete as having caused the injury. Symptom onset is usually gradual and it can take many weeks or months for the severity of the symptoms to significantly curtail sporting activity (Polglase, Frydman and Farmer, 1991). This suggests an overuse component to the aetiology of this condition. In many of the athletes who develop this condition there is a significant stiffness of one or both hips. Lumbar spine hypomobility and reduced flexibility of the hip musculature is also often encountered. If and how such hypomobility is linked to the development of inguinal disruption is unclear. However, it may be the case that the lower abdominal region, which is subjected to repetitive tension during many different sporting activities, may be exposed to extra loading if the adjacent joints and musculature are stiff. Such repetitive overload could then lead to tissue attenuation and breakdown.

Signs and symptoms   Pain is the chief complaint, and is experienced in the lower abdomen, often radiating to the medial upper thighs. Perineal and testicular pain is also frequently experienced. The nature of the pain ranges from a diffuse ache to severe sharp pain. It is usually elicited by running at speed, especially where explosive push-offs and quick changes of direction are involved. Kicking is also often limited by pain. Any increases in intra-abdominal pressure are also usually symptom-provoking, hence the frequently reported pain on coughing and sneezing and on resisted abdominal work. Another feature of this condition is the marked pain with associated stiffness in the inguinal and groin regions that is often encountered after strenuous physical exercise. Affected athletes often recount such symptoms as being particularly limiting when getting out of bed the morning following sports participation.

Cessation of sporting activity is usually forced upon the athlete by the eventual severity of the pain. After several days rest, the symptoms usually settle, but in cases where significant inguinal disruption is present the athlete rarely becomes completely asymptomatic. Resumption of sporting activity after a period of rest is usually followed by a rapid return of the symptoms. Failure of the damaged tissues to repair during these rest periods could be due to the fact that the significant pathology of the disrupted tissues is the inguinal ligament/conjoined tendon dehiscence and that healing is impossible because of the separation of the two structures (Gilmore, 1993).

Examination There is no one definitive test for this lesion. Dilation of the superficial inguinal ring may indicate the presence of an inguinal disruption and has been advocated as a useful examination procedure, the ring being examined via the scrotum with the little finger (Gilmore, 1993). In females there may be discomfort in the region of the superficial inguinal ring upon external palpation. However, tenderness in this region, with or without a dilation of the superficial inguinal ring, is not conclusive proof of the existence of inguinal disruption. Neither is the presence of a 'cough impulse' (a fibrillating pressure wave felt upon palpation of the inguinal region as the athlete coughs).

Because the complaint is of pain, which usually crosses a number of anatomical boundaries, it is mandatory to examine the lumbar spine, sacroiliac joints, hips and symphysis pubis, in order to determine if there is a clear link between the pain and an abnormal range of movement. Testing the abdominal musculature via a contraction test usually reproduces pain but placing it at end range stretch is infrequently asymptomatic. Tight and tender hip adductors are often associated with inguinal disruptions, but the fact that the pain is often experienced in the low abdomen and perineal/testicular region in addition to the adductor region gives a strong diagnostic clue that the adductors are not primarily responsible for the symptoms. Similarly, stiffness of the hips, towards the ranges of combined flexion and adduction and into combined flexion and medial rotation, often painfully occurs among athletes with this condition. These anomalies may pre-exist and are possibly contributory to the onset of the inguinal disruption.

The remaining tests are performed to rule out other pathology that could be causative or contributory to the symptoms, such as osteitis pubis and pelvic instability. Radiographic examination may be performed to ascertain this. The use of peritoneography (Ekberg, Blomquist and Ollson, 1981; Smedberg et al., 1985) or CT herniography (Hackney, 1993) to detect soft-tissue anomalies in the inguinal region has proved partially successful, but cannot be used as a conclusive test (Polglase, Frydman and Farmer, 1991). While a physical examination and radiographic investigations can indicate the presence of this type of lesion, it is usually a carefully detailed history, and an examination process that rules out other causes of the presenting symptomatology, that lead to a diagnosis of inguinal disruption.

Treatment Surgical repair of the soft-tissue defect gives a good chance (80–90%) of sports resumption (Hackney, 1993; Gilmore, 1993; Polglase, Frydman and Farmer, 1991). Postoperatively a period of 5–6 weeks has been advocated before sport is resumed (Hackney, 1993) and over this period the athlete's activities are gradually increased. However it is not unusual for the athlete to have a continuation of the symptoms following surgery and any progression in physical activities should be guided by any symptoms that are encountered. The 5–6 week time scale for a return to sport should be viewed as a bare minimum. Indeed, it invariably takes longer than this to rectify the previously mentioned vertebral and hip hypomobility with the associated muscular weakness and imbalances that usually present in such patients. Failure to address these anomalies could predispose the athlete to future injury to this region.

Treatment should be aimed at restoring restricted ranges of hip and trunk mobility and an active and passive mobilization programme should commence as soon as is practical. The surgical repair often stimulates vigorous scar tissue production and, after approximately 2 weeks, a programme of abdominal stretching work (guided by discomfort) can be instituted which will help to prevent unnecessary scar contracture. Gentle massage and the application of ultrasound to this area may facilitate this mobilizing and stretching process. Stretching the abdominals into straight extension positions (as described for the treatment of rectus abdominis strains) should also be performed to prevent contracture. The oblique abdominals should also be stretched by using positions of trunk rotation. It is also often necessary to mobilize and strengthen the hip adductors.

Abdominal strengthening and re-education is an important part of the postoperative rehabilitation. Initially, the emphasis should be on regaining control of the abdominals. One very effective way of achieving this is by the use of pressure biofeedback equipment to re-educate the abdominals to control the pelvis as regards posterior tilting and the associated neutral position of the lumbar spine. Adequate trunk muscle control should be achieved, particularly in relation to the ability of the athlete to stabilize the lumbar spine while simultaneously being able to use the hip musculature, before more vigorous and sport-specific abdominal and trunk work is introduced.

The traditional sit-up exercises that many athletes use to condition their abdominal musculature should be replaced with trunk curl exercises. The sit-up often overemphasizes hip flexor activity, especially when performed with foot fixation (Janda and Schmid, 1980) and this can place potentially injurious forces upon the lumbar spine, whereas the trunk curl, when performed without foot fixation, maximally recruits the abdominals and maintains a neutral lumbar spine position. The lower abdominals can be more specifically targeted with strengthening work by using modified bilateral straight leg raise exercises (Sallis and Jones, 1991). Performed from the supine lying position, by a subject with underconditioned abdominal muscles, this manoeuvre can exert potentially injurious forces on the lumbar spine. However, if the exercise is performed in reverse, i.e. the legs are lowered through a small arc of movement from a position of 90° while a neutral lumbar spine is maintained, then the potential negative effects of the manoeuvre can be avoided. Performing this exercise in a position where the heels can be lowered to rest against a wall is an ideal way of preventing too great a range of movement. This exercise and the previously mentioned trunk curl exercise can be performed with the trunk straight to emphasize the action of rectus abdominis, or can be performed with a partial rotation of the trunk to emphasize the oblique abdominals.

The sport-specific phase of abdominal conditioning is vital if sporting function is to be optimized (Norris, 1993). One particular type of abdominal activity that is employed in many sports and is frequently overlooked in rehabilitation protocols is outer range eccentric–concentric coupling. This involves eccentric abdominal work as the trunk extends, which places tension on the abdominal muscles as the trunk fully extends. This is followed immediately by a concentric abdominal contraction. This type of manoeuvre generates high forces in the involved muscles and their associated soft tissues (Komi and Bosco, 1979) and should therefore be incorporated into the rehabilitation programme so that the athlete is suitably conditioned and prepared. Functional sporting examples of this type of work are a soccer throw-in, bowling a cricket ball and a tennis serve or overhead shot.

The sporting actions of the athlete should be analysed to determine the type of abdominal muscle work involved and then exercises can be devised which match the postures, speeds, intensities and duration which the sport in question demands. The successful implementation of this type of abdominal training requires a full pain-free range of trunk extension and, in cases where there is hypomobility, particularly in the lumbar spine, passive mobilization should be used to regain the range before active end range movements are used to strengthen the abdominals.

6.3.5 The hip joint

The hip joint has a bony and ligamentous structure that permits relatively large ranges of movement without sacrificing stability. Because of its key role in bodyweight transmission and ambulation, the hip and its associated structures are prone to injuries occurring in many sports. The majority of these are chronic overuse problems rather than acute injuries. This is not surprising when one considers the fact that the forces transmitted through the hip during walking and running are equivalent to several times the bodyweight with each step (Oatis, 1990). This is because of the leverages involved in the alignment of the femoral neck to the femoral shaft (approximately 125° in the frontal plane – Warwick and Williams, 1973) and the vertical line of force that bodyweight imposes medially to the weightbearing surface of the hip. Because the body's centre of gravity falls medially to the weightbearing axis of the hip in double-leg standing, it is necessary for the pelvis to be shifted over the foot of the supporting leg when single lower limb stance positions are adopted. In order

to keep the pelvis horizontal during this manoeuvre, the hip abductors of the weightbearing side must work strongly to prevent the non-weightbearing side of the pelvis (which carries the weight of the head, arms trunk and opposite limb) from dropping (Oatis, 1990). It is clear therefore, that the hip abductors play a central role in the normal functioning of the hip in all weightbearing situations.

The injuries and conditions affecting the sporting hip that will be considered are stress fractures, slipped upper femoral epiphysis, tendinitis/bursitis, sprains and capsulitis.

(a) Stress fractures

The incidence of stress fractures has increased over recent years because of the increased number of individuals who regularly participate in sport (Kupke *et al.*, 1993). A stress fracture can be defined as a partial or complete break in a bone's structure due to its inability to withstand repeated loading (Sallis and Jones, 1991). Such loads may be imparted to the hip region in distance running events and jumping sports and can affect the femoral neck and the pubic rami. Stress fracture may result due to 'fatigue' or to 'insufficiency' (Packer, 1995). Here the term 'fatigue fracture' refers to the scenario where a stress fracture occurs after the application of an abnormal load (amount, frequency, unaccustomed or combination) to normal bone. In contrast, 'insufficiency fracture' refers to a stress fracture that occurs in bone of abnormal structure that is exposed to normal loading. In both scenarios the external force that is applied exceeds the bone's elastic range and microfractures result. Under normal loading situations there is a constant turnover of bony material, with new bone formation matching the rate of absorption. The continued application of excessive stresses to specific bony sites can result in the rate of tissue breakdown exceeding that of remodelling (Daffner and Pavlov, 1992). Certain systemic conditions can affect the inherent strength of bony tissue and predispose certain groups of athletes to stress fractures. Stress fractures are more commonly encountered in female athletes (Packer, 1995), and one explanation for this is that there is a high incidence of amenorrhoea among those athletes who are exposed to relatively high and long-term training loads, e.g. distance runners. In these athletes, low oestrogen levels have been linked to an increased risk of developing stress fractures as this results in decreased bone mass (Sallis and Jones, 1991).

Pelvic stress fractures

Signs and symptoms   Pain is usually the main or only complaint and is localized to the groin. An inflammatory periosteal reaction may affect the tendinous attachments of the adductors and abdominal muscles and result in painful stretching or contraction of these muscles. Stress fractures may be linked to an increase in the amount of the athlete's training load and the onset is usually gradual, with the severity of pain gradually increasing until it prevents sporting activity. There is invariably a direct link to the amount of pain experienced and the amount of provocative exercise undertaken.

Examination   This may be unremarkable: minimal or no pain may be reproduced on active or passive movement tests of the hip. Direct palpation of the pubic rami may elicit pain. The diagnosis is made by radiographic and bone scan examination.

Treatment   Single stress fracture of a pubic ramus does not affect the structural integrity of the pelvic girdle and so non- or partial weightbearing may only be required in the early acute stage, to control pain. Rest from pain-provoking activity is the treatment of choice and it may take from 2–6 months before sport can be resumed (Reid, 1992).

Femoral neck stress fracture

Femoral neck stress fractures have been classified as being either tension, compression or displaced fractures (Kupke *et al.*, 1993). Tension stress lesions are located on the upper aspect of the femoral neck and with repeated loading there is a risk of them becoming complete, displaced fractures. Compression stress fractures are located on the inferior aspect of the femoral neck.

Signs and symptoms   As with all stress fractures, pain is the principal complaint and is usually linked with activities that place repetitive weightbearing forces on the hips. When the pain increases in severity, the athlete may experience night pain (Sallis and Jones, 1991).

Examination   Because of the depth of the overlying tissues it is not possible to elicit specific tenderness with a palpatory examination, although there may be diffuse tenderness around the joint because of the presence of protective muscle spasm. No specific range of movement will be affected, although deep-seated pain may be elicited when overpressure is applied to some or all hip movements. A conclusive diagnosis of stress fracture can only be made following radiographic and bone scan investigations.

Treatment   As with all stress fractures, rest is the mainstay of treatment and is indicated for compression stress fractures of the femoral neck (Kupke *et al.*, 1993). In these cases, sport must only be resumed once repeat scans have demonstrated that healing has occurred and once the athlete is completely asymptomatic as regards activities of daily living. During the 'rest' period, the athlete will probably be able to follow a substitute training programme that avoids any significant hip impact loading. Activities such as deep water running are particularly suitable for athletes involved in running sports.

Tension stress fractures have a greater chance of becoming complete and possibly displaced femoral neck fractures than do compression fractures. Because of this and the fact that displaced femoral neck fractures have been associated with a high risk of avascular femoral head necrosis, it has been suggested that this type of stress lesion should be treated with internal fixation (Kupke *et al.*, 1993).

(b) Slipped upper femoral epiphysis

This condition affects children, before the epiphysis of the femoral neck unites in the mid- to late teens. It is more commonly seen in males between the ages of 11 and 15 years (Crawford, 1988). Slippage of the epiphysis may follow an episode of acute trauma such as a fall. However it may be a gradual and progressive process and in such cases the aetiology is unknown, although genetic and hormonal factors have been postulated (Rappaport and Fife, 1985). The femoral head is displaced in an inferior and posterior direction. If left untreated this condition can predispose the child to the development of avascular necrosis of the femoral head and osteoarthrosis.

Signs and symptoms The child usually complains of pain in the hip region but this may also be accompanied by knee pain (Corrigan and Maitland, 1994). The knee pain may even be the only area of pain. An antalgic gait, with associated decreased abductor strength when weightbearing (giving a Trendelenberg sign) may be present and the affected limb may be held in semiflexion and adduction.

Examination All hip movements may be limited by pain and stiffness and attempts to flex the hip may be accompanied by lateral hip rotation (Reid, 1992). Radiographic evidence reveals a widening of the epiphysis and a posteroinferior slippage of the femoral head.

Treatment Minimal slippage may be treated with bed rest and traction. Treatment of more obvious slippage may involve surgical pinning.

(c) Tendinitis and bursitis

These conditions will be considered together as, in the hip region, it is usually impossible to differentiate between the two. Tendinitis of adductor longus, rectus femoris and iliopsoas has already been covered. Here gluteal tendinitis/bursitis and trochanteric bursitis will be considered.

The trochanteric bursa is the most superficially placed bursa on the lateral aspect of the hip and lies between the underside of the tensor fascia lata and the lateral upper aspect of the greater trochanter. There is one more deeply placed bursae on the lateral aspect of the hip which lies between the tendons of gluteus minimus and medius. These tendons and bursae are probably the soft tissues around the hip most commonly affected by acute and chronic inflammation. This may result from single episodes of acute trauma, but usually involves overuse of the hips, as in distance running or cross-country skiing.

Signs and symptoms Pain is localized to the region of the greater trochanter and may radiate down the lateral aspect of the upper thigh. This is often felt as a 'burning' pain. Movements of repeated hip flexion and extension may be pain-provoking because the tensor fascia lata rides over the inflamed bursa. Forceful abduction of the hip may be painful in cases of gluteal tendinitis/bursitis. Swelling and tenderness may be evident in cases of inflammation of the more superficially placed trochanteric bursa. In cases where the injury has resulted from direct trauma such as a fall directly on to the greater trochanter, care should be taken to inspect the area for abrasions through which pathogens could pass and set up an infected bursitis. Signs of this would include a reddened, tense and exquisitely tender swelling over the greater trochanter, and possibly systemic signs of infection such as a raised body temperature, malaise and nausea.

Examination   Tenderness and swelling are often easily noted in cases of trochanteric bursitis. There may also be tightness of the iliotibial band/tensor fascia lata and pain in the region of the greater trochanter. Gluteal tendinitis/bursitis may be accompanied by pain at the greater trochanteric tendon insertion when resistance is applied to hip abduction or when it is stretched by adducting the hip. In acute cases the athlete may exhibit a Trendelenburg sign when walking because of pain inhibition of the glutei.

Treatment   Acute inflammation is treated with relative rest, ice and appropriate electrotherapy such as ultrasonics. Compression, in the form of a hip spica, may help to control swelling and ease pain. Taping may also be used for these purposes. Once the acute inflammatory stage has settled, it is important to mobilize the hip into any restricted ranges of movement and this may involve stretching the possibly shortened gluteal tendons and tensor fascia lata. Massage to the trochanteric region may also help to restore soft-tissue suppleness. Finally, a graduated programme of hip abduction strengthening work should be followed before sport is resumed.

(d) Sprained hip

The hip is a very stable joint, because of its bony architecture and the support it receives from its strong and extensive capsule and supporting ligaments. Anteriorly the pubofemoral ligament, and particularly the iliofemoral ligament, prevent excessive extension and are key stabilizers in this respect during ambulation. The ischiofemoral ligament, which supports the posterior aspect of the joint, has a spiral arrangement of fibres that are tightened by hip extension and by medial rotation. Despite the strength of the hip capsule and ligaments, the hip, like any other synovial joint, is susceptible to sprain injuries, although the frequency of such injuries is far less than for the other lower-limb weightbearing joints. Significant amounts of force are required to sprain the intrinsically strong passive hip stabilizers; these may occur in a wide variety of contact sports, or activities where high-speed falls can occur, such as downhill skiing.

Signs and symptoms   A definite history of a single traumatic injury is recalled by the athlete, which, in the case of moderate to severe sprains, prevents further sporting activity. Pain inhibition usually affects the glutei and a Trendelenburg gait results. Iliopsoas protective spasm is a common finding in many painful hip disorders and the affected hip may consequently be held semiflexed and in some degree of lateral rotation. Because of the depth of the hip joint, swelling may not be observable.

Examination   The range of movement that is most restricted by pain will depend upon which capsular/ligamentous structure has been damaged. When the athlete can recall the specific mechanics of the injury, this can help lead the physical examination in terms of the movements to be tested. As for any other type of joint sprain, the physical examination should measure any abnormal range of movement and relate this to associated pain responses. Testing the functional capacity of the glutei is important as they have a vital role in the normal functioning of the hip.

Treatment   Pain control is the first treatment goal and may be attained by the use of a walking aid plus the application of gentle accessory hip movements, ice and electrotherapy. Static hip abductor work should be commenced as soon as possible to overcome any inhibition. As the severity of the pain subsides, active and passive mobilizations should be administered to regain any lost range of movement. The direction of movement that was involved in the actual injury is frequently the most limited and specific attention should therefore be given to regaining this. A general programme of hip strengthening (particularly for the abductors) and proprioceptive re-education exercises appropriate to the sport of the injured athlete should be followed prior to a return to sport.

(e) Capsulitis

This term is frequently used in connection with the shoulder joint, where it is used to describe painful restriction of movement. It is less commonly used to describe the similar clinical pattern of pain and stiffness of the hip, which is made worse with activity and may follow a traumatic injury (Griffiths, Utz and Burke, 1985). All ranges of hip motion are usually affected, the most obvious restriction being into combined flexion and adduction. Rotation movements, particularly in a medial direction, are similarly affected. The diagnosis is made mainly on clinical grounds, although isotope bone scanning may reveal increased uptake, with arthrography not necessarily demonstrating capsular retraction (Chard and Jenner, 1988).

Over a period of weeks or months, resolution occurs spontaneously. The athlete should be reassured accordingly and a programme of active and passive mobilization into the most restricted ranges of movement should be implemented. The athlete should also be taught how to adopt positions that provide sustained stretches to the hip, especially variations of prone lying, which will help to counter flexion contracture. As the condition shows signs of resolution, sporting activity can be phased in.

6.3.6 Disorders of the symphysis pubis

The symphysis pubis is a cartilaginous joint between the two pubic bones and allows a small amount of movement between the two halves of the pelvis. In sporting situations it may be prone to inflammatory and instability problems. Diagnosis of these lesions is often difficult, and usually requires the elimination of other musculoskeletal (i.e. vertebral, pelvic and hip) causes.

(a) Osteitis pubis

This is an inflammatory disorder that affects the articulating bony ends of the pubic bones and their symphysis. In sports that impart repeated torsional forces through the symphysis pubis (e.g. by sudden changes in direction when running, or by kicking), mechanical irritation may set an inflammatory process in motion. An athlete with hypomobility of the hips or lumbar spine may be predisposed to the development of this lesion as a result of a functional overload being applied to the symphysis.

Signs and symptoms Pain is usually of insidious onset over a number of weeks or months. It may be experienced in the region of the symphysis pubis and may radiate to the groins and proximal thighs. Pain may be provoked by activity or movement that stresses the symphysis, such as vigorous or forceful trunk and hip work or running at speed or checking to sidestep or turn.

Examination This must include a test of all of the abdominal and hip musculature, although symptoms may be elicited on many of these tests when the condition is particularly acute. There is often tenderness upon palpation of the symphysis and pain may be reproduced with passive movements to the hemipelvis (forward and backward rotation) and to the symphysis (anteroposterior pressure). X-ray evidence may be inconclusive, because there are wide variations in the 'normal' appearance of the symphysis pubis. Radiographic evidence that goes some way to confirming the condition is a widening of the symphysis, sclerotic changes of the pubic bone ends and erosion (Reid, 1992).

Treatment   Rest is the basis of successful conservative management. This condition is usually chronic and recurrent and this can often be linked to the fact that any rest from sport has been for too short a period or the return to sport following rest has been too rapid. To be effective, the offending sport and any other pain-provoking activity must be completely stopped, in severe cases for a period of several weeks or even months. Substitute training during this time is usually possible but must not provoke any symptoms. Any stiffness of the hips or lumbar spine should be addressed by a suitable flexibility and passive mobilizing programme. Non-steroidal anti-inflammatory medication may be of help, as may steroid injections. However these treatments should not be used as a 'short cut' back to sport. They are useful only as adjuncts to rest and a graduated return to sport.

(b) Pubic symphysis instability

The types of athlete at risk of developing this condition are the same as those who are prone to osteitis pubis. The condition is usually due to overuse, with repetitive shear force over many months and years resulting in hypermobility of the symphysis (Gamble, Simmons and Fredman, 1986). The mode of symptom onset and the symptomatology are similar to osteitis pubis. Additionally, the athlete may occasionally be aware of a clicking or clunking sensation with certain movements such as kicking or turning over in bed. Diagnosis is made by excluding other musculoskeletal pathologies in this region and by the demonstration of actual instability of the symphysis on X ray. These are performed in alternate single-leg standing ('stork' views) and are positive when there is a significant difference between the pubic heights of the two sides.

Treatment is along the lines laid down for osteitis pubis and may take many months to settle and rehabilitate. Cases resistant to conservative treatment may require surgical fusion of the symphysis.

6.3.7   Hip and pelvic pain of nerve origin

While the majority of sports-related injuries to the hip and pelvic region involve musculoskeletal soft tissues, it is sometimes the case that nerve tissue can be a cause of pain and disability. In the region of the hip and pelvis the most commonly cited 'nerve cause' of pain is entrapment neuropathy that affects the lateral cutaneous nerve of the thigh. However, a number of nerves can be a cause of pain in this region and the reason does not have to be an entrapment. These 'nerve' conditions can occur together with the bony and soft-tissue pathologies that have been previously described, or they can occur in isolation. Nerve tissue may be damaged directly, or damage may affect nerve interface tissues such as the muscular and fascial tissues through which they pass and to which they are attached. Such nerve pathology does not necessarily result in a conduction block. The pathology involved is probably that of inflammation and associated swelling, tissue thickening and fibrosis and may result from mechanical irritation, e.g. tension or compression. The result may be a reduction in the range of movement of the nerve and an increase in its sensitivity to movement. Some of the pain areas that result from specific nerve involvement may be mistaken for the symptoms of musculoskeletal disorders. Some of these are listed in Table 6.4.

The implication of nerve pathodynamics in pelvic and hip conditions requires attention to detail in the subjective and objective examination of the athlete. Descriptions of symptoms that include the words 'burning', 'shooting', 'electric' or 'tingling' may give a clue as to the involvement of neural or neural-related tissues. Similarly, the provocation of symptoms by movements of remote body parts (e.g. foot/ankle movements or head, neck and trunk movements) should raise the suspicion of neural involvement. Objective testing to implicate nerves and their investments are based on neural tension tests such as straight leg raising, prone knee bending and the 'slump' position. The use of 'sensitizing' movements to these base tests may be used to differentiate between musculoskeletal and neural structures as causes of the presenting problem. An example of such an examination process is the differentiation of the lateral cutaneous nerve of the thigh (LCNT) from a local musculoskeletal cause of upper lateral thigh pain. If hip extension reproduces the pain, this could be due to tension in a pathological LCNT (which arises from the lumbar plexus, supplies the upper lateral thigh and is tensioned in positions of hip extension) or to irritation of a local musculoskeletal structure. If the hip extension is then performed while the head, neck and trunk are held in a 'slumped' position, a different pain response may be elicited if the LCNT is involved, i.e. more pain, because the slump position pretensions the LCNT via the lumbar plexus.

(a) Lateral cutaneous nerve of the thigh entrapment

This nerve originates from the L2 and L3 nerve roots and supplies the skin of the upper lateral thigh. It enters the lower limb by passing beneath the lateral portion of the inguinal ligament just medial to the anterior superior iliac spine. It is here that entrapment may occur and this may follow an episode of direct trauma.

Signs and symptoms The athlete complains of a 'burning' pain at the upper lateral aspect of the thigh. Numbness and paraesthesia in the same area may also be a complaint. Positions of hip extension provoke the symptoms and in moderate to severe cases,

simply extending the hip in the push-off phase of walking or running can cause symptoms.

Examination Positions of hip extension, as mentioned previously, reproduce the symptoms and can be linked with trunk 'slump' positions, which may emphasize the symptom severity. Pressure applied over the lateral portion of the inguinal ligament, approximately one fingerbreadth medial to the anterior superior iliac spine, may elicit tenderness and possibly reproduce lateral thigh symptoms. An assessment of lower limb sensation may reveal hypersensitivity or numbness of the upper lateral thigh.

Treatment Rest from aggravating activities, together with mobilization of the tissues in the area of entrapment, may bring about resolution. Infiltration of the same area with local anaesthetic and steroids may also be of help. In severe cases, where conservative measures fail to help, surgical decompression may be necessary.

(b) Non-musculoskeletal causes of pelvic and groin pain

While it is beyond the scope of this text to deal with non-musculoskeletal causes of symptoms in this area, a brief reference will be made to some of these pathologies (Table 6.5).

Table 6.5 should not be looked upon as a comprehensive list of pathologies upon which to base a differential diagnosis. The purpose of mentioning these conditions is to alert those clinicians such as physiotherapists, whose clinical remit does not include making a comprehensive differential diagnosis, to the fact that non-musculoskeletal pathologies should be considered. This is particularly true in cases where the symptoms have no specific traumatic origin, or are accompanied by signs and symptoms suggestive of a generalized illness.

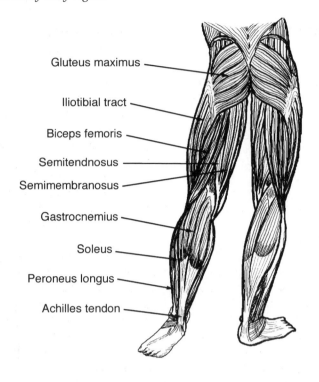

Gluteus maximus

Iliotibial tract

Biceps femoris

Semitendnosus

Semimembranosus

Gastrocnemius

Soleus

Peroneus longus

Achilles tendon

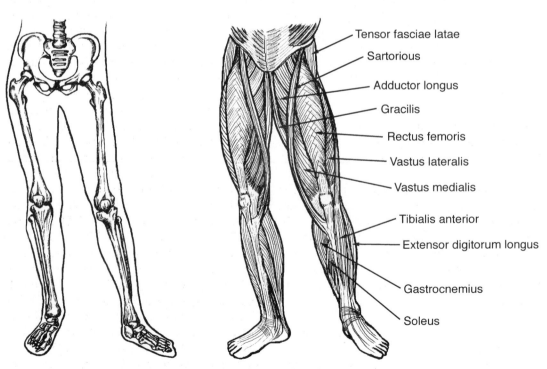

Tensor fasciae latae

Sartorious

Adductor longus

Gracilis

Rectus femoris

Vastus lateralis

Vastus medialis

Tibialis anterior

Extensor digitorum longus

Gastrocnemius

Soleus

Figure 6.4   Anatomy of the lower limb.

6.4 LOWER LIMB MUSCLE INJURIES

6.4.1 Introduction

Acute and chronic muscle pathology probably accounts for the majority of sports injuries (Renstrom, 1983; Benazzo *et al.*, 1989). Of these, the hamstrings, rectus femoris and gastrocnemius are probably the most frequently injured. In this section, these muscles will be considered, particularly in relation to episodes of acute injury. Some basic guidelines for examination, treatment and management will then be covered and it should be possible to apply this information to other muscle injuries.

The rectus femoris, hamstrings and gastrocnemius share physical and biomechanical properties, which could account for their apparent predisposition to injury. All these muscles have a high percentage of type II muscle fibres and are therefore well suited to the production of rapid, forceful movements (Richardson, 1992). This may, on occasions, expose them to potentially damaging levels of force. Some of their shared anatomical and functional characteristics will be reviewed and discussed in relation to running, as the majority of injuries to these muscles occur during running or running-related activities.

Perhaps the most obvious similarity between these muscles is the fact that they cross the boundaries of two joints (Figure 6.4).

This means that, during ambulation, the muscles will at some stage be either stretched or shortened over two joints and will subsequently be exposed to greater length changes than single joint muscles. These muscles are able to produce both single joint movements and simultaneous movements at adjacent joints.

- The hamstrings flex the knee and extend the hip.
- The rectus femoris flexes the hip and extends the knee.
- The gastrocnemius flexes the knee and plantarflexes the foot.

This analysis concentrates only on the concentric action of the muscles in question. To fully appreciate the role that these muscles play in the running cycle, attention must also be given to their eccentric actions. These are particularly evident, in terms of force production, during fast-paced running. During the mid- to late swing phase, the hamstrings work eccentrically to decelerate the extending knee and to prevent knee hyperextension. At foot strike, they then work concentrically, i.e. from a position of stretch, to generate a forward push-off. After the foot has contacted the ground and propelled the body forwards, the hip is prevented from being overextended by the eccentric action of the rectus femoris and this eccentric action also controls knee flexion. From the position of hip extension, which stretches the rectus femoris, it contracts to aid the other hip flexors in swinging the limb forwards. The gastrocnemius works concentrically to produce a plantarflexing 'push-off' but immediately prior to this, i.e. at the initial foot-strike, it works eccentrically in order to control foot dorsiflexion.

As well as controlling and preventing specific ranges of joint movement, this eccentric muscular activity provides a source of force production additional to that which the muscle can produce through an isolated concentric contraction. This is achieved by utilizing the elastic properties of the non-contractile elements of the muscle. These consist of the series elastic component (SEC) and the parallel elastic component (PEC). These non-contractile tissues (which are the fascial/connective tissue investments of the muscle fibres and the aponeurotic/tendinous attachments respectively) are stretched during the process of eccentric muscle lengthening and this in effect momentarily stores elastic energy. This energy can then be used to augment the force from the concentric contraction of the muscle that immediately follows its eccentric prestretch. In this way significantly larger force values can be generated than can be achieved through isolated concentric muscle work (Komi and Bosco, 1979; Thys, 1972). While this system of concentric and eccentric coupling provides an efficient means of generating fast, high-force output movements, which are fundamental to many sporting situations, it may also place the lower limb musculature under potentially injurious loads.

The previously mentioned running action is a complex activity which requires a finely tuned neuromotor control mechanism to ensure that the muscles in question fire synchronously during high-speed eccentric lengthening and active shortening. A failure of this control system (e.g. as a result of fatigue), could result in a poorly timed concentric muscle contraction, which, if occurring at the time when external forces are imposing a stretch upon the muscle, could result in damage to the muscle's contractile and/or non-contractile tissues (Ganett *et al*, 1984).

6.4.2   Prevention of lower limb injuries

The prevention of muscular injury has included attention to the following topics:

- Flexibility training
- Strength training
- Agonist/antagonist strength ratios.

(a) Flexibility training

Over the years there has been widespread support for the belief that muscles which have optimum flexibility are less likely to be injured, than muscles that are not conditioned in this way (Beaulieu, 1981; Anderson, Beaulieu and Cornelius, 1984). This is based upon the premise that reduced muscular stiffness will allow greater force dissipation and thereby reduce the likelihood of injury. However, to date there is no clear scientific evidence to suggest that this is actually the case.

Despite this, it is probably advisable for the sportsperson to follow an ongoing flexibility programme and to integrate this with a programme of exercises that condition the muscles to the specific demands of their sport. When undertaking a programme of flexibility training, it is important to concentrate on the quality of the stretches that are being undertaken rather than just on the quantity of the stretch. For example, the actual range of movement that is attainable when stretching the hamstrings is of less importance than the quality of the stretch. A good-quality stretch has an end feel that is resilient and elastic, as opposed to a poor-quality stretch which, has a hard, unyielding end feel. It is a frequently encountered clinical finding that poor-quality stretches are associated with muscle groups that are prone to strain injury. Consequently, attention should be made to optimize this 'quality' aspect of stretching and this may be achieved by emphasizing through-range movements rather than vigorous end-range stretching.

(b) Strength training

One form of 'strengthening' work that fits in well with a flexibility training programme and for the vast majority of sports imposes functional, if not sport-specific muscular loading is free weight training. This type of training has the disadvantages of requiring relatively specialized weight lifting equipment and having to be performed under expert guidance. However, when performed correctly, many of the lifting techniques encourage patterns of flexibility and strength that are relevant to many sporting situations. A suitable strength training programme will not only improve and/or maintain the contractile strength of muscle but will also improve and maintain the tensile strength of the muscle's non-contractile tissues (Curwin and Standish, 1984). This is of vital importance in the prevention of strain injuries, as most of these occur at the interface of the muscle's contractile elements and the non-contractile tissues, e.g. musculotendinous junctions. Where possible, some form of functional and sport-specific strength training should be incorporated into training programmes. While there is no conclusive evidence that strength training programmes can prevent muscle injury, a study by Hejna and Rosenberg (1982) demonstrated a significant reduction in injury rates among a trained group of high-school athletes as opposed to an untrained group. The means by which this protects the athlete from injury is unclear. Possible explanations could be a combination of increased musculotendinous strength which allows higher force values to be absorbed, and improved endurance, which delays the onset of exercise-induced fatigue (Glick, 1980).

(c) Agonist/antagonist ratios

Opposing muscle groups have a 'natural' balance of strength. If changes occur to this 'normal' ratio (e.g. as a result of injury or the selective strengthening effect of a particular sport), then there may be a predisposition to injury (Grace, 1985). In relation to the quadriceps and hamstrings, strength deficits in excess of 10% between the muscle groups of opposite sides of the body have been identified as being a predisposition to injury (Jarvinen, 1994). It has also been stated that hamstring strength values of less than 60% of the quadriceps similarly raise the risk of injury (Kibler and Chandler, 1993). However the relevance of some of the methods of determining normal and abnormal strength data to real-life sporting situations has been questioned (Grimby, 1982). For example the frequently cited 'normal' ratio of hamstring strength to quadriceps strength is a measurement of peak concentric torque (usually measured by non-functional isokinetic evaluation). As these peaks occur in different ranges of knee flexion for each muscle group, the functional relevance of the 'normal' figure could be called into question.

A more functional approach would be to compare the agonist/antagonist strength values at the same joint angle, or to measure force production through range rather than an angle-specific torque value.

Another factor that should be borne in mind when attempting to ascertain normative data of this kind is the fact that, in many sports situations, one muscle works concentrically while its antagonist works eccentrically. A comparison of agonist–concentric/antagonist–eccentric strength may therefore be of greater functional relevance.

6.4.3 General principles of rehabilitation

As with other soft-tissue injuries, the initial management of muscle strains, which result in tissue disruption and subsequent swelling and bruising, is to minimize the amount of post-traumatic exudate and to provide optimum conditions for the healing process. The healing process can be divided into the three stages of inflammation, repair and remodelling. Some form of rest is usually required during the initial inflammatory stage in order to prevent further tissue damage, but this should be kept to a minimum, as early mobilization has been shown to reduce the degree of postinjury disability (Lehto, Duance and Restall, 1985). In the repair and remodelling phases, exposure of the injured muscle to contractile and tensile forces improves the quality and strength of the connective tissue that forms to breach the gap at the injury site (Jarvinen, 1994). It also optimizes the penetration and orientation of regenerating muscle fibres (Benazzo *et al.*, 1989). In the remodelling phase, particular attention should be given to achieving and maintaining the flexibility of the scar tissue that has been laid down. This type of connective tissue has the propensity to contract many weeks and months after the actual injury and failure to prevent this could result in reinjury.

The contractile forces that the muscle is exposed to should be progressed from

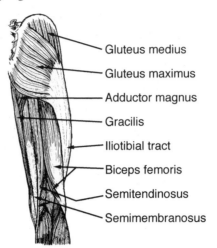

Figure 6.5 The hamstring muscles.

isometric to isotonic (initially stressing concentric work over eccentric), finally emphasizing concentric–eccentric coupled activities specific to the action of the sport in question. This approach to strengthening muscles following injury ensures that they are subjected to eccentric loads that should, in the final progression, replicate the forces to which they will be subjected when sport is resumed. This should:

- improve the muscle's contractile strength;
- improve the tensile strength of the series elastic component and parallel elastic component;
- improve neuromotor control with regard to high-speed eccentric–concentric coupling.

Such a progression should be made with broad reference to healing time scales and with close reference to the presenting signs and symptoms, particularly pain responses to contractile and tensile forces.

6.4.4 Injuries to specific muscles

(a) Hamstrings

The hamstrings are composed of the medially placed semitendinosus and semimembrano-

sus and the laterally placed biceps femoris (Figure 6.5).

They attach proximally to the ischial tuberosity and distally the medial two attach into the upper tibia. The biceps femoris attaches into the fibula head. These three muscles work together to extend the hip and to flex the knee. They also produce rotation of the knee, the biceps femoris producing lateral rotation and the semitendinosus and semimembranosus medial rotation. Injuries to the hamstrings are common across all sports that are running-based or impart explosive and/or repetitive forces to the lower limbs. As pain in the posterior thigh can, and often does, arise from sources other than the hamstrings, it is vital that all presentations of 'hamstring' pain are subjected to a comprehensive examination which should include the vertebral column, hips, sacroiliac joints and sciatic nerve. These structures may be the cause of the symptoms, may contribute to them, or may be affected as a consequence of a primary hamstring problem.

Signs and symptoms The onset of symptoms may be gradual or sudden. When the athlete presents with posterior thigh pain that came on gradually and was not linked to a specific injuring episode, suspicion should fall upon remote structures, particularly the vertebral column, or on local/remote structures such as the sciatic nerve as being causative. Symptoms of gradual onset can of course be caused by a local hamstring problem but there must be a reason for this, such as an overload of training/playing or some unaccustomed or unusually prolonged activity that has overloaded the hamstrings, such as bouts of hill running or plyometric training. There may be a predisposing factor to such an overload, e.g. neural pathodynamics.

Acute injuries are always linked to a specific episode of trauma. This is usually one that imparts high forces to the muscle, such as sprinting, or driving bodyweight off forcefully through the lower limb. Pain is experienced suddenly and is associated with immediate weightbearing disability. In the case of all but the most minor strains, the athlete is unable to continue sporting participation and the usual signs of soft-tissue trauma (swelling, tenderness, heat and bruising) will be evident either immediately or within a few hours. In the case of deep-seated tears, it may take a number of days for bruising to become evident. In the first few days following the injury any activity that stretches the hamstrings or makes them contract will be painful. As the inflammatory response subsides, so does the pain. The length of time that this takes depends upon the extent of the injury but it invariably takes several days. In contrast, episodes of hamstring pain secondary to sciatic nerve pathodynamics very often improve relatively quickly, with pain responses to stretch and contraction abating or even disappearing within a few days. In such circumstances, the main cause of pain is probably protective local hamstring spasm in the absence of muscle/connective tissue disruption. Presentations of this type of hamstring 'strain' are very similar to those of a true muscle fibre disruption, with the exception that there is no swelling or bruising.

Examination Where muscle and connective tissue have been disrupted, there will be an area of acute local soreness and possibly of swelling. Protective muscle spasm may be evident and a static or manually resisted hamstring contraction usually provokes pain. Static tests are best performed from the lying position, prone lying giving the advantage of being able to visualize the muscle bulk. This may reveal a defect in the muscle at the site of the tear, which is not evident when the muscle is relaxed. Testing the extensibility of the hamstrings should be done using a straight leg raise (SLR) manoeuvre. In the case of acute injury, the limit of this passive movement would be pain onset. The standard SLR test can then be modified in a number of ways, so that the emphasis of tension is placed on different structures. This may help to differentiate between neural and musculotendinous tissues as the cause of the pain. For example, hamstring pain that is experienced at a position of, say, $50°$, which is then increased in severity by dorsiflexing the foot of the same limb (while holding the $50°$ SLR position) could indicate a neural pathodynamic component to the pain. Other neural tissue 'sensitizing' movements, which could be added to or subtracted from the base SLR test to differentiate between muscle and neural structures, include hip adduction and/or medial rotation. Another example of changing the basic SLR test for the purposes of differentiation is to compare the pain onset/range response of the base SLR test with that produced when the SLR is performed with the pelvis anteriorly tilted (perhaps with a rolled towel beneath the lumbosacral area). This anteriorly tilted position of the pelvis prestretches the hamstrings by proximally moving their ischial attachment and it also reduces the tension on the sciatic nerve. An increased pain response or a decrease in the range of SLR before the onset of pain, compared to that obtained in the basic SLR test, would implicate muscle pathology ahead of neural pathodynamics.

Another test that can be used to differentiate between muscle and nerve tissue as the cause of pain in these cases is the slump test (section 4.3.4(b)). Its inclusion in the examination of all 'hamstring' pain should be mandatory as it frequently gives positive results in cases of 'hamstring tears' (Butler, 1991).

Treatment   The treatment of acute soft-tissue injuries has been outlined previously and so, in this section, the restoration of muscular strength and extensibility, which are the two key elements of hamstring rehabilitation, will be considered. In practice it is usually possible to institute treatment, exercise and manual therapy, in order to affect both strength and stretch, simultaneously. However, it is probably most effective to stress the mobilizing work initially and, depending upon the extent of the trauma, this may be commenced at the third or fourth day following the injury. This is best done passively, the stretch being gently applied by a therapist in such a way as to avoid the provocation of pain or spasm. Some form of SLR stretch may be used to do this. It may also be effective to stretch the hamstrings by performing knee extension, which is performed with the hip flexed at right angles. Increased hamstring tension may be gained by tilting the pelvis anteriorly. The use of such pelvic positioning has been shown to increase the efficacy of hamstring stretching programmes (Sullivan *et al*, 1992). Sustained stretches can be applied in these positions and PNF techniques can also be used. Stretching the hamstrings in weightbearing positions (e.g. variations on the toe-touching manoeuvre) utilize upper body weight to achieve the stretch, and these should be avoided in the early stages, as they are not as sensitive to pain or resistance as the previously described stretching manoeuvres and can result in further injury. In cases where there is no obvious nerve involvement it is still preferable to include some nerve mobilizing procedures to ensure that the sciatic nerve/ muscle interface is not compromised by

bleeding and/or scar tissue, which may arise as a consequence of the injury (Kornberg and Lew, 1989).

As pain reduces and extensibility of the hamstrings increases, the initial static muscle exercises can be augmented by through-range exercises. Initially these can be performed across one joint at a time, e.g. resisted hip extension or knee flexion so as not to impart too high a force on the healing tissues. At this stage the weight of the limb may be sufficient resistance, or light elastic bandage resistance may be used. It is important that none of the active exercises provoke pain, as this will inhibit normal muscle function and be counterproductive in bringing about strength gains. Combined hip extension and knee flexion would then be a logical progression and again could use elastic bandage resistance or part-bodyweight resistance, as in the lifting of bodyweight from the supine position (Figure 6.6).

Once the athlete is able to perform slow, pain-free concentric knee flexion combined with hip extension and then return the limb to the starting position by painlessly controlling (eccentrically) the lengthening hamstrings, speed can be increased. This will place greater loads on the muscle and is

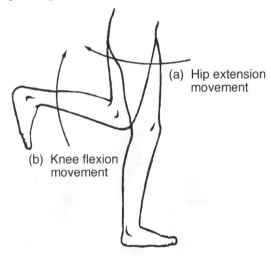

(a) Hip extension movement

(b) Knee flexion movement

Figure 6.6   Combined hip extension and knee flexion.

sport-specific for many running-based activities. It was mentioned previously that the hamstrings are exposed to high forces when the athlete runs at speed. During late swing phase (i.e. as they decelerate the lower limb), these have been measured to be in the region of 250 Nm at the hip and 150 Nm at the knee. At early stance phase (i.e. as concentric–eccentric coupling occurs) these forces increase to 300 Nm at the hip and to 160 Nm at the knee (Moffroid and Whipple, 1972). The exercises used in the latter stages of hamstring rehabilitation need therefore to replicate these forces and as training effects are very specific to joint angle and limb velocity (Sale and MacDougal, 1981; Worrell and Perrin, 1992), the mechanics of high-speed running (see above) must be taken into account when formulating appropriate strengthening exercises.

The very simple, yet highly effective prone lying 'catch' exercises devised by Stanton and Purdam (1989) for this purpose are recommended. These can be performed in the more functional standing position but were originally described in the prone position. In order to replicate the position of hip flexion, as occurs at the end of the swing phase of sprinting, the athlete lies over the edge of a treatment couch, supporting the upper body on the forearms. This position prestretches the hamstrings at the hip. A pillow is placed beneath the foot of the limb to be exercised so as to prevent the terminal 20–30° of knee extension. The subject then performs repeated knee flexion and extension. This latter movement involves eccentric hamstring work, which terminates at a 'catch' some 20–30° from full knee extension, at which point the hamstrings work concentrically to flex the knee. Progression is made by increasing the speed of the 'catches' and by the addition of ankle weights (up to a maximum of 5 kg). These exercises have been shown to replicate the previously encountered hip and knee forces to which the hamstrings are subjected during high-speed running. Before the athlete returns to sprinting, it is vital that such exercises are practised, progressed and mastered so that sufficient strength (in both the contractile and non-contractile muscle tissues) is restored and adequate neuromotor control is re-established.

(b) Rectus femoris

This muscle, which is the most anteriorly placed component of the quadriceps, has its proximal attachment at the anterior inferior iliac spine (the 'straight' head), with a 'reflected' head just below at a point just above the acetabulum (Figure 6.7). Distally, it inserts into the quadriceps tendon.

Rectus femoris, therefore, has a flexing action at the hip as well as contributing to the movement of extension at the knee. Rectus femoris has a high proportion of fast twitch muscle fibres (type II) and is suited to the production of high-speed movement (Richardson, 1992). In contrast, iliopsoas (which acts with rectus femoris to flex the hip) and vastus medialis (which acts with rectus femoris to extend the knee) have properties associated with slow twitch muscle fibres (type I) (Richardson, 1992). This includes the ability of the muscle to control low forces over long periods of time. If, therefore, fast hip flexion

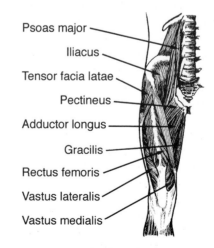

Figure 6.7 The quadriceps muscles.

or fast knee extension movements are performed, as is the case during many different running and kicking sports, rectus femoris will be preferentially recruited ahead of the iliopsoas and vastus medialis muscles. This fact may go some way to explain why rectus femoris injuries are associated with speed and power activities such as sprinting and kicking.

Signs and symptoms   With acute injuries, there will be localized tenderness and possibly swelling, bruising and a palpable gap. Any contraction or stretching of the muscle produces pain and initially, following injury, this may be provoked simply by walking, as the affected hip is flexed to swing the non-weightbearing lower limb forwards and again as the affected limb is extended at the hip during 'push-off'. Less irritable symptoms, as frequently occur in many chronic conditions, may only be provoked with quicker movements such as running at speed, when the pain is usually experienced as the knee of the affected side is flexed quickly. Forceful movements such as kicking are also usually pain-provoking.

Examination   Static testing of the muscle should include isometric testing of rectus femoris as a hip flexor and as a knee extensor. Stretching the muscle by performing combined knee flexion and hip extension usually demonstrates a restriction, by stiffness and pain. It is often useful to perform this stretch in two ways. The first is by applying the hip component before the knee component and the second a reverse of this process. Each method may reproduce subtly different stretch and pain responses, as may the addition of rotation at the hip. The response most comparable to the patient's symptoms would be used in treatment. Adopting different testing positions to evaluate the muscle's contractile ability is also useful as this can influence the site and degree of symptom response. For example, a test of knee extension with

the hip flexed, as occurs in the sitting position, may give a different pain/range response than if resisted knee extension is performed with the hip extended, e.g. with the patient lying supine with the knees flexed over the end of the treatment bench. The position which most closely replicates the patient's symptoms presumably stresses the muscle/tendon in the damaged area and could be used as a position in which to perform strengthening exercises.

Treatment   Active exercise and passive stretching should commence after the initial inflammatory response has subsided. The specific stretches used should be those that most closely replicate the patient's symptoms as these will presumably stress the muscle/tendon in the appropriate region. For the same reason, the actual exercises used to strengthen the muscle should be progressed (as the severity of the pain response diminishes) to include those movements and positions that similarly reproduce relevant signs and symptoms. Initially the usual progression from pain-free isometric exercise through to the various types of isotonic muscle work should be made. Due to the high force production that occurs in rectus femoris during high-speed movements, it is important to progress the speed of the strengthening exercises to those relevant to the sport in question.

(c) Gastrocnemius

This muscle has two heads, the medial and lateral heads, which are attached proximally to the medial and lateral femoral condyles respectively. Distally they unite and insert with the soleus into the Achilles tendon (Figure 6.8).

The gastrocnemius works hard in all activities where bodyweight needs to be propelled quickly, both in vertical and in horizontal directions. When running it contributes to the forwards propulsive effort by generating ankle plantarflexion, and at foot-strike it

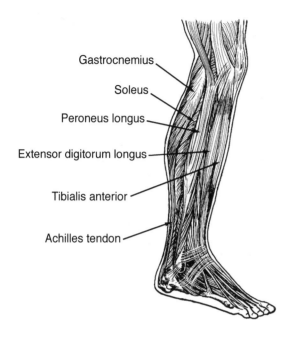

Gastrocnemius

Soleus

Peroneus longus

Extensor digitorum longus

Tibialis anterior

Achilles tendon

Figure 6.8   The muscles of the lower leg.

helps prevent excessive ankle dorsiflexion. Acute injuries are often experienced when running or jumping and are frequently sustained when suddenly changing direction, e.g. from travelling backwards to pushing off vigorously in a forwards direction. They most commonly involve the musculotendinous junction of the medial head and middle-aged athletes are frequently affected (Corrigan and Maitland, 1994). One explanation for this could be the histological and biochemical changes that have been documented in the gastrocnemius muscle, which seem to be linked with the ageing process (Coggan, 1992). These changes consist of a reduction in the proportion of type II muscle fibres and in the muscle's capillary density. It should be noted that this study dealt with sedentary individuals. Whether physical training can halt or slow down these changes has not been investigated.

Signs and symptoms   As with hamstring problems, any onset of calf pain that is gradual and accounted for by a relatively insig-

nificant episode of trauma or amount of exercise should be viewed with suspicion as far as muscular pathology is concerned. In such cases, a careful examination of the vertebral and nerve structures must be performed. Acute muscle injury invariably affects the medial head of the gastrocnemius and the superficial position of the muscle makes it easy to ascertain the amount and degree of swelling and bruising, which are often quite marked, even in mild to moderate tears. Walking is usually severely affected, because of the painful limitation of dorsiflexion due to protective spasm of the calf.

Treatment   Following the treatment and gentle early exercise in the acute phase, efforts should be made to restore full stretch to the muscle. This can be achieved by passively mobilizing the ankle into dorsiflexion while maintaining full knee extension. It is also beneficial to mobilize the tibial nerve by using SLR and slump mobilizing positions to ensure that its mobility is not compromised by traumatic exudate and subsequent scar tissue formation.

Once the extensibility of the muscle has been regained, so that a weightbearing plantargrade position of the foot can be achieved, efforts should be made to regain a normal gait pattern. This is an important functional activity to re-establish and, once mastered, can be progressed to 'power walking'. This is simply a walking gait with an exaggerated emphasis on stride length and push-off. Power walking places a functional strengthening load upon the gastrocnemius and should be mastered as a precursor to the commencement of running. A wide variety of weightbearing exercises can be used to strengthen the calf musculature. Most of these are variations on the 'toe-raise' manoeuvre. The most demanding of these, as far as the gastrocnemius is concerned, involves the shifting of bodyweight from a position of full stretch to a position of maximum contraction while maintaining full knee extension.

However this type of exercise is not functional in terms of lower limb push-off activities as it does not incorporate combined active knee extension. The coupling of ankle plantarflexion and knee extension does not specifically target the gastrocnemius, but it is functional as regards the stance/push-off phase of running and as such should be practised before strenuous running is introduced. As many sports require explosive lower limb push-off ability, it is often necessary to incorporate hopping and bounding activities into the final stages of the rehabilitation programme.

6.5 THE KNEE COMPLEX

6.5.1 Introduction

Injuries to the knee are common occurrences across many different sports (Albert, 1983; Howe and Johnson, 1982; Marans *et al.*, 1988) and probably account for the majority of all sporting injuries. They can also be the most profound in terms of subsequent disability, whether they are of traumatic origin or caused by overuse. This susceptibility of the knee to injury should not be surprising, however, given its central role in the function of most sports and the fact that at times it is subjected to extreme loading and also to repetitive loading. The anatomy of the knee complex will be covered briefly and then some of the more commonly encountered traumatic and overuse injuries will be discussed.

6.5.2 Anatomy

The knee complex can be divided into the patellofemoral and the tibiofemoral articulations (Figure 6.9). The tibiofemoral articulation can be further divided into medial and lateral compartments.

(a) The tibiofemoral joint

The tibiofemoral joint (TFJ) is formed by the medial and lateral femoral condyles, which are convex from front to back and from side to side. They are of unequal size, the medial condyle being longer anteroposteriorly and more curved than the lateral femoral condyle. These condyles articulate, via the medial and lateral menisci, with the medial and lateral tibial condyles. The medial tibial articular surface is reciprocally shaped to the medial femoral condyle while the lateral tibial condyle is concave from side to side but is convex from front to back. The bony configuration of the tibiofemoral joint permits a complex combination of joint surface sliding, gliding and rolling movements to occur during the apparently simple activity of knee flexion,

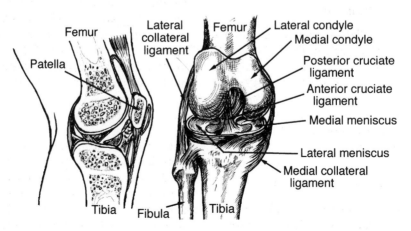

Figure 6.9 The knee joint.

extension and rotation. These accessory joint movements are controlled in direction and range by the capsular and ligamentous structures of the joint. The four main ligaments of the joint are the medially placed tibial collateral ligament, the laterally placed fibular collateral ligament and the centrally located posterior and anterior cruciate ligaments.

(b) The patellofemoral joint

The patellofemoral joint (PFJ) is formed by the articulation of the femoral trochlea, which has lateral and medial articulating surfaces, and the posterior aspect of the patella, which has corresponding articular facets. The medial patella facet can be subdivided to include a medially placed 'odd facet'. This portion of the patella only comes into direct contact with the femur in positions of extreme flexion. The patella serves to increase the mechanical advantage of the quadriceps by up to 50% (Ficat and Hungerford, 1977) and the PFJ transmits and dissipates forces acting through the knee. These forces can amount to over three times bodyweight during stair-climbing (Ficat and Hungerford, 1977) and considerably more when higher-speed sporting activities are performed.

(c) The collateral ligaments

The passive stabilizing structures of the medial and lateral aspects of the tibiofemoral joint are composed of structurally and functionally inter-related capsular and ligamentous tissues. The collateral ligaments are individual components of these capsulo-ligament complexes and should not therefore be described in isolation.

(d) Medial capsulo-ligament complex

The medial aspect of the tibiofemoral joint can be divided into anterior, middle and posterior thirds, with the joint capsule covering all

three. In the anterior portion the capsule is relatively loose and in the middle third it is reinforced by the tibial collateral ligament. This has superficial and deep components. The superficial fibres pass between the medial femoral and tibial condyles, while the deeper fibres attach the tibial and femoral condyles to the outer surface of the medial meniscus. The posterior third of the medial capsulo-ligament complex (MCLC) is composed of the posterior oblique ligament (an expansion of the superficial portion of the tibial collateral ligament), the posteromedial capsule and expansions from the semimembranosus. This portion of the joint is dynamically stabilized by the adjacent pes anserinus tendon.

(e) Lateral capsulo-ligament complex

The lateral capsulo-ligament complex (LCLC) of the knee joint can also be divided into anterior, middle and posterior thirds. The joint capsule covers all three areas and in the anterior third is reinforced by the patellar retinaculum and by expansions from the quadriceps tendon. In the middle third the capsule is supported by the iliotibial band and in the posterior third it is supported by the fibular collateral ligament (FCL) and the arcuate ligament (AL). Both of these attach distally to the fibular head, with the FCL attaching proximally to the lateral epicondyle of the femur and the AL attaching into the posterolateral part of the femoral condyle. The posterolateral corner of the tibiofemoral joint also receives dynamic support from the tendons of biceps femoris and popliteus.

(f) Posterior capsule

The posterior joint capsule is reinforced in the posterolateral corner by the previously mentioned, Y-shaped arcuate ligament and more centrally and medially by the oblique popliteal ligament (a thickening of the posterior capsule into which the semimembranosus attaches). The popliteus muscle has connections with the arcuate ligament, the lateral meniscus and the posterior capsule and supports the posterior aspect of the joint, particularly in positions of flexion. Dynamic support of the posteromedial corner of the joint is provided by semimembranosus and the medial head of gastrocnemius, while the lateral head of gastrocnemius and biceps femoris dynamically stabilize the posterolateral corner.

(g) Anterior cruciate ligament

The anterior cruciate ligament (ACL) has a central position in the knee, passing from the anterior tibial intercondylar region upwards, laterally and posteriorly to attach to the medial aspect of the lateral femoral condyle. It has a spiral arrangement of its fibres which ensures that it is tensioned through varying degrees of knee flexion. It is most taut at terminal extension and contributes to the passive resistance of hyperextension. It also resists excessive anterior tibial translation and internal rotation. The ACL is therefore multifunctional in its role as a passive stabilizer of the knee, but it plays an equally important role in maintaining joint stability by relaying proprioceptive information to the central nervous system. The ACL is richly innervated, neural tissue accounting for up to 2.5% of its total volume (Schutte *et al.*, 1987). In addition to nocioceptive sensory endings, the ACL has mechanoreceptors which, via reflex pathways, affect the motor control and therefore the stability of the knee (Kennedy, Alexander and Hayes, 1982; Schultz *et al.*, 1984).

(h) Posterior cruciate ligament

The posterior cruciate ligament (PCL) has its distal attachment on the posterior portion of the tibial intercondylar region and from here it passes upwards, anteriorly and medially to its femoral attachment on the laterally facing portion of the medial femoral condyle. The PCL is thicker and stronger than the ACL

and restrains the tibia from being displaced posteriorly. It also contributes, with the ACL, to controlling the complex tibiofemoral joint surface movements of rolling, sliding and gliding that occur when the joint flexes and extends.

6.5.3 Traumatic injuries

Episodes of sporting trauma can affect many structures of the knee complex. However, this discussion will focus on ligament injuries as these are probably the most commonly encountered and often prove particularly debilitating. Many of the principles of treatment that will be described are transferable to other knee injuries.

For the sake of clarity, injury to individual ligaments will be described. However, in practice, combined ligament injuries are commonly encountered and may result in combinations of the clinical instabilities. It is important to have an appreciation of the complex interaction that takes place between all the knee joint's stabilizing structures. Under normal circumstances the forces the knee complex is subjected to are absorbed and dissipated by an inter-related system of active and passive stabilizers. The active knee stabilizers are the lower limb muscles, which act directly and indirectly upon the knee joint, while the passive stabilizing system consists of the articulating bony surfaces, menisci, capsular and ligamentous structures. Efficient knee function is dependent upon an intimate, dynamic relationship between these two systems. For example, during vigorous sporting activities, the knee's ligaments and capsular structures are frequently subjected to levels of force that exceed potential injury levels (Kuo, Louie and Mote, 1983). These potentially injurious forces are resisted only in part by the mechanical properties of the ligaments. Muscular activity is responsible for the majority of knee joint stability (Johansson, Stolander and Sojka, 1991). However, this muscular activity can only be effective if there is an efficient control system that can initiate appropriate and well-timed muscular contractions, i.e. before the passive stabilizers are overloaded. This system is based on 'ligamentomuscular reflexes', which come into play when sufficient tension is applied to the passive stabilizers. Sensory nerve endings within the knee ligaments are sensitive to tension and their stimulation has a powerful effect upon the muscles acting on and around the knee joint (Johansson, Stolander and Sojka, 1991). Normal knee function is therefore dependent upon an overlap of function between individual passive stabilizers and an intimate interaction between these passive stabilizers and the active stabilizers. An appreciation of this fact is important when evaluating specific injuries and when formulating treatment and rehabilitation programmes.

(a) Knee instability

The term 'instability' refers to the frequently encountered clinical finding of excessive joint movement (either accessory, physiological or combinations of the two), evident on examination and usually relates to an episode of trauma. The presence of instability does not necessarily mean that the joint in question will be functionally impaired. It is a frequent finding among even elite sporting competitors for full asymptomatic knee function to be possible in the presence of marked clinical instability (Gauffin *et al.*, 1990). The opposite scenario may also be encountered – a sportsperson who experiences functionally restricting episodes of knee instability but exhibits little or no clinical instability.

In order to avoid confusion, the term 'instability' should be defined as being either 'clinical instability' or 'functional instability'. The functionally unstable joint may give rise to numerous symptoms. The most dramatic are episodes of the knee giving way when loaded with bodyweight. The direction in which the knee gives way and the activities that precipitate such incidents depend upon the type and direction of instability that is present.

The classification of knee instabilities can be confusing. They are classified either in relation to the direction of movement of the instability in question, or to the location of the incompetent capsulo-ligamentous structures responsible for the excessive joint mobility. For example, 'anterior instability' refers to the direction of movement in a knee that exhibits excessive anterior tibial translation (due to ACL insufficiency), whereas 'medial instability' refers to the structurally incompetent MCLC structures that allow excessive valgus knee motion (i.e. tibial abduction).

Instability tests are sometimes referred to as stress tests. This title can give an inaccurate impression of how they should best be applied. By oscillating the test movement instead of applying it instantly, the examiner will obtain a better appreciation of the amount of movement present. In addition, combining an oscillatory test movement with a gradual summation of end-of-range pressure will facilitate the task of determining the type of end feel that is present. This assessment of 'end feel' is an important qualitative measurement. The functional prognosis for a joint exhibiting a range of instability that has a firm end feel may be better than for one with a poorly defined end point to the range of movement being tested.

Knee instabilities are classified as either straight, rotary or combined.

Straight instability

These occur in isolation or in combination. They are classified as medial, lateral, anterior and posterior. They are named in relation to the position of the capsulo-ligamentous structures that are functionally incompetent, i.e. in stabilizing the tibiofemoral joint.

Medial instability   Medial instability occurs when the MCLC fails to function in passively resisting gapping of the medial tibiofemoral joint line. The structural integrity of the MCLC is best tested with the knee in a position that reduces the tension of the cruciate ligaments, i.e. 10–20° from terminal extension. The thigh is then stabilized and the leg is abducted to impart a valgus force to the knee. The same test can then be carried out with the knee fully extended. Significant laxity in the semiflexed position indicates MCLC damage while significant laxity elicited in full extension indicates combined MCLC and cruciate damage.

Lateral instability   Lateral instability occurs when the LCLC fails to function in passively resisting gapping of the lateral tibiofemoral joint line. The test is similar to that previously described for testing the MCLC, except that a varus force (tibial adduction) is imparted to the knee. This test should also be performed with the knee in 10–20° of flexion (to test the integrity of the LCLC in isolation) and also in terminal extension (to test the LCLC in combination with the cruciates).

Anterior instability   Anterior instability is present when the anterior cruciate ligament fails to passively resist anterior tibial subluxation at the knee. The most sensitive test for this is Lachman's test, which involves supporting the knee in a few degrees of flexion, usually by supporting the distal femur with one hand, and then with the other hand displacing the upper tibia anteriorly in an attempt to sublux it at the tibiofemoral joint. This test will only be valid if the patient is completely relaxed, as even minimal tension in the hamstrings will prevent tibial subluxation. Although relatively simple, this test requires a high degree of joint handling skills if it is to be performed satisfactorily. Anterior instability can also be tested by performing an anterior drawer test. This is performed with the patient in supine lying, with the knee in a position just short of 90° flexion and the sole of the foot resting on the treatment couch. The lower leg is stabilized by the examiner partially sitting against the front of the resting foot. The upper tibia is then grasped and subluxed in an anterior direction. A comparison is made, if possible, with the non-affected side. This test must also be performed with the limb relaxed. This test is not as sensitive as Lachman's test and can be negative in the presence of a complete ACL tear because of the restraining effect upon the tibia of the collateral ligaments.

Posterior instability   Posterior instability can very often be detected by observation alone. The limb is placed in the same position as that described for the anterior drawer test and if this instability is present the upper tibia will be seen to sag posteriorly under the influence of gravity. This indicates injury to the PCL but it can only be ascertained if the limb is relaxed. Comparison with the non-affected side should be made and a reverse of the technique described for the anterior drawer test can be performed to ascertain the extent of the hypermobility and the end feel.

Care should be taken when interpreting the findings of the drawer tests. If the examiner does not realize that a posterior sag of the upper tibia is present (indicating a PCL lesion), then it might appear that there is excessive anterior tibial displacement. A diagnosis of ACL injury might then be made, when in fact all that has happened is that the test has reduced the tibiofemoral joint back to a neutral position.

Rotary instabilities

These can be classified as anteromedial, anterolateral, posteromedial and posterolateral. They are named in relation to the portion of the tibial condyle that maximally subluxes.

Anteromedial instability   Anteromedial instability is present when there is an abnormal amount of tibial lateral rotation. This can be tested for by modifying the anterior drawer test described for the testing of anterior instability. The basic anterior drawer test position is changed by placing the tibia in a position of lateral rotation. This pretensions the MCLC and the test is performed by attempting to anteriorly sublux the upper tibia and simultaneously draw the medial tibial condyle into further lateral rotation. This test may be positive in the presence of MCLC injuries. Combined cruciate and MCLC injury would give rise to more pronounced instability.

Anterolateral instability This movement involves the forward displacement of the anterior portion of the lateral tibial condyle with combined medial rotation and may be an indication of ACL insufficiency, as the ACL limits the degree of internal tibial rotation at the tibiofemoral joint. It can be tested for by performing a modified anterior drawer test (the modification being the pretensioning of the tibiofemoral joint into some medial rotation) or by modifying Lachman's test. This involves performing Lachman's test as previously described but with pressure applied in such a way as to draw the anterior tibial condyle into internal rotation as well as forwards.

Anterolateral instability may also be elicited by the lateral pivot shift test. There are a number of variations in the way that this test is applied. Perhaps the least traumatic for the joint is the method that commences with the knee in an extended position with the examiner supporting the lower limb just clear of the examination couch beneath the heel. The entire lower limb is held in some degree of internal rotation and the examiner's other hand places a firm but gentle pressure against the lateral aspect of the tibiofemoral joint. This places a valgus force on the joint, which is maintained as the knee is flexed. The test is positive if, at approximately 30° of flexion, the lateral tibial condyle is felt to 'jerk' anteriorly. Continued flexion of the knee will then almost immediately reduce the tibial

condyle. This test involves rotary tibiofemoral joint subluxation and, if it is performed with too much force, it is conceivable that joint trauma could result. The maxim of 'don't hurt the patient' when examining should be followed. The degree of anterolateral instability may be magnified if the LCLC is damaged as well as the ACL.

Posteromedial instability Posteromedial instability is most noticeable when combined PCL and MCLC injuries exist. The method of identifying this instability is similar to that for determining posterior instability. It would be suspected if, in the drawer test position, the upper tibia was seen to sublux posteriorly and the posterior portion of the medial tibial condyle fell backwards into some medial rotation. The handling procedure is similar to that described for the posterior instability test but attempts would be made to correct the rotational subluxation of the posterior medial tibial condyle. The tibia would then be repeatedly moved from the subluxed position to the reduced position in order to assess the degree of instability and the end feel of the movement.

Posterolateral instability Posterolateral instability is indicative of a failure of the capsule and ligaments at the posterolateral corner of the tibiofemoral joint, particularly the arcuate ligament complex. It involves the subluxation of the posterior tibial condyle into a posterior and laterally rotated direction. It can be detected by observing the knee in the drawer position in a similar way to that described for the detection of posteromedial instability. It may also be demonstrated by performing the 'big toe test'. This involves lifting the weight of the relaxed lower limb by the toes while observing and feeling for a change in the resting posture of the knee. The test is positive if the tibiofemoral joint is seen to fall into a slight varus position (tibial adduction) and to simultaneously hyperextend and laterally rotate. These postural changes may be discrete and the test requires a high degree of expertise. A simpler way of eliciting this direction of instability is to perform a combined posterior glide and lateral rotation of the tibial condyles with the patient in prone lying and the knee in 20–30° of flexion. The hand positions for this manoeuvre are similar to those for Lachman's test.

Causes of knee instability

Overuse may be a factor in the development of clinical and functional instability. However, most cases are directly due to episodes of trauma. Such injuries are common across many sports, especially those with elements of body contact. Forceful movements that tension the passive stabilizing structures of the knee can result in ligament and capsular stretching or rupture. These injuring movements may be caused by an opponent, as in a tackle, or may be the result of sudden deceleration or acceleration manoeuvres, which generate high joint forces. Certain types and degrees of instability may give rise to episodes of the knee collapsing. Pain during and following exercise is also a common complaint, together with swelling. These signs and symptoms are probably due to joint irritation resulting from the overload placed on the remaining passive stabilizers.

Following many cases of moderate to severe ligament injury, it is common to find combinations of the instabilities described previously when the knee is clinically tested.

(b) Medial capsulo-ligament complex injury

Mechanisms of injury Forceful valgus and/or rotational forces (especially lateral tibial rotation) to the knee, can result in rupture of the MCLC. The MCLC is relatively lax in positions of knee flexion, and this explains the reason why most injuries to it occur with the knee semiflexed. Injuring forces may be sustained when the knee is non-weightbearing, as in a block tackle in soccer, or when the foot is fixed to the ground, as occurs when twisting and turning. Another common mechanism of injury occurs in contact sports, when a medially directed force is applied to the lateral aspect of the knee, as frequently occurs during soccer and rugby tackles. The fact that the deep fibres of the tibial collateral ligament are connected to the medial meniscus has been used to explain the high incidence of associated injury between the medial meniscus and MCLC structures.

Signs and symptoms Pain localized to the medial aspect of the knee is usually the main complaint. The degree of pain and associated disability is of course proportional to the degree of injury that has been sustained. Localized medial knee swelling and tenderness may be evident and in cases of second degree sprains there may be an associated synovial effusion. Running activities, particularly those involving rapid cutting manoeuvres or speed sessions, may be pain-provoking. Kicking with the instep is also often pain-provoking, as is block tackling in soccer.

Examination Careful observation and palpation will determine the amount and exact location of swelling and tenderness. Relatively small amounts of joint cavity swelling caused by bleeding and/or synovial effusion may be detected by performing a patellar tap test or a stroke test. The former involves compressing the suprapatellar pouch to disperse any fluid into the centre of the joint. This fluid pushes the patellofemoral joint surfaces apart. The suprapatellar pressure is maintained and the test is positive if rhythmical, posteriorly directed pressure applied to the patella causes it to 'tap' against the femoral condyles. The 'stroke test' is performed by first applying posteriorly applied pressure to the patellofemoral joint and to the adjacent medial and lateral portions of the knee. This displaces any fluid within the joint superiorly. The lateral or medial aspect of the knee is then firmly 'stroked' with the hand in a proximal to distal direction and any fluid within the joint will be dissipated away from the examiner's hand and be seen to make the opposite patellar gutter area bulge. Injury to the tendon of pes anserinus is commonly encountered in tandem with MCLC injury.

Any joint positions that place the MCLC under tension will provoke pain in cases of partial rupture and can be used to determine the extent of instability. These joint positions are extension, lateral tibial rotation and tibial abduction (valgus knee motion). Testing the MCLC with such tension tests is done to elicit pain responses and to determine the presence and extent of any instability. Relatively little pain associated with gross amounts of medial tibiofemoral compartment gapping and a soft end feel are indicative of marked grade two sprains or of complete rupture (grade three). Following such injuries, there may be little or no swelling. This can occur if the complete MCLC rupture provides a route for the traumatic exudate to escape from the joint cavity.

Treatment   Minor MCLC sprains are treated along the lines of any other soft-tissue injury. Conservative or surgical methods of treatment may be undertaken following avulsion injuries or for extensive ruptures. It is common for complete MCLC ruptures to occur in combination with anterior cruciate ligament damage. This associated cruciate ligament injury may be the dictating factor when deciding between operative or conservative treatment. Whichever type of management is employed, it will be necessary to protect the MCLC for a period of time while it heals. Complete immobilization of the knee has the disadvantages of postimmobilization joint stiffness and of reducing the tensile strength of the healing ligament (Burroughs and Dahners, 1990; Gomez and Woo, 1989). The use of some form of functional bracing, which permits knee flexion and extension but which prevents undue strain being placed upon the MCLC (valgus and lateral rotational

forces), minimizes postimmobilization joint stiffness and allows the healing ligament to be subjected to controlled amounts of stress, which will stimulate the healing process. Following the protection phase, knee mobility, strength and coordination must be restored. Before vigorous sporting activity is commenced it will be necessary to regain full extensibility of the MCLC. In this respect, regaining the movements of full pain-free tibiofemoral extension and lateral tibial rotation are particularly important. Regaining full pain-free passive knee abduction is also important before any kicking activities are resumed. Strengthening the thigh musculature is also often necessary so that strength deficits that have resulted from inactivity are made good. It may also be beneficial to specifically strengthen the muscles that share the pes anserinus tendon (sartorius, gracilis and semitendinosus), as this provides dynamic support to the medial aspect of the joint.

(c) Lateral capsulo-ligament complex injury

Mechanisms of injury   Damage to the lateral structures usually follows exposure of the knee to a varus force (tibial adduction). Associated injury to the iliotibial band and to the biceps femoris is commonly encountered (DeLee, Riley and Rockwood, 1983; Grana and Janssen, 1987) and although the incidence of LCLC injury is less than that for injury to the medial side of the knee, the resulting disability is often greater (Grana and Janssen, 1987).

Signs and symptoms   Laterally located tibiofemoral tenderness and swelling are similar to the findings described for MCLC injuries.

Treatment   This is along the same lines as described for MCLC injuries. Specific strengthening for the dynamic stabilizers of the lateral aspect of the knee (the iliotibial

and the biceps femoris) may also be
l.

(d) Anterior cruciate ligament injury

The ACL passively stabilizes the knee in multiple directions and provides proprioceptive information to the central nervous system that is vital to normal knee function. It is clear, therefore, that injury to such a key structure may result in profound disability.

Mechanism of injury Any knee movement or combinations of movement, if taken to forceful extremes, may cause ACL injury. The more usually encountered injury movements are probably twisting and valgus movements.

Signs and symptoms The overwhelming majority of knee haemarthroses indicate the presence of an ACL tear. A haemarthrosis can be identified by the occurrence of knee swelling, either immediately after or within a few hours of an episode of trauma. The sportsperson may also recount a feeling of the knee momentarily 'separating' or of 'one bone moving on the other'. Severe pain may be experienced at the instant of the injury but this often passes quickly. Immediately following the injury, the athlete is usually unable to continue sport due to weightbearing disability or may be able to walk and to jog in a straight line but experience functional instability when attempting to turn.

Examination Swelling and muscle spasm may make an immediate postinjury diagnosis difficult or impossible. However, it may be possible to perform Lachman's test, which, in the hands of a skilled practitioner, can elicit small amounts of anterior and anterolateral instability. To perform more vigorous tests such as the lateral pivot shift test at an early acute stage is inappropriate because of the potential for further damage (ligamentous or meniscal) to the joint. Associated injury to other knee structures is common with ACL injuries and signs such as restricted terminal extension and joint line tenderness may be present which could indicate collateral ligament and meniscal damage. Presentations of chronic ACL deficiency are usually associated with wasting of the quadriceps, especially vastus medialis, and this may be present despite attempts by the athlete to 'build the muscles up'. One of the key features of the examination process to determine the presence of ACL insufficiency should be careful questioning of the patient as regards their own feelings of security and confidence in the affected knee. Persistent and recurrent feelings of insecurity regarding the ability of the knee to support, control and propel bodyweight is probably the most important indicator of ACL deficiency. Although such information is purely subjective, it should raise a high degree of suspicion about the functional integrity of the ACL.

Treatment The type of management implemented for injuries to the ACL depends upon the degree of injury that has been sustained (both directly to the ACL and to other joint structures) and the resultant disability. It has been previously mentioned that the presence of clinical instability does not necessarily mean that the athlete will have a functionally unstable knee. This can pose a difficult dilemma when making the decision between surgical and conservative management. The proponents of surgical management, in the form of reconstructive surgery, point to the fact that sports-active competitors who are ACL-deficient succumb to progressive joint deterioration (Hawkins, 1987; Kannus and Jarvinen, 1987) and that reconstruction will preserve joint structures such as the articular surfaces and menisci (Feagin et al., 1995). This discussion will focus on the key issues of rehabilitation following ACL reconstruction. It should be possible to extrapolate this information to help formulate a conservative approach to ACL-deficient knee management.

ACL reconstruction may be performed in numerous ways (both intra- and extra-articularly) and may involve the use of different graft materials. These factors need to be taken into consideration when formulating specific features of the rehabilitation programme. For example, the use of a bone–patella–bone autograft involves surgical trauma to the patella/extensor apparatus of the knee. Appropriate patellofemoral mobilizing and strengthening work would therefore be indicated to prevent the development of patellofemoral pain syndrome and episodes of tendinitis. If a semitendinosus autograft was used to reconstruct the ACL, then the hamstrings would need specific attention to regain and/or maintain their flexibility and strength.

Whatever method is chosen to perform the reconstruction, the key aim should be to regain full knee extension as soon as possible, preferably within the first two postoperative weeks. Without full (full with manual over-pressure) pain-free extension the knee will not have optimal strength nor weightbearing function. Passive extension mobilizations are therefore a vital part of the early rehabilitation protocol and their early, safe application is made possible by accurate graft placement and sound surgical fixation. This approach has been termed 'accelerated rehabilitation' (Shelbourne and Nitz, 1990) and also involves the application of unrestricted knee motion from the first postoperative week. A failure to achieve full knee extension may be due to fibrosis of the ACL graft, which causes impingement in the femoral intercondylar notch. The restricted range of terminal extension may be accompanied by crepitus and clicking. This lesion is sometimes referred to as a 'Cyclops lesion' (due to its appearance on arthroscopy) and arthroscopic excision of the nodule yields good results (Marzo *et al.*, 1992; Fisher and Shelbourne, 1993).

In the early stages after reconstruction it is important that the graft is not unnecessarily tensioned and overstretched. Care is therefore necessary with the types of exercise that are given to restore thigh strength, as some forms of exercise, particularly for the quadriceps, have been shown to impart potentially damaging shear forces to the ACL graft site (Yack, Collins and Whieldon, 1993). These exercises involve resisted quadriceps work in non-weightbearing, where the leg is lifted, possibly against an external resistance (e.g. the seated knee extension manoeuvre). This type of exercise has been termed 'open kinetic chain exercise' and has been shown to cause anterior tibial translation at the knee, which could be potentially injurious to the ACL graft (Renstrom *et al.*, 1986; Yack, Collins and Whieldon, 1993). Open kinetic chain exercises should be avoided for this reason and also for the equally important reason that, for the majority of everyday activities and for most sporting activities, they are not functional. The functional weightbearing activities of semisquatting do not impose damaging forces on the ACL graft (Yack, Collins and Whieldon, 1993; Ohtoshi *et al.*, 1991) and, because they involve the control of bodyweight, they can be used both to improve knee strength and to re-educate proprioception. Open kinetic chain exercises for the hamstrings (e.g. prone lying hamstring curls) do not impose any potentially damaging shear forces on the newly reconstructed knee but they should not be used as the mainstay of the hamstring strengthening programme. This is because they are not functional and any strength gains achieved through their use would therefore probably not transfer to the functional and sport-specific activities to which the sportsperson is striving to return (Palmitier *et al.*, 1991). Exercises in which the hamstrings work across both the hip and the knee are more functional and should be practised. The role of the hamstrings as knee stabilizers should also be borne in mind when devising suitable conditioning exercises.

While strengthening the knee musculature is a key aim of the rehabilitation process, any gains in strength will be of minimal value if the knee's proprioceptive ability is diminished. The use of proprioceptive training has been shown to significantly enhance the functional outcome of patients recovering from ACL injury (Beard, 1994). Because the previously mentioned closed kinetic chain exercises involve weightbearing positions, they can have a beneficial effect upon joint position control. These activities should initially be performed slowly and in a controlled fashion and the athlete should be encouraged to compare their bodyweight control through the affected knee with the non-affected side. The use of trampettes and balance boards can be used to enhance proprioceptive ability.

Once adequate strength and weightbearing control have been regained, agility and coordination training should be emphasized. The types of activity appropriate for this stage of rehabilitation will depend upon the sport of the athlete in question. Field sport athletes would need to practise side-to-side, cutting manoeuvres and rotational running drills once they had mastered straight-line running. These types of sport-specific activity should initially be practised at submaximal speeds and be thoroughly mastered before being progressed. When the athlete's weightbearing activities are progressed it is frequently the case that slight restrictions in the range of terminal knee extension occur postexercise. In addition the athlete may also lose some of their ability to slowly control their bodyweight when stepping and semisquatting. It is therefore important for the therapist to educate the athlete to continually monitor these aspects of knee range and function so that any aberrations can be immediately identified and corrected.

Sport-specific training, like coordination training, is based upon the activities that the athlete's sport requires and is the final part of the rehabilitation programme. The therapist must analyse the key movements and activities that are required by the sport in question and, where they consist of complex movement patterns, they should be broken down into simpler subcomponents. These can than be practised by the athlete and then reconstituted. This process not only prepares the athlete physically by restoring the final degrees of strength, coordination and agility, but also prepares them mentally and helps to restore their confidence prior to a return to full competition. The timing of this return obviously depends upon the athlete's functional ability, but this is only one part of the equation that must be taken into account when advising on functional time scales. The other part is the biological time scale, which relates to the maturity of the ACL graft material and its point of fixation within the knee. It is currently impossible to accurately predict the exact time scales that operate for individual athletes in respect to ACL graft maturation (Fu, Woo and Irrgang, 1992). However, the success of the ACL reconstruction procedure should not be measured simply in terms of how quickly the athlete can return to his/her sport. More important factors to bear in mind are the level of sporting ability that is attainable and the length of time that the athlete is able to maintain this performance. A period of between 6 and 12 months following reconstructive surgery is probably required for the athlete to regain sufficient functional ability and graft maturity before a return to competitive sport is feasible.

(e) Posterior cruciate ligament injury

Injury to the PCL is probably not as common an occurrence as is injury to the ACL. However, the true extent of PCL injuries is difficult to quantify, as the PCL-deficient knee is invariably fully functional as regards sporting participation and consequently many episodes of knee injury that result in PCL injury may not come to light. While the PCL-deficient athlete may be able to continue to participate in sport, the onset of degenerative joint changes within 5 years of injury has been reported (Keller *et al.*, 1993).

Mechanism of injury Direct trauma to the upper anterior border of the tibial condylar area often results in PCL injury. Falls on to this area or impacts sustained in contact sports are frequently the cause of PCL rupture.

Signs and symptoms Pain inhibition rather than actual functional instability usually prevents the athlete from continuing sport immediately following the injury. Because of the intimate relationship of the PCL to the posterior capsule of the tibiofemoral joint, capsular damage is usually associated with PCL trauma. This may be evident by the appearance of popliteal swelling and deep bruising. There may also be an increased range of knee extension. In chronic cases of PCL insufficiency, the athlete may be able to actively demonstrate large excursions of tibial anteroposterior gliding, when sitting with the knee flexed to 90°. This is done by alternately tightening and relaxing the quadriceps, which draws the posteriorly subluxed tibia forwards and back beneath the femur.

Examination The tests for posterior instability have already been described. Care must be taken in interpreting the results of tests to determine the presence of anterior instability (Lachman's and anterior drawer tests) when the PCL-deficient knee is examined. Because the lack of the PCL's restraining action on the tibia results in the tibial condyles subluxing posteriorly when the athlete is positioned in supine lying, it may seem that there is excessive anterior tibial translation when the ACL's structural integrity is tested. However, where the ACL is undamaged, the anteriorly directed forces merely reduce the tibial condyles to a neutral position. Excessive hyperextension of the tibiofemoral joint is a common finding which in chronic cases is usually pain-free.

Management The broad aims of regaining lost ranges of knee movement, regaining muscular strength and control around the knee and the restoration of sport-specific agility and coordination are the same as for post-ACL-reconstruction rehabilitation. The means by which these are achieved, which have been outlined for the rehabilitation of the ACL-reconstructed knee, apply to the conservative management of PCL-deficient knees. As with the rehabilitation of any joint, it will not be possible to restore optimal strength and control in the PCL-deficient knee if there are ranges of pain and hypomobility. Following PCL rupture, restrictions of terminal knee flexion due to pain and associated stiffness are frequently encountered. This is probably due to associated posterior capsular trauma. In addition to limiting knee flexion, this may also cause popliteal pain when the hamstrings contract forcefully. Massage techniques and passive mobilizations should be used to restore adequate posterior capsular mobility and to regain limited ranges of knee flexion.

The problems of open kinetic chain exercises for the quadriceps, as regards potentially damaging anterior tibial shear forces, does not apply to rehabilitation of isolated PCL injuries. However, closed chain kinetic exercise should be the mainstay of the strengthening programme because of its inherently functional nature and the fact that it can be used to improve proprioception, unlike its open chain counterpart. The effect of open kinetic chain exercise for the hamstrings (e.g. prone-lying hamstring curl exercises) on the PCL-deficient knee is unclear. However it would seem that their application could induce excessive posterior tibial translation, which may place excessive and unnecessary strain on the posterior capsule of the knee and on other passive stabilizers such as the menisci. The use of closed kinetic chain hamstring exercises (i.e. where there is weightbearing pressure through the foot) would presumably overcome these potential problems.

6.5.4 Overuse conditions

The conditions which will be covered are patellofemoral pain syndrome, tendinitis/

bursitis (patellar tendinitis, biceps femoris tendinitis and pes anserinus bursitis) and pulling osteochondritis (Osgood–Schlatter's disease and Sinding-Larsen–Johansson disease). This list is not intended to be exhaustive but it includes some of the more commonly encountered problems that have an overuse factor in their aetiology. The principles of management that apply to these conditions can easily be applied to those conditions that are less commonly encountered and which are not covered in this text.

(a) Patellofemoral pain syndrome

The term patellofemoral pain syndrome (PFPS) has been chosen to describe the commonly encountered complaint of anterior knee pain, because it does not signify a particular pathological process. Other titles that are sometimes used to describe this commonly encountered complaint, e.g. chondromalacia patellae (CP), can give an oversimplified and possibly misleading impression of the underlying cause of the problem. Such names should only be used to classify known pathological changes as their presence does not necessarily have any bearing on the pain problem the athlete presents with. PFPS is a frequent complaint among sportspeople of all ages and levels of ability and is seen across many different sports.

PFPS can have a multifactorial pathology but this discussion will concentrate on what is probably the most common cause of PFPS – lateral patellar tracking (Shelton, 1991; Doucette and Goble, 1992; McConnell, 1987). A lateral deviation of the patella in relation to the femoral trochlea can result in excessive pressure being applied to the lateral portion of the patellofemoral joint (PFJ). This will lead to medial PFJ hypopressure and lateral PFJ hyperpressure. Pain is usually the result, although the exact mechanism of pain production is unclear. Because the amount of compression that is transmitted between the patella and femoral articular surfaces

increases in proportion to the amount of knee flexion, it is positions of weightbearing knee flexion that tend to provoke anterior knee pain in the athlete with PFPS. These forces can amount to approximately five times bodyweight when running and seven times bodyweight when squatting (McConnell, 1986; Ficat and Hungerford, 1977).

The alignment of the patella can be affected by bony anomalies affecting the articular surfaces of the patella and femur and by tightness of the passive stabilizers such as the lateral retinaculum and the iliotibial band, both of which attach to the lateral patella border. Lower limb malalignments may also result in excessive lateral PFJ deviation. These include femoral anteversion, genu valgum and excessive foot pronation. Imbalance between the functional strength of vastus lateralis and vastus medialis has also been identified as being contributory to lateral patellar maltracking (McConnell, 1987; Fulkerson and Shea, 1990; Hughston, 1968). Vastus lateralis has a laterally inclined as well as a proximally inclined line of pull on the patella. Vastus medialis (VM) also pulls the patella proximally, but it also exerts a medially directed pull on the patella and this movement is more specifically facilitated by the action of vastus medialis oblique (VMO). Theoretically, these opposing force vectors are resolved into a 'straight' proximal pull on the patella. Selective weakness/inhibition of either the medial or lateral portion of the quadriceps will result in the patella being subjected to an asymmetrical pulling force and patellar deviation toward the stronger side will result. Clinically, the overwhelming proportion of athletes who present with PFPS have observable and measurable (via electromyography) VM/VMO atrophy, weakness/inhibition. Whether such selective muscle anomalies occur as a consequence of PFPS or as a consequence of the previously mentioned soft-tissue contractures and limb malalignments, or whether they are in themselves directly causative of PFPS, is unclear. However, a logical and systematic approach to the identification of the possible causative and contributory factors to PFPS, invariably gives the clinician sufficient information on which to base an effective treatment and rehabilitation programme. The treatment and rehabilitation strategies that are frequently effective in the treatment of PFPS will be discussed in relation to exercise, manual therapy and corrective taping. But first, some of the signs and symptoms indicative of PFPS will be described together with some of the key examination points.

Signs and symptoms The athlete's complaint is chiefly one of pain, which is usually identified as being 'behind the knee cap'. The pain is usually most pronounced when the knee is loaded in some degree of flexion with bodyweight. Consequently, squatting and negotiating stairs frequently causes pain. Quick weightbearing movements such as checking, to push off and run from the affected knee or to quickly decelerate the running gait, are also usually limited by retropatellar pain. This pain can occasionally be severe enough to cause sensations of 'giving way'. These episodes of weightbearing dysfunction should not be confused with episodes of true functional instability. Careful questioning usually differentiates between these two very different scenarios. Occasionally the athlete may also experience episodes of the knee seizing in a position of flexion. This usually follows a period of rest, where the knee has been kept in a semiflexed position for some time, as in sitting. Careful questioning will differentiate these complaints from episodes of true mechanical locking of the knee, i.e. those that are due to some form of internal derangement.

Examination A general observation of total body posture and more specifically of lower limb alignment (in standing and in lying) should be made and any of the previously mentioned anomalies should be noted. The bulk of the lateral and medial components of the quadriceps should also be observed and compared to the non-affected side so as to determine the presence of asymmetry, which could indicate the presence of muscular imbalance. Finally, the position of the patella in relation to the femur must be assessed both in extension and also in varying degrees of flexion (both non-weightbearing and weightbearing). Commonly encountered patellar positional anomalies associated with PFPS are lateral gliding and lateral tilting of the patella.

Passive testing of the PFJ should be performed to identify movement anomalies. These frequently consist of painful hypomobility of the patella when it is moved medially, longitudinally (in a caudal direction) or in combinations of the two. These PFJ movements should be tested in positions of knee flexion as well as in extension and compared to the non-affected side. The extensibility of the iliotibial band (ITB) should also be tested. This can be done by performing passive hip abduction. The effect that any identified ITB tightness has upon the lateral PFJ soft tissues should also be assessed. A method of doing this is to compare the amount of medial patellar excursion that is available in the neutral position and then compare it to the amount that is available in a position of ITB stretch. A reduction of medial patellar displacement in a position of ITB tension (as compared to the opposite limb) could indicate PFPS-contributory ITB tightness. The flexibility of the hamstring and calf muscles should also be assessed, as tightness in these groups could lead to flexed knee postures being adopted This would increase patellofemoral forces.

Testing functional activities that reproduce the pain is vital if a diagnosis of PFPS is to be confirmed and if the efficacy of later treatment is to be properly ascertained. These movements involve bodyweight control through the semiflexed knee. In cases of PFPS where the symptoms are relatively irritable, simply squatting through a few degrees of knee flexion may be all that is required to elicit a pain response. Less irritable cases may require activities such as deep squat positions, hopping or lunging to reproduce the symptoms. The use of electromyography to measure the activity in the VMO during weightbearing activities can also provide useful information on the presence and amount of weakness/inhibition.

Management The management of PFPS often requires attention to a number of factors such as posture/limb malalignments, joint hypomobility, soft-tissue tightness and muscular weakness/inhibition.

The presence of postural defects or limb malalignments among those athletes who present with PFPS and their relevance to the presenting condition must be evaluated with care. The majority of these findings are present to some degree in sportspeople competing at all levels who are completely asymptomatic. Such anatomical and postural conditions should therefore be viewed as 'normal abnormalities'. However, the possible contribution of these anatomic factors to the aetiology and pathology of PFPS should be borne in mind and it is frequently the case that their relevance to PFPS can only be ascertained by retrospectively evaluating the effect of correcting them (where possible), e.g. by using an orthotic devise to counter an over-pronating foot.

Painful and hypomobile ranges of PFJ mobility must be rectified by suitable passive mobilizing procedures and tight lateral structures such as the lateral patella retinaculum and ITB should be stretched. This is done with the aim of reducing PFJ loading and associated pain. Improvements in medial patellar mobility may also allow the VMO to work more efficiently and any reduction in pain will reduce VMO inhibition. A similar result may also be achieved by corrective taping of the patella (McConnell, 1986, 1987). This procedure consists of correcting patellar position abnormalities (most commonly lat-

eral gliding and/or tilting) with rigid adhesive tape. This corrective taping can give immediate and sometimes significant reductions in pain with concomitant improvements in weightbearing lower-limb function and its effectiveness in rectifying lateral deviations of the patella, both pre- and postexercise has been demonstrated (Larsen *et al.*, 1995). The use of this type of corrective taping enhances the programme of exercise (particularly for strengthening and re-education of the VMO) and joint and soft-tissue mobilization that should be central to the treatment programme.

The VMO strengthening and re-education exercises should not cause any pain or any joint reaction such as swelling. These responses will inhibit VMO activity and simply compound problems of muscular imbalance. The central thrust of the VMO programme should be functional exercises (weightbearing) that are performed with the intention of re-educating precise patterns of movement rather than simply strengthening. For the exercises to be functional, they must in the majority of instances be weightbearing exercises. The widely used seated knee extension exercises (open kinetic chain exercise), where the quadriceps work in isolation, expose the PFJ to greater reaction forces and stresses than do leg press or similar closed kinetic chain exercises (Steinkamp *et al.*, 1993). The use of closed chain exercises to retrain VMO function is therefore preferable so as to avoid overstressing the PFJ and to ensure that improvements in muscular and neuromotor control transfer to functional weightbearing activities. Combining isometric hip adduction with quadriceps exercises (both closed and open kinetic chain) has been advocated as a way of emphasizing the work of the VMO, as this portion of the quadriceps has an attachment to the tendon of adductor magnus. Theoretically this would enhance VMO activity by improving its stability. This however has not been substantiated by electromyographic evaluation (Karst and Jewett, 1993).

Integrated programmes of taping, stretching, mobilizing and taping have been reported to have 86–96% success rates (Gerrard, 1989; McConnell, 1987) in the treatment of PFPS.

(b) Tendinitis/bursitis

Inflammation of the tendons and bursae around the knee may result from acute injuries or from overuse situations. The former are usually linked to a single specific injury and are relatively straightforward conditions to manage, as long as adequate rest is implemented and suitable treatment and exercise are undertaken to modulate the inflammatory response and to restore strength. In contrast, chronic tendinitis problems can give rise to sport-limiting symptoms for protracted periods of time. Chronic inflammation of the patellar tendon, biceps femoris and pes anserinus bursa will be considered.

Patellar tendinitis

Failure to address pain from an inflamed patellar tendon with appropriate activity modification and treatment can result in persistent and recurrent pain, which, in the most severe cases, can be career-threatening. The cause may be some form of overload such as an unaccustomed amount or intensity of plyometric exercise, or may be due to repetitive episodes of minor trauma. Chronic inflammation may also arise from an episode of acute tendinitis that is not managed with suitable rest and a graduated exercise programme.

Some form of focal degeneration within the tendon could predispose it to overuse. The cellular changes that occur in these instances are probably similar to those changes that have been described in relation to cases of Achilles tendinitis. The result may be a reduction of the tensile strength of the tendon.

Signs and symptoms Pain is localized to the affected patellar tendon and may take the form of severe sudden pain when the tendon is exposed to sudden high loading such as jumping or kicking. An ache and associated stiffness may also be experienced, particularly towards the end of and after bouts of exercise. Tenderness and pain are often experienced when any pressure is applied directly to the tendon, e.g. when kneeling.

Examination Tenderness is often easy to elicit by palpation of the tendon, usually at the inferior patellar pole. Cystic areas of mucoid degeneration within the patellar tendon have been described (Scranton and Farrar, 1992) and are associated with relatively localized areas of tenderness rather than diffuse tenderness. The latter can affect the whole patellar tendon and is more characteristically associated with cases of acute tendinitis. Non-weightbearing resisted quadriceps work is frequently pain-provoking and stretching the tendon by performing passive prone knee bending may also reproduce pain. A full evaluation of the PFJ should be undertaken as there are often ranges of movement that are painfully hypomobile.

Treatment A conservative treatment approach will be outlined. This is broadly similar to the treatment that would be appropriate for cases that are managed operatively. Most sportspeople present with chronic patellar tendinitis after the symptoms have been present for weeks or months, and have finally progressed to the stage where training and competition are severely affected. In these cases, a complete cessation of sport and any activity that provokes the symptoms must be enforced if treatment is to succeed. Electrotherapy and ice applications to modulate pain and swelling may be of help and can be used to supplement the manual therapy and exercises which are the key elements of the rehabilitation programme. Restricted ranges of motion that could affect the normal dynamics of the patellar tendon should be treated with mobilizing and stretching techniques. This may involve PFJ mobilizations and stretches to improve limitations of prone knee bending. Specific soft-tissue mobilizing techniques, as described by Hunter (1984), may be applied directly to the tendon in an attempt to optimize its extensibility. Improvements in the extensibility of the patellar tendon in particular, and the extensor mechanism in general, could result in a reduction in the amount of force that the patellar tendon is subjected to.

The exercise programme should aim to restore relevant muscular strength as well as tensile strength of the patellar tendon. Improvements in tendon tensile strength may be achieved by implementing an exercise programme that exposes the tendon to progressively increasing loads (Curwin and Standish, 1984). Such a programme has been described in the section on the Achilles tendon. For the majority of sports, the patellar tendon will be exposed to relevant training stimuli by the predominant use of closed kinetic chain exercises. The use of open kinetic chain exercise for the quadriceps/patellar tendon places potentially large localized loads on the tendon, which, in the early stages of rehabilitation, may provoke pain. Where kicking is an integral part of the injured athlete's sport, open kinetic chain exercises will need to be performed to ensure that full sport-specific function is restored. However, the propensity of these exercises to aggravate the condition means that they should be used as a final exercise progression. Taping the tendon to provide support or to pull it either laterally or medially may reduce the pain associated with exercise, possibly by altering its line of pull and 'unloading' the symptomatic portion.

Biceps femoris tendinitis

This is a relatively common condition, usually brought on by an excessive amount of hamstring-specific activity such as sprint training. However, pain localized to the posterolateral aspect of the knee and adjacent lower thigh is commonly caused by neural pathodynamics, either alone or in association with a musculotendinous inflammatory lesion. A careful differential diagnosis is therefore important with such pain presentations.

Signs and symptoms Biceps tendinitis is characterized by very localized soreness and tenderness. Pain in this area due to neural pathodynamics (probably affecting the common peroneal nerve) may be less precisely localized to the actual tendon of the biceps femoris and may radiate into the adjacent upper posterolateral calf. Activities such as sprinting, or any movements that entail rapid or stretching forces to the tendon, will elicit pain.

Examination SLR and slump testing should be performed to confirm or rule out a neural component to pain production. Careful palpation of the biceps tendon, and of the common peroneal nerve, which runs along its medial border and is easily palpable, should also be carried out. Nerve tenderness is a common finding in cases of relevant neural pathodynamics and the pain response can be compared in and out of tension positions (e.g. SLR and slump) This may help to confirm or rule out the presence of a neural component to the presenting problem. Static tests involving resistance to combined knee flexion and lateral rotation are usually positive, in terms of pain reproduction, in the presence of tendinitis.

Treatment Stretching work for limitations of hamstring flexibility should be performed and coupled with more specific mobilizing techniques directed specifically to the tendon. The superficial position of the biceps femoris tendon makes it an ideal structure for the application of these techniques, which can be performed with the tendon relaxed and in some degree of tension. These techniques are described in section 6.6.3. Strengthening exercises as described for hamstring injuries should be implemented and progressed along the lines proposed by Curwin and Standish (1984). These are also described in section 6.6.3. Exercises to specifically target the biceps femoris consist of combined knee flexion and lateral rotation. The use of an elasticated exercise band makes such exercises easy to administer.

Pes anserinus bursitis

The tendon and bursa, while distinct anatomical entities, form a functional unit. For this reason it is impossible and unnecessary to differentiate between the pathologies of tendinitis and bursitis. The pes anserinus ('goose-foot') tendon is a shared insertion for sartorius, gracilis and semitendinosus. It is therefore subjected to tensile stresses during any activities that involve active forceful hip adduction, knee flexion and medial tibial rotation. It is also tensioned by passive forces that stress the tibiofemoral joint into valgus positions or into lateral rotation. There is therefore significant potential for acute and overuse pes anserinus injury in many different sports. These often occur in association with MCLC injuries.

Signs and symptoms The symptoms of pain are usually provoked by the activities described in section 6.5.3(b). However, the location of pain and swelling will be more inferiorly and, at the level of the tibiofemoral joint line, more posteriorly located.

Examination Swelling and pain at the location of the bursa/tendon insertion (i.e. the upper anteromedial portion of the tibia) can usually be identified by observation and palpation. Passive stretching of the tendon by abducting the tibia (in slight knee flexion) or by laterally rotating the tibia may also reproduce pain. Both of these manoeuvres stress the MCLC and so a differentiating test

is required (other than that of palpation). This could be manually resisted combined knee flexion–medial rotation.

Treatment Passive mobilizations as described for MCLC injuries should be used to regain any lost extensibility. Resisted exercises should be used to strengthen the tendon. These may use individual or combined movements of hip adduction or extension and knee flexion or medial rotation. Because the pes anserinus functions as a dynamic stabilizer of the medial side of the tibiofemoral joint, closed kinetic chain exercises should be featured in the exercise programme so that this function is rehabilitated.

(c) Pulling osteochondritis

Children (particularly boys) are affected, usually between the ages of 10 and 15. The lesion is an inflammatory one of the apophyses at the tibial tuberosity (Osgood–Schlatter's disease) or at the inferior pole of the patella (Sinding-Larsen–Johansson disease). It is caused by repetitive traction imparted by the quadriceps via the patellar tendon.

Pain is the chief complaint and is often associated with exquisite tenderness. In the case of Osgood–Schlatter's disease there may be a firm swelling at the tibial tuberosity. Resisted quadriceps work may provoke the pain.

As the cause is overuse against a background of immature skeletal tissue, rest from aggravating activity is the only cure. This rarely necessitates a complete lay-off, but rather a reduction in the amount of sport that is played or the avoidance of excessive knee forces, e.g. by avoiding hard surfaces and wearing suitable shock-absorbing footwear. These measures will need to be implemented as necessary, i.e. until the inflammation settles or the epiphysis starts to close. 'Exercise within the pain' is the basic advice that should be given. Ice and non-steroidal anti-inflammatory medication may be of some help in reducing pain but reliance on such treatment to 'get through' training and competition should not be encouraged. A full examination of the PFJ should be made. Corrections of abnormal PFJ movements (by taping and or passive mobilizations) and of associated lower limb malalignments may be helpful. Taping of the patellar tendon as described for patellar tendinitis may also alleviate discomfort.

6.6 SELECTED INJURIES OF THE LOWER LEG, ANKLE AND FOOT

6.6.1 Introduction

The injuries and conditions selected are those that are most frequently encountered and/or can be particularly troublesome from the perspective of both athlete and clinician.

These disorders have been classified as either musculotendinous, joint, bony or neural.

- Musculotendinous
  - Chronic compartment syndrome
  - Achilles tendon disorders
  - Medial tibial stress syndrome
- Joint
  - Ankle sprain
  - Ankle instability
- Bony
  - Stress fracture
  - Talotibial exostoses.

6.6.2 Compartment syndromes

Compartment syndromes are either chronic or acute. Chronic compartment syndrome (CCS) refers to pain that occurs as a consequence of a pressure increase within a musculofascial compartment that is exercise induced. Acute compartment syndromes (ACS) are relatively rare occurrences and, while they may also be related to sessions of exercise, some form of trauma is usually responsible (Allen and Barnes, 1994). ACS are medical emergencies, as they involve the build-up of intracompart-

mental pressure to the point where the arterial circulation is compromised. The consequence can be limb loss if surgical decompression is not performed. In contrast to ACS, the pressure increase in CCS never affects the arterial blood supply to the involved muscles but is sufficient to compromise capillary blood flow (Allen and Barnes, 1994). It is this that causes the ischaemic pain.

CCS most frequently affects the muscles of the lower leg (Figure 6.10). The muscles of this region are situated within one of four fascial compartments (Table 6.6)

CCS usually (approximately 80% of cases) affects the anterior compartment and in the majority of cases the condition is bilateral

Table 6.6 The myofascial compartments of the lower leg

Compartment	Muscles
Anterior	Tibialis anterior Extensor hallucis longus Extensor digitorum longus
Medial	Tibialis posterior Flexor hallucis longus Flexor digitorum longus
Lateral	Peroneus longus Peroneus brevis
Posterior	Gastrocnemius Soleus Plantaris

(Allen and Barnes, 1994; Styf and Korner, 1986; Turnispeed, Detmer and Girdley, 1989).

While the cause of the pain in CCS is an increase in intracompartmental pressure, it is not clear why this happens. A decrease in the extensibility of the muscular fascia, an increase in muscle bulk as a result of exercise and alterations in the muscle blood supply have all been put forward as possible explanations (Allen and Barnes, 1994).

Signs and symptoms   Pain associated with exercise is the primary complaint. Runners or

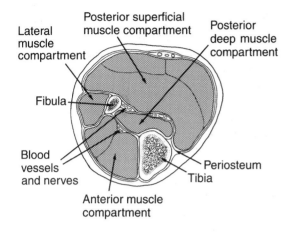

Figure 6.10 Lateral section of the compartments of the lower leg.

sportspeople from running-based sports are most commonly affected and usually complain of a dull diffuse ache with associated tightness. This comes on after a bout of running-based exercise and may become so severe that exercise has to be curtailed. Rest from running relieves the symptoms. Over a period of weeks or months the severity of the symptoms may increase and the amount of activity required to trigger them may reduce.

Examination There is usually nothing of relevance on objective testing. A provisional diagnosis of CCS is made on the basis of the symptomatology and by excluding other conditions. The vertebral column, hips, knee complex and superior tibiofibular joints should be excluded by appropriate active and passive testing. The peripheral and central nervous system should also be examined to ascertain the presence of any relevant neural pathodynamics (by SLR, PKB and slump testing). Conditions such as medial tibial stress syndrome and stress fracture also need to be discounted. A conclusive diagnosis of CCS can only be made if intracompartmental pressures are measured, i.e. by catheterization.

Treatment Modification of pain-provoking exercise is an obvious starting point. This could take the form of a reduction in the amount or intensity of training and playing and could be linked to the use of shock-absorbing insoles and the avoidance of hard training and playing surfaces. Anatomical and postural anomalies may also be implicated and the use of postural re-education and orthotics to counter malalignments such as overpronated feet may be of help. Failure of conservative treatment would be an indication for surgical decompression of the offending compartment. Such fasciotomies should be immediately followed by an active exercise programme so that the decompressed fascia does not heal in a manner that could once more compromise the compartment (Allen and Barnes, 1994).

6.6.3 Achilles tendon disorders

Most sporting activities impose large tensile forces upon the Achilles tendon (tendo achillis – TA). The magnitude of these forces during activities such as running and jumping, together with the repetitive nature of many sports, means that the TA is prone to both acute and chronic injuries.

The two TA pathologies that are probably the most frequently encountered are inflammation (due both to acute and overuse injury) of the superficial portion of the TA and focal degeneration of the tendon substance. These are referred to as peritendinitis and tendinosis respectively (Kannus and Josza, 1991). These conditions may occur in isolation but are frequently encountered in combination. They will therefore be discussed together and, following this, TA ruptures will be considered.

(a) Peritendinitis and tendinosis

Peritendinitis may result from a single episode of direct trauma, such as a kick, which sets up an acute inflammatory reaction in the TA paratenon. Continued exercise in the presence of such an inflammatory response may perpetuate the condition and set up a chronic cycle of repetitive mechanical irritation and continued inflammation. Chronic peritendinitis may also arise as a result of continual minor irritation of the TA e.g. by the rubbing of poorly positioned heel tabs or by excessive training on hard surfaces. Tendinosis may also be related to an overuse scenario, but any inflammation is usually subclinical. The condition is characterized by focal degeneration of the tendon substance. Relative avascularity of parts of the TA may be the cause of tendinosis (Corrigan and Maitland, 1994).

Aetiology   Numerous factors have been postulated as being causative or contributory to the TA disease processes of peritendinitis and tendinosis. Some of these have been summarized in Table 6.7.

Table 6.7 Postulated aetiological factors in Achilles tendon disease (adapted from Reid, 1992)

Training errors
- Sudden increase in running mileage
- Sudden increase in running intensity
- Hill running
- Recommencement of training after period of inactivity

Surface and equipment
- Repetitive jumping on hard floors
- Running on uneven terrain
- Shoes with inadequate shock absorption
- Pressure from shoe on to tendon
- Soft/loose fitting heel counter
- Excessively narrow or flared heel base

Anatomical factors
- Age and tendon collagen changes
- Poor tendon blood supply
- Thin heel pad
- Rear foot valgus in flexible foot
- Rear foot varus in rigid foot
- Tibial varum
- Proximal limb and pelvic malalignments
- Gastrocnemius/soleus strength-to-tendon-size imbalances

Direct trauma
- Kick or laceration to tendon

Signs and symptoms   Peritendinitis is usually characterized by pain and associated tenderness along the TA. Crepitus may also be elicited by repeated dorsiflexion and plantarflexion of the foot. Resisted plantarflexion is also usually pain-provoking. In contrast, tendinosis is invariably asymptomatic. It may only be diagnosed following soft-tissue scanning investigations or exploratory TA surgery.

Examination   It is not possible to make a firm diagnosis of tendinosis purely on the basis of a standard clinical examination. Some form of soft-tissue scanning or exploration of the TA would be required to do this. However the clinician might be suspicious of the existence of such pathology if the TA exhibited signs of chronic swelling and thickening. Such signs may also be associated with peritendinitis, but in such cases the swelling would probably be diffuse. Nodular swelling of the TA substance would be more indicative of tendinosis pathology. These two types of swelling can sometimes be differentiated by palpating the swollen tissues while the TA is moved (actively and/or passively). If the swelling is felt to be relatively well localized and moves as one with the tendon, then it is probably a thickening of the actual tendon substance. Conversely, any swollen/thickened tissues that are felt to statically overly the moving tendon are probably associated with peritendinous structures such as the paratenon. In cases of peritendinitis, palpation or squeezing the tendon usually elicits acute tenderness and it may be possible to palpate crepitus when the foot is repeatedly dorsi- and plantarflexed. Activities such as standing on the toes or hopping on the spot are also usually pain-provoking. Stretching the TA may produce pain but is frequently asymptomatic. The proximity of the sural nerve to the lateral aspect of the TA may result in its dynamics being adversely affected by inflammatory and associated soft-tissue thickening of the tendon. The tests previously described for nerve pathodynamics should therefore be routinely performed, i.e. SLR and/or slump positions with the sural nerve pretensioned with inversion and dorsiflexion of the foot (Butler, 1991). An assessment of the nerve's sensory distribution (lower posterolateral aspect of the foot and lateral aspect of the foot and ankle) should also be undertaken.

Treatment   The usual physical therapies for the modulation of pain and swelling may be of help in both acute and chronic cases of paratendinitis. However it is pointless to institute such therapies without simultaneously addressing any of the relevant predisposing factors listed in Table 6.7. The return to sporting activities should be a phased one with a graduated programme of sport-specific exercises preceding full sports participation. The type of graduated exercise programme for increasing the tensile strength of the tendon outlined by Curwin and Standish (1984) should be implemented. This exercise programme is based upon the premise that tendon tissue, like all other connective tissue, can be positively affected (in terms of increased tensile strength) by external forces that act upon it. If too much tension is applied to the tendon, then tissue breakdown can occur. For this reason isometric exercises are the first to be introduced and are administered and progressed in relation to any symptom production. Initially these exercises should be performed pain-free. They are then progressed to involve isotonic muscle work, which in the initial stages consists of concentric activity. The more demanding (in terms of force production) eccentric isotonic exercise is then introduced as a progression. If necessary these exercises can be performed in non-weightbearing against a relatively low resistance such as an elastic bandage and can be progressed to weightbearing where partial and then full bodyweight is used as the resistance. Finally, external resistance in the form of free weights can be used and the final progression would be to introduce high-speed plyometric activities, where the tendon is exposed to an eccentric contraction of the calf/prestretch, before having to transmit a forceful concentric, foot-plantarflexing contraction. The timings of the progressions and the overall length of such a programme would of course vary from case to case but would probably take a minimum of 6–8 weeks to administer safely. Attempts to condense the programme into a shorter time scale would run the risk of overloading the tendon and achieving the opposite of the treatment goal, i.e. tissue breakdown.

(b) Achilles tendon rupture

Achilles tendon ruptures (both partial and complete) are relatively rare occurrences in sport (Mahler, 1992). However, they usually have a significant functionally limiting impact, both in the short and long term, for those unfortunate enough to sustain them. The incidence of TA rupture seems to be increasing (Nillius, Nilsson and Westlin, 1976), particularly among sports participants over the age of 30 (Josza, Kvist and Balint, 1989). Sports that involve sudden acceleration, deceleration and jumping are usually associated with these injuries. A significant number of TA ruptures occur in soccer (33.5% in one study) (Josza, Kvist and Balint, 1989).

Pathoanatomy

Uncertainty exists as to the factors that predispose some individuals to TA rupture. Hypotheses citing only mechanical factors have been proposed (Barfred, 1973), but others have linked degenerative tendon conditions (tendinosis) to episodes of TA rupture (Kannus and Josza, 1991; Landvatter and Renstrom, 1992; Puddu, Ippolito and Postacchini, 1976). Both scenarios probably apply, i.e. rupture due to abnormally high forces placed on a normal tendon and rupture of an abnormal tendon exposed to normal stresses.

Proponents of degenerative TA pathology as contributory to tendon rupture point to the fact that a high proportion of TA ruptures are located between 2 cm and 6 cm above the calcaneal insertion (Josza, Kvist and Balint, 1989). From a biomechanical perspective, this is unexpected, given that the tensile strength of a healthy TA at its midpoint is greater than at its insertion (Landvatter and Renstrom, 1992). An explanation for this is the relatively poor blood supply to the TA in this 2–6 cm zone. There is an increase in this relative avascularity with age and as a result the area becomes relatively hypoxic and prone to degenerative changes (Langergren and Lindholm, 1958/59). These changes would reduce the tensile strength of the TA and increase the likelihood of mechanical failure when under load. The fact that tendinosis occurs gradually and is usually pain-free explains why up to two-thirds of patients who sustain complete spontaneous TA rupture are asymptomatic prior to the rupture (Kannus and Josza, 1991).

The use of injected corticosteroids (into the tendon), has been identified as a cause of TA rupture (Puddu *et al.*, 1994; Renstrom, 1988). However, while corticosteroids have been shown to have a devitalizing effect upon tendon tissue, the link between their use in the treatment of certain inflammatory TA conditions and tendon rupture is tenuous (Mahler, 1992). Most of the individuals who sustain acute TA rupture are asymptomatic prior to rupture and have therefore never been injected with corticosteroids (Mahler, 1992). However injections of corticosteroids directly into tendons is not recommended (Leadbetter, 1990).

The freshly ruptured TA may be treated conservatively or operatively. The proponents of each method point to satisfactory functional outcomes with the main advantage of conservative treatment being the avoidance of postoperative complications such as deep infections, fistulae formation, tendon necrosis and nerve damage (Landvatter and Renstrom, 1992). Those who prefer surgical management cite the main advantages as being a lower incidence of tendon re-rupture (Landvatter and Renstrom, 1992) and a greater chance of being able to resume preinjury-level sport (Cetti *et al.*, 1993).

Rehabilitation

Whatever method of management is chosen, the process of rehabilitation will be similar, although invariably less protracted in the surgically managed ruptures that are mobilized early. Such early mobilization uses a functional orthosis that limits dorsiflexion, so protecting the repair while allowing plantarflexion and thereby limiting postoperative stiffness and weakness (Carter, Fowler and Blokker, 1992). Such a device would be used for a similar length of time to an orthodox cast, i.e. 6–8 weeks. The implementation of early postoperative motion results in less functionally limiting stiffness and weakness but even this group will require an intensive programme of mobilizing, strengthening and conditioning work before sporting activity can be resumed.

For descriptive purposes, the rehabilitation programme can be divided into the four phases listed below. However it should be realized that, in practice, there are no clearly defined boundaries between the phases of rehabilitation.

1. Immobilization/protection phase
2. Mobilizing and strengthening phase
3. Functional rehabilitation phase
4. Performance rehabilitation phase.

Immobilization/protection phase If a full and/or below-knee cast is used to protect the TA repair for the immediate postoperative period, there is a limited amount that can be done to minimize the amount of foot and ankle stiffness and weakness that will inevitably occur. During this period regular strengthening exercises can be given for the uninvolved limb and this could include single-leg cycling and rowing, which would have the dual benefits of maintaining local muscular strength and cardiovascular fitness. The affected side can be exercised isometrically, and to prevent undue stress to the repair site this would involve simultaneous isometric contractions of the anterior tibials and calf muscles, which should be performed submaximally and should not cause any discomfort. A cardiovascular substitute training programme should also be instituted as soon as possible to maintain general cardiovascular conditioning and to keep the athlete in a positive frame of mind.

If some form of functional brace is fitted, active plantarflexion can be used as a strengthening and mobilizing exercise within the constraints of the cast, which will probably limit dorsiflexion to the plantargrade position. Such functional braces can usually be removed and, once the surgical wounds have healed, soft-tissue massage techniques can be used around the foot and ankle joints, together with active and passive foot and ankle movements to reduce swelling and improve/maintain ranges of plantarflexion, inversion and eversion.

Mobilizing and strengthening phase   As soon as the cast or brace has been removed, mobilizing work can begin in earnest. By this time (approximately 6–8 weeks) the repair should be strong enough to withstand modest tension and it will be possible to mobilize actively and passively into dorsiflexion. Initially these mobilizations should be aimed primarily at the ankle joint. By performing the dorsiflexion movements while keeping the knee flexed, the TA will receive relatively little tensile stressing. An example of such an exercise, which is functionally important as far as ambulation is concerned, is the walk standing lunge. Here partial bodyweight is used to push the knee over the foot (which is kept flat) and to thereby mobilize into a position of weightbearing dorsiflexion. While it will be possible and desirable to institute

some early strengthening work at this time, it should be realized that gaining mobility must be the prime concern.

Non-weightbearing strengthening exercises against low resistance, e.g. using an elastic bandage for all of the foot/ankle movements, are appropriate for the early rehabilitation phase. Walking, initially with crutches, can also be used as a functional strengthening exercise, but this should only be progressed in terms of duration and speed if it is of good quality.

Functional rehabilitation phase   It was mentioned earlier that there are in practice no clear boundaries between the various phases of the rehabilitation process and this is particularly the case with 'functional' rehabilitation activities. For example, walking, which is obviously a functional activity, can be used from the earliest stages of rehabilitation to improve strength and coordination. In the mid- and late stages of rehabilitation, walking can be progressed (as soon as sufficient mobility and strength have been regained) from walking with crutches to walking without to power walking. Power walking can be a particularly effective way of functionally strengthening the calf musculature and preparing the patient for running activities and is simply a normal walking gait performed at speed and emphasizing the push-off phase. Walking backwards can also be a useful functionally strengthening activity and should be looked upon as a progression from forward ambulation as it involves the more challenging muscular work of eccentric calf activity in lowering the heel to the floor. When this activity is first introduced, care should be taken to ensure that good technique is possible at slow speeds before allowing quicker movements. This is one of the basic principles of all rehabilitation exercise, particularly functional exercises.

Other functional activities that are often of value are proprioceptive single-leg standing activities, which can be progressed by the

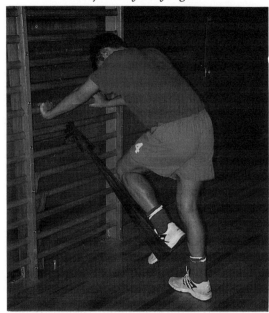

Figure 6.11   The use of an elastic bandage for resistance exercises involving combined knee extension and plantarflexion.

use of elastic bandage resistance, and combined knee extension and ankle plantarflexion exercises, which use partial or complete body-weight as a resistance (Figure 6.11). Because of its similarity to the push off phase of running, the ability to perform such an exercise satisfactorily, should be a pre-requisite before running activities are introduced

Performance rehabilitation phase   This phase of rehabilitation refers to the process of introducing the athlete to exercises that directly relate to the actual activities they will have to perform on returning to their sport. Failure to progress the patient through this stage may mean that the final degrees of strength and coordination are not restored and that as a consequence substandard performances and reinjury result. The process of performance rehabilitation involves breaking down complex sporting activities into subcomponents, practising these as individual exercises and then reconstituting them and practising the actual sporting activity.

As far as TA rehabilitation for the field-sports player is concerned, the activities that usually require particular attention are:

- short-distance sprints from a stationary position, e.g. to intercept a ball or make a tackle;
- running backwards, e.g. to shadow an opposing player;
- jumping and landing, e.g. to avoid a tackle or to catch or head a ball.

6.6.4   Medial tibial stress syndrome

This condition is most prevalent in running or in sports where running is a major physical component. The complaint is of exercise-related pain along the medial border of the tibia. As the name suggests, this condition is one of overuse, but it is unclear whether the bony tenderness that results is due to weightbearing forces or to the traction of attached muscles, i.e. tibialis posterior, soleus and flexor digitorum longus (Fredricson *et al.*, 1995). This bony tenderness results from periosteal oedema and may be associated with vigorous new periosteal bone production i.e. not in the presence of actual stress fractures (Lee, Zhang and Chen, 1985). It has been postulated that medial tibial stress syndrome is an initial response to imposed stress which could progress to stress fractures of the tibia (Fredricson *et al.*, 1995).

Signs and symptoms   Medial tibial border pain is linked directly to episodes of running-based activity and may persist as a dull ache for some time afterwards. At its most severe, the pain can prevent exercise. There is usually accompanying soreness to the touch, and this can take the form of exquisite tenderness.

Examination   Tenderness of the medial tibial border and of the adjacent soft tissues is easily identified and percussion of the tibia may also be pain-provoking. The extensibility of the long toe flexors and of the soleus and tibialis posterior may be reduced and stretching them may reproduce pain. Plain X-rays do not reveal any abnormality but bone scans reveal a diffuse 'tubular pattern' of isotope uptake as opposed to a focal area in cases of stress fracture (Allen and Barnes, 1994). Postural anomalies and malalignments of the lower limb should be noted (Fredricson *et al.*, 1995).

Treatment As with all overuse conditions, modification of aggravating training and competition forms the basis of successful management. Restrictions in muscular extensibility, usually involving tibialis posterior, soleus and flexor digitorum longus should be made good and any correctable postural or malalignment anomalies should be rectified. Failure of conservative treatment and accompanying rest may be an indication for surgical management which could consist of soft-tissue release.

6.6.5 Ankle sprains

Sprains of the ankle ligaments, particularly the lateral ligament complex, are commonly encountered across all sports (Nicholl, Coleman and Williams, 1991). In sports where running and jumping are key physical elements, ankle injuries have been shown to account for a quarter of all injuries. Of these, three-quarters are sprains, the overwhelming majority of these being inversion sprains (Mack, 1982).

Minor sprain episodes may cause only minimal disruption to training and playing routines. Moderate and severe sprains can, however, result in lengthy periods of sporting disability and can lead to recurrent and long-term disability, especially if they are poorly managed at the time of and immediately after the injury.

Sprain injury of the ankle usually affects the lateral ligaments. Inversion sprains will therefore be covered here, but the principles of examination and treatment can be easily transferred to eversion sprains.

Functional anatomy The joint is formed between the superior articular surface of the talus and the lower ends of the tibia and fibula (Figure 6.12).

The medial malleolar projection of the tibia provides a laterally facing articular surface and the fibular component of the joint provides a medially inclined joint surface. This tibial and fibular bony arrangement has been likened to a mortise joint. The ankle articulation allows the physiological movements of plantarflexion and dorsiflexion. As the width of the superior articular surface of the tibia is greater anteriorly than posteriorly, there has to be some compensatory mechanism within the joint to accommodate the relatively wide anterior portion of the talus in positions of full foot dorsiflexion. This is achieved by a degree of flexibility in the inferior tibiofibular joint. The structural stability of the joint relies on bony surface congruence, collateral ligament support and active muscular support.

The lateral ligament complex is composed of three ligaments, which support the joint capsule. These are the anterior talofibular ligament (ATFL), the calcaneofibular ligament (CFL) and the posterior talofibular ligament (PTFL). All these structures limit excessive inversion of the talus, but it is usually the ATFL that is involved in inversion sprain injuries. It may also be damaged by forceful end-range plantarflexing movements of the foot. Although not part of the ankle joint, the ATFL should be considered in any functional analysis of this joint. This ligament is frequently injured in moderate to severe lateral ankle sprains, probably because excessive movements of the talus forces the inferior tibiofibular joint apart. This is thought to occur when the injuring movement involves rotation of the talus (Taylor and Bassett, 1993).

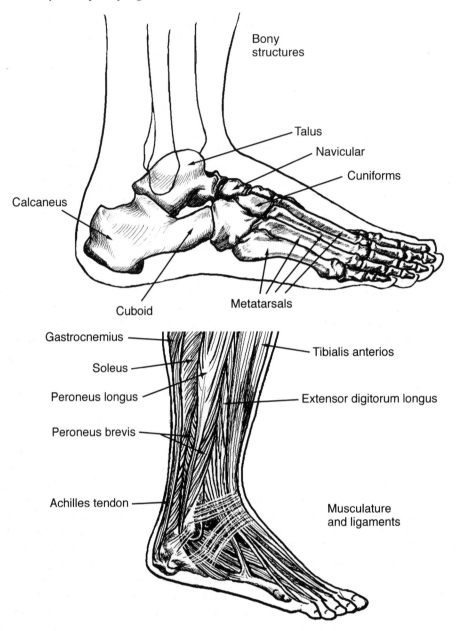

Figure 6.12 Anatomy of the ankle joint.

Signs and symptoms Swelling localized to the lateral ankle joint line is usually present and proportional to the degree of injury. Moderate to severe inversion sprains usually result in a generalized joint effusion. Weight bearing disability is usually experienced, with pain being produced by inversion and/or plantarflexion of the foot.

Examination Active movements of the ankle are often inhibited and passive movements, particularly into inversion and plantarflexion, are usually limited by pain. Gross amounts of foot inversion, in the absence of pain or with minimal discomfort, could indicate a complete ligamentous rupture. Tenderness is usually elicited on palpation of the lateral joint line, especially anterolaterally over the ATFL. There may also be medial ankle discomfort on palpation, probably due to impingement of the medial ankle soft tissues at the time of the injury. Testing the range of calcaneal inversion (by tilting the talus) with the foot in a plantargrade position is said to specifically stress the CFL, while the frequently injured ATFL is best tested by performing an anterior drawer test (Baumhauer *et al.*, 1995). This can be done with the patient in prone lying and the knee in 90° of flexion. The examiner stabilizes the lower tibia just above the ankle with one hand and, with the other, performs an anterior gliding movement of the foot via pressure to the heel. This is best done in approximately 20° of plantarflexion. Excessive draw of the talus in the mortise of the ankle joint indicates ATFL injury.

In moderate to severe cases of inversion sprain, the stability of the inferior tibiofibular joint should be tested. Mechanisms of injury that involve foot/talar rotation may cause additional ligament injury at the inferior tibiofibular joint (Taylor and Bassett, 1993). Any excess movement of the distal fibula in an anteroposterior or posteroanterior direction could indicate the presence of such injury. A positive squeeze test (the application of firm compression across the tibiofemoral joint line), indicated by a pain response, may also indicate inferior tibiofibular joint injury. The true extent of instability at this joint will only be ascertained by carrying out stress radiographs. Identification of significant inferior tibiofibular joint involvement usually means that there will be a protracted rehabilitation period.

Tests to determine the pathodynamics of the sural nerve (which may be subjected to traction injury when inversion sprains occur) should be undertaken and simply involve performing SLR and slump tests with the sural nerve pretensioned by dorsiflexing and inverting the foot (Butler, 1981).

Treatment For minor and moderate inversion sprains, ice compression and elevation are the initial first aid therapies that should be instigated. Compression applied in such a way as to provide it focally, i.e. specifically to the traumatized structures, is more effective than a general compression bandage (Wilkerson and Horn-Kingery, 1993). This may be applied with felt stirrups and elasticated strapping or by proprietary supports, which provide their compression via air-filled cushions or sponge-like material positioned over the affected area and held in place by plastic side pieces and straps. An initial period of non- or partial weightbearing (depending upon the severity of the injury) is helpful to prevent further trauma and control swelling and pain. Non-weightbearing active mobilizing exercises can commence within the first 48 hours and compression and ice treatment should continue until the swelling is under control.

Passive mobilizations should be used to augment active mobilizing exercises; initially, regaining the range of dorsiflexion is a priority so that an even walking gait can be established. After this, the ranges of plantarflexion and inversion must be restored. In tandem with this mobilizing work, exercises to improve the control and strength of the foot/ankle musculature should be performed and progressed from non- to full weightbearing as soon as pain allows. Peroneal strengthening work is a key component of successful rehabilitation, as is coordination training (Karlsson and Faxen, 1994). The eccentric action of the ankle stabilizing muscles, especially the peronei, should be stressed in the exercise programmes. Weightbearing activities specific to the sport of the athlete are an important final progression, so that full function is restored prior to a return to competition.

Complete lateral ligament complex ruptures may be treated with primary surgically repair but functional conservative management has been shown to give equally good results (Karlsson and Faxen, 1994; Sommer, Pauschert and Thomsen, 1995). This approach uses functional braces that protect the injured lateral joint structures by preventing inversion and extreme plantarflexion but permit other ranges of motion. These braces are removable and allow treatment such as ultrasonics, ice and manual therapies (e.g. massage) to be given, in an attempt to reduce swelling and promote healing. The controlled amount of early movement that is permitted by the use of such braces has the effect of stimulating the injured ligamentous structures and this optimizes their tensile strength (Long *et al.*, 1982).

In cases where there is associated inferior tibiofibular joint instability, it may be prudent to enforce a longer period of non- or partial weightbearing. This is done in an attempt to allow the joint to settle and prevent early weightbearing forces from overstressing the injured ligaments. These initial weightbearing forces may be controlled across the inferior tibiofibular joint with the use of external support such as strapping. Persistent pain or swelling associated with weightbearing exercise, in the presence of inferior tibiofibular joint instability, would be an indication for surgical stabilization.

6.6.6   Ankle instability

Functional instability of the ankle is the most serious residual disability following serious lateral ligament ankle injuries. It is characterized by persistent pain, swelling and giving way, which is experienced with physical activity, particularly if this involves twisting and checking manoeuvres or ambulation across rough terrain. The cause of such instability is probably multifactorial in most cases, overstretched lateral ligaments, reduced proprioception and weak ankle muscles (especially the peronei) being the main com-

ponents (Karlsson and Faxen, 1994). Inhibition of the active ankle stabilizers by pain and swelling is also probably contributory.

Conservative treatment should be given along the lines mentioned for treatment of lateral ligament sprains. The key areas are control of swelling and pain and functional exercises to re-establish adequate muscular (particularly the peronei) control and strength. Such an approach will probably take a minimum of 3 months to achieve optimum results and the athlete should continue with a programme of strengthening and proprioceptive maintenance exercises for the remainder of their sporting career. For a small proportion of athletes, surgical reconstruction, usually in the form of a tenodesis (using peroneus brevis or longus) may be required. The need for a rehabilitation programme, as already outlined, applies in these cases.

6.6.7   Stress fractures

These can be defined as partial or complete fractures of bone due to its inability to withstand repetitive submaximal forces (Sallis and Jones, 1991). Stress fractures have been described as being due to fatigue or to insufficiency. Fatigue fractures occur to bone with a normal structure when it is subjected to abnormal loads. Sportspeople may succumb to such injuries when training loads are rapidly increased or when new, vigorous training methods are introduced. Insufficiency fractures can be caused by normal forces that act upon bone which has abnormal mineral content or reduced elastic resistance (Packer, 1995).

Risk factors   Sports that impart repetitive loading over long periods and with high frequency probably carry a relatively high risk for stress-fracture development. Running is one such sport. Among such athletes the presence of narrow tibiae, low arches and externally rotated hips may be predisposing factors (Giladi *et al.*, 1991). Errors in training programme formulation may also cause or contribute to stress-fracture development, a commonly encountered scenario being a marked increase in training and playing loads over a relatively short period of time. Female athletes are also more prone to stress lesions than their male counterparts (Packer, 1995). One explanation for this is the fact that there is a high incidence of amenorrhoea among endurance athletes, particularly distance runners, and the resulting decreased oestrogen levels cause reduced bone mass (Giladi *et al.*, 1991).

Signs and symptoms Pain associated with exercise and relieved by rest is the basic subjective picture. Tenderness of the bone in cases where the fracture is superficial may also be noted. If the lesion is close to a joint there may be associated stiffness.

Examination There are no specific clinical tests for stress fractures that give conclusive evidence of their presence. Careful questioning about the onset of the problem and the training routine leading up to it is often enlightening. A high index of suspicion regarding the presence of a stress fracture is usually arrived at after eliciting a history of atraumatic pain onset associated with some form of training-induced skeletal overload and linking this to an objective examination that excludes muscular and joint pathology. Conclusive proof of a stress fracture can only be obtained through radionuclide bone scanning, CT scanning or magnetic resonance imaging (Fredricson *et al.*, 1995; Sallis and Jones, 1991).

Treatment Rest from all pain-provoking activities is mandatory. The duration of this relative rest period will be dependent upon the site of the lesion and the degree of injury. Several weeks will probably be required before sport can be resumed and this will need to be gradually progressed over a number of weeks with constant reference to any pain that is encountered.

6.6.8 Talotibial exostoses

Exostoses or bony growths that form at the anterior and posterior margins of the ankle (on both the talus and tibia) are encountered in athletes from many different sports. In the majority of instances they are asymptomatic, but they may give rise to symptoms of pain and localized swelling. They form as a response to traction and/or compression between opposing bony joint margins. For example, they may result from kicking (causing anterior ankle traction) in a footballer or from landing on the feet with the ankles in a fully dorsiflexed position (causing anterior ankle compression) in a gymnast.

Signs and symptoms Sharp momentary catches of pain may be experienced with ankle movements that tension or compress the portion of the joint affected by the exostosis.

Examination There may be localized joint line/margin tenderness and thickening and pain may be reproduced by overpressuring dorsiflexion or plantarflexion of the foot.

Treatment Passive movements to optimize ranges of movement (especially to dorsiflexion and plantarflexion) should be given together with electrotherapy and ice to treat any localized areas of pain and inflammation. Injections of local anaesthetic and corticosteroids may also be of help (Corrigan and Maitland, 1994).

6.7 REFERENCES

Albert, M. (1983) Descriptive three year data study of outdoor and indoor professional soccer injuries. *Athletic Training*, **18**, 218–220.

Allen, M.J. and Barnes, M.R. (1994) Chronic compartment syndromes. *Sports Exercise and Injury*, **9**, 36–40.

Anderson, B., Bealieu, J.E. and Cornelius, W.L. (1984) Roundtable: flexibility. *National Strength and Conditioning Association Journal*, **6**, 10–73.

Balduini, F.C. (1988) Abdominal and groin injuries in tennis. *Clinical in Sports Medicine*, 7(2), 349–357.

Barfred, T. (1973) Achilles tendon rupture. *Acta Orthopaedica Scandinavica Suppl.*, **152**, 1–126.

Baumhauer, J.F., Denise, M., Alosa D.M. *et al.* (1995) A prospective study of ankle injury risk factors. *American Journal of Sports Medicine*, **23**, 564–570.

Beard, D.J. (1994) Proprioception enhancement for ACL deficiency. A prospective randomised trial of two physiotherapy regimes. *Journal of Bone and Joint Surgery*, **76B**, 654–659.

Beaulieu, J.E. (1981) Developing a stretching programme. *Physical Sports Medicine*, **9**, 59–69.

Benazzo, F., Barnabei, G., Monti, G. and Ferrario, A. (1989) Current thinking on the pathogenesis, progression and treatment of muscle haematomas in athletes. *Italian Journal of Sports Traumatology*, **11**, 273–304.

Burroughs, P. and Dahners, L.E. (1990) The effect of enforced exercise on the healing of ligament injuries. *American Journal of Sports Medicine*, **18**, 376–378.

Butler, D.S. (1991) *Mobilisation of the Nervous System*, Churchill Livingstone, Edinburgh.

Carter, T.R., Fowler, P.J. and Blokker, C. (1992) Functional post operative treatment of Achilles tendon repair. *American Journal of Sports Medicine*, **20**, 459–462.

Cetti, R., Christensen, S.E., Ejsted, R. *et al.* (1993) Operative versus non operative treatment of Achilles tendon rupture. *American Journal of Sports Medicine*, **21**, 791–799.

Chard, M.D. and Jenner, J.R. (1988) The frozen hip: an underdiagnosed condition. *British Medical Journal*, **297**, 596–597.

Codman, E.A. (1934) *The Shoulder*, T. Todd, Boston, MA.

Coggan, A.R. (1992) Histochemical and enzymatic comparison of the gastrocnemius muscles of young and elderly men and women. *Journal of Gerontology*, **47**, B71–B76.

Conway, J.E., Jobe, F.W., Glousman, R.E. and Pink, M. (1992) Medial instability of the elbow in throwing athletes: treatment by repair or reconstruction of the ulnar collateral ligament. *Journal of Bone and Joint Surgery (Am)*, **74A**, 67–83.

Corrigan, B. and Maitland, G.D. (1994) *Musculoskeletal and Sports Injuries*, Butterworth-Heinemann, Oxford.

Crawford, A.H. (1988) Slipped capital femoral epiphysis. *Journal of Bone and Joint Surgery*, **(70)** 1422–1427.

Curwin, D. and Standish, E. (1984) *Tendinitis: Its Etiology and Treatment*, Heath and Co., Lexington, MA.

Daffner, R.H. and Pavlov, H. (1992) Stress fractures: current concepts. *American Journal of Roentgenology*, **159**, 245–252.

De Lee, J.C., Riley, J.B. and Rockwood, C.A. (1983) Acute straight lateral instability of the knee. *American Journal of Sports Medicine*, **11**, 404–411.

Doody, S.G., Freedman, L. and Waterland, J.C. (1970) Shoulder movements during abduction in the scapular plane. *Archives of Physical Medicine and Rehabilitation*, 595–604.

Doucette, S.A. and Goble, E.M. (1992) The effect of exercise on patellar tracking in lateral patellar compression syndrome. *American Journal of Sports Medicine*, **20**, 434–440.

Ekberg, O., Blomquist, P. and Ollson, S. (1981) Positive contrast herniography in adult patients with obscure groin pain. *Surgery*, 532–535.

Feagin, J.A., Levy, A.S., Linter, S.A. and Zorilla, P.A. (1995) Current concepts in anterior cruciate ligament surgery. *Sports Exercise and Injury*, **1**, 176–182.

Ficat, R.P. and Hungerford, D.S. (1977) *Disorders of the Patellofemoral Joint*. Williams & Wilkins, Baltimore, MD.

Fisher, S.E. and Shelbourne, K.D. (1993) Arthroscopic treatment of symptomatic extension block complicating anterior cruciate ligament reconstruction. *American Journal of Sports Medicine*, **21**, 558–564.

Fredricson, M., Bergman, A.G., Hoffman, K.L. and Dillingam, M.S. (1995) Tibial stress reaction in runners. *American Journal of Sports Medicine*, **23**, 472–481.

Fu, F.H., Woo, S.L.Y. and Irrgang, J.J. (1992) Current concepts for rehabilitation following anterior cruciate ligament reconstruction. *Journal of Orthopaedic and Sports Physical Therapy*, **15**, 270–278.

Fulkerson, J.P. and Shea, K.P. (1990) Current concepts review, disorders of patellofemoral alignment. *Journal of Bone and Joint Surgery*, **72A**, 1424–1429.

Gamble, J.G., Simmons, S.C. and Fredman, M. (1986) The symphysis pubis: anatomic and pathologic considerations. *Clinical Orthopaedics and Related Research*, **203**, 261–272.

Garrett, W.E., Callif, J.C. and Bassett, F.H. (1984) Histochemical correlates of hamstring injuries. *American Journal of Sports Injury*, **12**(2), 98–103.

Gauffin, H., Petterson, Y., Tegner, Y. and Tropp, H. (1990) Function testing in patients with old rupture of the ACL. *International Journal of Sports Medicine*, **11**, 73–77.

Gerrard, B. (1989) The patellofemoral pain syndrome: a clinical trial of the McConnell programme. *Australian Journal of Physiotherapy*, **35**, 71–80.

Giladi, M., Milgrom, C., Simkin, A. and Danon, Y. (1991) Stress fractures: identifiable risk factors. *American Journal of Sports Medicine*, **19**, 647–652.

Gilmore, O.J.A. (1993) Gilmore's groin: a previously unsolved problem in sportsmen, in *Intermittent High Intensity Exercise, Preparation Stresses and Damage*, (ed. MacLeod), E. & F. Spon, London, pp 477–486.

Glick, J.M. (1980) Muscle strains; prevention and treatment. *Physician and Sports Medicine*, **8(2)**, 73–77.

Glousman, R. (1993) Electromyographic analysis and its role in the athletic shoulder. *Clinical Orthopaedics and Related Research*, **288**, 27–34.

Gomez, M. and Woo, L.Y. (1989) The advantages of applied tension on healing medial collateral ligament. *Transactions of the Orthopaedic Research Society*, **14**, 184.

Gordon, H.M. (1975) Physiotherapy of muscle strains of the lower limb. *Physiotherapy*, **61**, 4.

Grace, T.G. (1985) Muscle imbalance extremity injury: a perplexing relationship. *Sports Medicine*, **2**, 77–82.

Grana, W.A. and Janssen, T. (1987) Lateral ligament injury of the knee. *Orthopaedic*, **10(7)**, 1039–1044.

Griffiths, H.J., Utz, R., Burke, J. *et al.* (1985) Adhesive capsulitis of the hip and ankle. *American Journal of Roentgenology*, **144**, 101–105.

Grimby, G. (1992) Clinical aspects of strength and power training, in *Strength and Power in Sport*, (ed. P. V. Komi), Blackwell, Oxford.

Hackney, R.G. (1993) The sports hernia: a cause of chronic groin pain. *British Journal of Sports Medicine*, **27**, 58–62.

Hawkins, R.J. (1987) Follow up of the non operated isolated ACL tear. *American Journal of Sports Medicine*, **14**, 205–210.

Hejna, W.F and Rosenberg, A. (1982) The prevention of sports injuries in high school students through strength training. *National Strength and Conditioning Association Journal*, **4**, 28–31.

Howe, J. and Johnson, R.J. (1982) Knee injuries in skiing. *Clinical Sports Medicine*, **1(2)**, 277–288.

Hughston, J.C. (1968) Subluxation of the patella. *Journal of Bone and Joint Surgery*, **50A**, 1003–1026.

Hunter, G. (1994) Specific soft tissue mobilisation of soft tissue lesions. *Physiotherapy*, **80**, 15–21.

Janda, V. and Schmid, H.J.A. (1980) Muscles as a pathogenic factor in back pain. *Proceedings of the International Federation of Orthopaedic Manipulative Therapists 4th Conference, New Zealand*, 17–18.

Jarvinen, M. (1994) Muscle injuries, in *Clinical Practice of Sports Injury Prevention and Care*. (ed. P. A. F. H. Renstrom), Blackwell, Oxford.

Johansson, H., Stolander, P. and Sojka, P.A. (1991) Sensory role for the cruciate ligaments. *Clinical Orthopaedics and Related Research*, **268**, 161–178.

Josza, L., Kvist, M. and Balint, B.J. (1989) The role of recreational sport activity in Achilles tendon rupture. *American Journal of Sports Medicine*, **17**, 338–343.

Jull, G.A. and Janda, V. (1987) Muscles and motor control in low back pain: assessment and management, in *Physical Therapy of the Low Back*, (ed. L.T. Twomey), Churchill Livingstone, Edinburgh.

Kamkar, A., Irrgang, J.J. and Whitney, S.L. (1993) Non operative management of secondary shoulder impingement syndrome. *Journal of Orthopaedic and Sports Physical Therapy*, **17(5)**, 212–224.

Kannus, P. and Jarvinen, M. (1987) Conservatively treated tears of the ACL long term results. *Journal of Bone and Joint Surgery*, **69A**, 1007–1012.

Kannus, P. and Josza, L. (1991) Histopathological changes preceding spontaneous rupture of a tendon. *Journal of Bone and Joint Surgery*, **73A**, 1507–1525.

Karlsson, J. and Faxen, E. (1994) Chronic ankle injuries, in *Clinical practice of Sports Injury Prevention and Care*, (ed. P. Renstrom), Blackwell Scientific Press, Oxford.

Karlsson, J., Sward, L., Kalebo, P. and Thomec, R. (1994) Chronic groin injuries in athletes: recommendations for treatment and rehabilitation. *Sports Medicine*, **17(2)**, 141–148.

Karst, G.M. and Jewett, P.D. (1993) Electromyographic analysis of exercise proposed for differential activation of medial and lateral quadriceps femoris muscle components. *Physical Therapy*, **73**, 286–299.

Keller, P.M., Shelbourne, K.D., McCarroll, J.R. and Rettig, A.C. (1993) Nonoperatively treated isolated posterior cruciate ligament injuries. *American Journal of Sports Medicine*, **21**, 132–136.

Kennedy, J.C., Alexander, I.J. and Hayes, K.C. (1982) Nerve supply of the human knee and its functional importance. *American Journal of Sports Medicine*, **10**, 329–335.

Kibler, W.B. and Chandler, T.J. (1993) Sport-specific screening and testing, in *Sports Injuries. Basic Principles of Prevention and Care*, (ed. P.A.F.H. Renstrom), Blackwell, Oxford.

Komi, P.V. and Bosco, C. (1979) Potentiation of the mechanical behaviour of human skeletal muscle through prestretching. *Acta Physiology Scandinavica*, **106**, 467–472.

Kornberg, C. and Lew, P. (1989) The effect of stretching neural structures on grade I hamstring injuries. *Journal of Orthopaedic and Sports Physical Therapy*, **June**, 481–487.

Kuo, C.Y., Louie, J.K. and Mote, C.D.J. (1983) Field measurements in snow skiing injury research. *Journal of Biomechanics*, **16**, 609–615.

Kupke, M.J., Kahler, D.M., Lorenzoni, M.H., and Edlich, R.F. (1993) Stress fracture of the femoral neck in a long distance runner: biomechanical aspects. *Journal of Emergency Medicine*, **11**, 587–591.

Kvitne, R.S. and Jobe, F.W. (1993) Diagnosis and treatment of anterior instability in the throwing athlete. *Clinical Orthopaedics and Related Research*, **291**, 107–123.

Landvatter, J. and Renstrom, P. (1992) Complete Achilles tendon ruptures. *Clinics in Sports Medicine*, **11**, 741–758.

Langergren, C. and Lindholm, A. (1958/59) Vascular distribution in the Achilles tendon. *Acta Chirurgica Scandinavica* 116, 491–495.

Larsen, B., Anderson, E., Urfer, A. *et al.* (1995) Patellar taping: a radiographic examination of the medial glide technique. *American Journal of Sports Injury*, **23**, 465–471.

Leadbetter, W.B. (1990) Corticosteroid injection therapy in sports injuries, in *Sports Induced Inflammation: Clinical and Basic Science Concepts*, (ed. W. B. Leadbetter), American Academy of Orthopaedic Surgery, New York.

Lehto, M., Duance, V.C. and Restall, D. (1985) Collagen and fibronectin in a healing skeletal muscle injury: an immunohistochemical study of the effects of physical activity on the repair of injured gastrocnemius muscle in the rat. *Journal of Bone and Joint Surgery*, **67B**, 820–828.

Li, G., Zhang, S. and Chen, G. (1985) Radiographic and histologic analyses of stress fracture in rabbit tibias. *American Journal of Sports Medicine*, **13**, 285–294.

Lifield, F.W. (1992) Can stroke modification relieve tennis elbow. *Clinical Orthopaedic*, **276**, 182–186.

Long, M.L., Frank, C., Schachar, N.S. and Dittrich, D. (1982) *The Effects of Motion on Normal and Healing Ligaments*, Orthopaedics Research Society, New Orleans, LA.

Lovell, G., Malycha, P. and Pieterse, S. (1990) Biopsy of the conjoined tendon in athletes with chronic groin pain. *Australian Journal of Science and Medicine in Sport*, **December**, 102–103.

McConnell, J.S. (1986) The management of chondromalacia patellae: a long term solution. *Australian Journal of Physiotherapy*, **32**, 215–223.

McConnell, J.S. (1987) Training the vastus medialis oblique in the management of patellofemoral pain, in *Proceedings of the 10th International Congress of the World Confederation of Physical Therapists, Sydney, Australia*, vol. 2, pp 412–415.

Mack, R.P. (1982) Ankle injuries in athletics. *Clinical Sports Medicine*, **1**, 71–84.

Mahler, F. (1992) Partial and complete ruptures of the Achilles tendon and local corticosteroid injections. *British Journal of Sports Medicine*, **26**, 7–14.

Maitland, G.D. (1991) *Peripheral Manipulation*, 3rd edn, Butterworth-Heinemann, Oxford.

Marans, H.J., Kennedy, D.K., Davanagh, T.C. and Wright, T.A. (1988) A review of intra articular knee injuries in racquet sports diagnosed by arthroscopy. *Canadian Journal of Surgery*, **31**, 199–201.

Marzo, J.M., Bowen, J.K., Warren, R.F. *et al.* (1992) Fibrous nodule as a cause of loss of extension following anterior cruciate ligament reconstruction. *Arthroscopy*, **8**, 10–18.

Moffroid, M and Whipple, R. (1970) Specificity of speed of exercise. *Physical Therapy*, **50**, 1692–1700.

Neer, C.S. (1983) Impingement lesions. *Clinical Orthopaedics*, **173**, 70–77.

Nicholl, J.P., Coleman, P. and Williams, B.T. (1991) *Injuries in Sport and Exercise*. Sports Council Fact Sheet, SC/169/5M/4/93.

Nillius, S.A., Nilsson, B. E. and Westlin, N.E. (1976) The incidence of Achilles tendon rupture. *Acta Orthopaedica Scandinavica*, **47**, 118–121.

Norris, C.M. (1993) Abdominal muscle training in sport. *British Journal of Sports Medicine*, **27**(1), 19–27.

Norris, C.M. (1995) Spinal stabilisation: muscle imbalance and the low back. *Physiotherapy*, **81**(3) 127–138.

Norwood, L.A., Shook, J.A. and Andrews, J.R. (1981) Acute medial elbow ruptures. *American Journal of Sports Medicine*, **9**, 16.

Oatis, C.A. (1990) Biomechanics of the hip, in *Physical Therapy of the Hip*, Churchill Livingstone, Edinburgh.

O'Brien, S.J., Neves, M. C., Arnoczky, S.P. and Warren, R.F. (1990) The anatomy and histology of the inferior glenohumeral ligament complex of the shoulder. *American Journal of Sports Medicine*, **18**, 449–456.

Ohkoshi, Y., Yasuda, K., Kaneda, K. *et al.* (1991) Biomechanical analysis of rehabilitation in the standing position. *American Journal of Sports Medicine*, **19**, 605–611.

Packer, G. (1995) Stress fractures in athletes. *Sports Exercise and Injury*, **1**(2), 64–69.

Palmitier, R.A., An, K.N., Scott, G. and Chao, E.Y.S. (1991) Kinetic chain exercise in knee rehabilitation. *Sports Medicine*, **11**, 402–413.

Peterson, L. and Renstrom, P. (1986) *Preventative Measures. in Sports Injuries: Their Prevention and Treatment*, (ed. W. A. Grana), Yearbook Medical Publishers, Chicago, IL.

Polglase, A.L., Frydman, G.M. and Farmer, K. C. (1991) Inguinal surgery for debilitating chronic groin pain in athletes. *Medical Journal of Australia*, **155**, 674–677.

Puddu, G., Ippolito, E. and Postacchini, F.A. (1976) Classification of Achilles tendon disease. *American Journal of Sports Medicine*, **4**, 145–150.

Puddu, G., Scala, A., Cerullo, G. *et al.* (1994) Achilles tendon injuries, in *Clinical Practice of Sports Injury Prevention and Care*, (ed. P. Renstrom), Blackwell Scientific Publications, Oxford.

Rappaport, E.B and Fife, D. (1985) Slipped capital femoral epiphysis in growth hormone deficient patients. *American Journal of Diseases in Children*, **139**, 396–399.

Regan, W., Woo, L.E., Coonrad, R. and Morrey, B.F. (1992) Microscopic histopathology of chronic refractory lateral epicondylitis. *American Journal of Sports Medicine*, **20**, 746–749.

Reid, D.C. (1992) *Sports Injury Assessment and Rehabilitation*, Churchill Livingstone, Edinburgh.

Renstrom, P. (1983) Muscle injuries in sport, in *Sports Medicine in Track and Field Athletics*. Proceedings of the First IAAF Medical Congress, Finland.

Renstrom, P. (1988) Diagnosis and management of overuse injuries, in *The Olympic Book of Sports Medicine*, (ed. A. Dirix), Blackwell Scientific Press, Oxford.

Renstrom, P. (1992) Tendon and groin injuries in the groin area. *Clinics in Sports Medicine*, **11**(4), 815–831.

Renstrom, P. and Peterson, L. (1980) Groin injuries in athletes. *British Journal of Sports Medicine*, **14**(1), 30–36.

Renstrom, P., An, M.S., Stanwick, T.S. *et al.* (1986) Strain within the ACL during hamstring and quadriceps activity. *American Journal of Sports Medicine*, **14**, 83–87.

Richardson, C.A. (1992) Muscle imbalance: principles of treatment and assessment. *Proceedings of the New Zealand Society of Physiotherapists Challenges Conference, Christchurch New Zealand.*

Sale, D. and MacDougal, D. (1981) Specificity in strength training. A review for the coach and athlete. *Canadian Journal of Applied Science*, **6**(2), 87–92.

Sallis, R.E. and Jones, K. (1991) Stress fractures in athletes. *Postgraduate Medicine*, **89**, 185–191.

Schenkman, M. and De Cartaya, V.R. (1987) Kinesiology of the shoulder complex. *Journal of Orthopaedic and Sports Physical Therapy*, **8**(9), 438–450.

Schultz, R.A., Miller, D.C., Kerr, C.S. and Micheli, L. (1984) Mechanoreceptors in human cruciate ligaments. A histological study. *Journal of Bone and Joint Surgery (American)*, **66**, 1072–1076.

Schutte, M.J., Dabezies, E.J., Zimny, M.L. and Happel, L.T. (1987) Neural anatomy of the anterior cruciate ligament. *Journal of Bone and Joint Surgery*, **69A**, 243.

Scranton, P.E and Farrar, E.L. (1992) Mucoid degeneration of the patellar ligament in athletes. *Journal of Bone and Joint Surgery (American)*, **74A**, 435–437.

Shelbourne, K.D. and Nitz, P. (1990) Accelerated rehabilitation after anterior cruciate ligament reconstruction. *American Journal of Sports Medicine*, **18**, 292–299.

Shelton, G.L. (1991) Rehabilitation of patellofemoral dysfunction: a review of literature. *Journal of Orthopaedic and Sports Physical Therapy*, **14**, 243–249.

Silvermetz, M.A. (1990) Pathokinesiology of supine double leg lifts as an abdominal strengthener and suggested alternative exercises. *Athletic Training*, **25**, 17–22.

Smedberg, S.G.G., Broome, A.E.A., Elmer, O. and Gullmo, A. (1985) Herniography in the diagnosis of obscure groin pain. *Acta Chiropody Scandinavica*, **151**, 663–667.

Sommer, H.M., Pauschert, R. and Thomsen, M. (1995) Functional treatment of ruptures of the fibular ligaments of the ankle from a medical and economic point of view. *Sports Exercise and Injury*, **1**, 76–82.

Stanton, P. and Purdam, C. (1989) Hamstring injuries in sprinting – the role of eccentric exercise. *Journal of Orthopaedic and Sports Physical Therapy*, **3**, 343–349.

Steinkamp, L.A., Dillingham, M.F., Market, M.D. *et al.* (1993) Biomechanical considerations in patellofemoral joint rehabilitation. *American Journal of Sports Medicine*, **21**, 438–444.

Stroyan, M. and Wilk, K.E. (1993) The functional anatomy of the elbow. *Journal of Orthopaedic and Sports Physical Therapy*, **17**, 279–288.

Styf, J.R. and Korner, L.M. (1986) Chronic anterior compartment syndrome of the leg. *Journal of Bone and Joint Surgery*, **68A**, 1338–1347.

Sullivan, M.K, Dejulia, J.J. and Worrell, T.W. (1992) Effects of pelvic position and stretching method on hamstring flexibility. *Medicine and Science in Sport and Exercise*, **24**, 1383–1389.

Taylor, D.C. and Bassett, F.H. (1993) Syndesmosis ankle sprains: diagnosing the injury and aiding recovery. *Physician and Sportsmedicine*, **21**, 39–46.

Thys, H. *et al.* (1972) Utilisation of muscle elasticity in exercise. *Journal of Applied Physiology*, **32**, 491–494.

Turnispeed, W., Detmer, D.E. and Girdley, F. (1989) Chronic compartment syndrome: an unusual cause for claudication. *Annals of Surgery*, **210**, 557–563.

Warner, J.P., Deng, X.H., Warren, R.F. and Torzilla, P.A. (1992) Static capsuloligamentous restraints to superior–inferior translation of the glenohumeral joint. *American Journal of Sports Medicine*, **20**, 675–685.

Warwick, R. and Williams, P.L. (eds.) (1973) *Gray's Anatomy*, 35th edn. Longman, Harlow.

Watrous, B.G. and Ho, G. (1988) Elbow pain. *Primary Care*, **15**, 725–735.

Wilk, K.E. and Arrigo, C. (1993) Current concepts in the rehabilitation of the athletic shoulder. *Journal of Orthopaedic and Sports Physical Therapy*, **18**(1), 365–378.

Wilkerson, G.B and Horn-Kingery, H.M. (1993) Treatment of the inversion ankle sprain: comparison of different modes of compression and cryotherapy. *Journal of Orthopaedic Sports Physical Therapy*, **17**, 240–246.

Worrell, T.W. and Perrin, D.H. (1992) Hamstring muscle injury: the influence of strength, flexibility, warm up and fatigue. *Journal of Orthopaedic and Sports Physical Therapy*, **16**, 12–18.

Yack, H.J., Collins, C.E. and Whieldon, T.T. (1993) Comparison of closed and open kinetic chain exercise in the anterior cruciate deficient knee. *American Journal of Sports Medicine*, **21**, 49–54.

7. Injuries in team sports

7.1 INTRODUCTION

The physical demands and stresses of each sport tends to result in certain injuries occurring with a greater or lesser frequency, and hence each sport has a particular injury profile. This can also be the case within a sport, where particular playing positions are vulnerable to certain types of injury because of their role within the game. The following chapter will discuss the injury profiles of a number of popular team sports and a list of the most common injuries is provided in the section on each sport. However the list cannot be totally comprehensive since almost any injury can occur in any sport and if more information is needed the reader should refer to the specific sections on diagnosis and treatment in Chapters 3–6. In this chapter a number of sports are sometimes linked together for the purpose of discussion because of their similar injury profiles.

A brief description of the physical nature of each sport included in this chapter is provided. This is not intended to be a detailed description of the sport's rules and how to play it, but simply to provide any therapist who is unfamiliar with the sport with an insight into its physical nature and hence the potential causes of injury. This can then be used by the practitioner or coach when considering how to rehabilitate the individual and minimize the risk of the injury recurring.

7.2 INJURIES IN RUGBY AND AMERICAN FOOTBALL

Both rugby and American football are aggressive physical contact sports involving frequent collisions between players and impact with the ground. The nature of the injuries that occur in these sports tend to reflect this aspect of the game and are often of a 'traumatic' nature (Figure 7.1). Within each sport, specific playing positions have particular tasks that influence their susceptibility to various injuries; thus a representative injury profile can be made up for the various playing positions.

7.2.1 The background to rugby football

There are two forms of rugby football: Rugby Union and Rugby League. In both games the overall objectives are similar, although some of the phases, such as rucks, mauls and line-outs, are not used in Rugby League. However, in general the over-riding similarities between the two games result in a similar pattern of injuries, enabling them to be discussed together.

In both codes of rugby points are scored by touching the ball down behind the opponent's try line (scoring a try) or kicking the ball over the bar between the goal posts. The latter may be achieved through a conversion after a try, a drop goal or a penalty goal. During the game the ball may be moved towards the opponent's try line by running with the ball or kicking it forwards. The ball can, however, only be passed backwards. A team's progress with the ball may be stopped by the opponents who will attempt to tackle the player in possession of the ball. In the interests of safety tackling can only occur below the neck and 'high' tackles are penalized. The general open play of running with the ball and passing is punctuated by various forms of play that result from a player being tackled, the ball going out of play

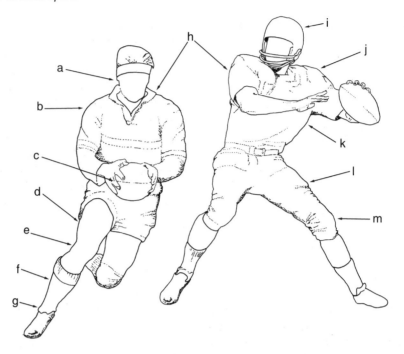

Figure 7.1 Common injuries occurring in rugby and American football.
(a) Orofacial Injuries. (b) Fractures to upper limbs, particularly the clavicle. (c) Stubbed fingers.
(d) Pulled hamstring muscles. (e) Knee ligament damage. (f) Pulled calf muscles. (g) Sprained ankle.
(h) Spinal injuries. (i) Concussion. (j) Dislocated shoulder. (k) Cracked ribs. (l) Bruised muscles from
collisions. (m) Knee meniscal damage.

or foul play resulting in a penalty. In the case of Rugby Union these phases of play include rucks, mauls and line-outs, during which each team attempts to obtain possession of the ball, thereby enabling them to progress further towards the opponent's goal. Both codes also use scrums, which again have the potential to cause injury. Each of these are discussed in more detail later, along with the injury risk that they present.

Minor injuries such as bruises and cuts are relatively common in rugby football due to the contact nature of the sport. However the game can also cause more serious injuries, especially to the head, neck and spine. It is suggested that the incidence of certain injuries has been on the increase due to a rise in foul play and recklessness within the game. Indeed, some authorities would suggest that

around 30% of injuries are caused by deliberate foul play. To combat this, rules are constantly being revised in order to protect the participants from deliberate or unintentional injury, the indications being that these changes have been successful in reducing the frequency of such injuries.

In rugby, injuries can occur to any part of the body, both the upper and lower body being affected. Examples include concussion, bruised muscles, dislocated shoulders, sprained ankles, torn knee cartilages, fractures of the clavicle, cracked ribs and orofacial and cervical spinal injuries. It is a feature of rugby football that protective clothing is restricted and typically only includes the quilting of the shirts which provides a slight amount of cushioning upon body contact, binding around the head to protect the ears (for forwards in the scrum), shin pads and mouthguards.

7.2.2 The occurrence of injuries in Rugby Union

In Rugby Union the type and incidence of injuries vary between playing positions and the phases of the game, with other factors such as the state of the pitch also contributing. On the pitch the players can be classified as either forwards or backs, each tending to participate in different phases of the game. The forwards tend to be ball winners who participate in phases such as scrums, line-outs, rucks and mauls. They are large, powerful individuals who are involved in close, aggressive play, such as pushing back opponents and trying to rip the ball from an opponent's possession. Such activities cause them to collide forcefully with the opposition and they can also be trodden on while on the ground. The backs or three-quarters tend to be slighter individuals whose function is to run with the ball or prevent the opposing backs from running with it. This makes them vulnerable to injury when tackled by the opposition or attempting to tackle them. Many of the injuries experienced by this group are therefore related to tackling and open play. In addition to this general division of players' roles, specialist positions such as front-row forwards are particularly vulnerable to injury in the 'scrum', while the scrum half and full back also have particular injury profiles due to the specialist nature of their playing positions.

7.2.3 Injuries related to phases of play in Rugby Union

(a) The kick-off

The kick-off is used to start the game at the beginning of each half and to restart the game after each score. The ball may be kicked as far as possible into the opponent's half or alternatively it may be kicked diagonally into the opponent's half towards the sideline, where both sets of forwards will compete for it. In the first instance the full back who catches a ball deep in his own half of the pitch may be struck by opponents charging after the ball. Such collisions, which may be legitimate or not, can result in injury to almost any part of the player's anatomy. In the latter case injuries can occur through the collision of opposing forwards, especially to the player who catches the ball, since s/he will attempt to turn and shield the ball from the opponents, making him/her susceptible to charges in the back.

(b) The maul

A maul occurs when the player carrying the ball is stopped but remains on his feet. When this happens s/he will attempt to turn away from his/her opponents, thus shielding the ball and making it available to his/her own players. Players from both sides will then form up on opposing sides of the player with the ball in an attempt to get the ball and/or push the player with the ball towards the opponent's try line. Players participating in the maul situation therefore tend to be the forwards, plus the player with the ball who may be a back. Players charging into the maul in a reckless or violent manner can cause injury to other players. Head and neck injuries can occur if the maul collapses into a pile.

(c) The scrum

The scrum is a set play involving both sets of eight forwards. Each set of forwards has a front row consisting of three players: a hooker and two prop forwards, who are positioned on either side of the hooker. The remaining forwards form up behind the front row in set positions. Each player is positioned with his back flexed so as to be parallel with the ground, enabling him/her to push against the player in front. Each player holds on to his neighbour by wrapping an arm around his/her body, which enables a tight binding of the pack. This, combined with the appropriate positioning of heads and linking with other players, produces a tight scrummaging unit that can drive forward in unison, pushing against the opposing pack. The opposing front rows of each pack are positioned with their heads alternating and push against the opposing front row with their shoulders. The ball is put into the scrum by the 'scrum half' and the front row attempts to hook it back with their feet. At the same time the opposing packs push against each, other attempting to drive the opponents backwards.

Injuries may occur in the scrum for a number of reasons: foul play may occur, where a player punches an opponent (the front-row forwards are especially vulnerable to this). Collapsing the scrum can also cause injuries, the back and neck being particularly at risk. Cervical spinal injuries caused by hyperflexion are of particular concern in rugby and may occur if the scrum collapses; deliberately collapsing the scrum is an offence. The binding of the forwards in the scrum can result in the outer ear experiencing a considerable friction/pressure, which can cause haematoma and the condition of 'cauliflower ear'. The kicking action used by front-row forwards attempting to direct the ball back through the scrum can also cause injury to the opposition (deliberate or otherwise) and shin pads are therefore essential for these players.

(d)   The ruck

A ruck takes place when the player in possession of the ball is grounded. In being grounded s/he must release the ball but in doing so will attempt to fall on the opponent's side of the ball, thus shielding it from them while making it available to his/her own players. In many respects the formation of a ruck is similar to the scrum but since it takes place in open play rather than being a set play, it is less organized and structured. The essence of the ruck is to drive the oppos-

ing players backwards, revealing the ball and thereby obtaining possession. In a ruck it is often the case that several players are grounded and it is these individuals who are most vulnerable to injury.

Injuries in the ruck can occur through aggressive or violent play as opponents attempt to obtain the ball. Deliberate foul play can also occur in this phase. Players may also be hurt as other players drive over them: injuries caused by studs are not uncommon, some of which may be deliberate. During a ruck players may also attempt to free the ball from the ruck by dragging it back with their boot; this can result in the 'raking' of opponents with the studs. In such aggressive play facial injuries and damage to the fingers can occur.

(e)   The line-out

In a line-out the ball is thrown in from the sideline between two rows of opposing forwards. The forwards will jump for the ball and either try to tip it back to their scrum-half or catch it. If they do catch the ball they will attempt to turn away from the opposing forwards and shield the ball, as in a maul. Injuries in the line-out may be due to elbowing opponents or players being hit while airborne and therefore falling awkwardly.

(f)   Tackling

Tackling is used to stop an opponent's forward progress. Tackles are only permitted on the player with the ball and must be below the neck. Typically the player making the tackle will attempt to envelope the opponent's body or legs with both arms. This may cause them to fall heavily. Poor tackling technique may injure both players. For example, when making a tackle around the legs the player should position his/her head behind the opponent's knees; positioning the head in front is likely to result in being kicked or kneed in the head.

When a player falls to the ground, an awkward fall may result in damage to the hand, arm or shoulder. The impact of collision may also cause damage to the menisci of the knee and/or ligaments of the knee and ankle. In this respect hard pitches that offer no give upon landing cause more injuries; furthermore hard pitches, which do not permit the foot to move upon collision but cause it to lock in the ground, are also likely to cause more injuries to the knees and ankles than soft pitches, which allow the foot to move.

7.2.4 Injuries associated with particular playing positions in Rugby Union

While all players are susceptible to injury a number of pieces of research indicate that the full back is the most vulnerable. The full back represents the last line of defence and therefore has to often make 'try saving' tackles. S/he also has to catch high balls kicked towards him/her; such catches are often made in the face of charging opponents. Of all the playing positions full backs are therefore most prone to injuries such as concussion.

The backs are prone to injury while being tackled or tackling; this may often occur at high speed and rapid explosive movements such as sidestepping can cause injury to the knee and ankle joints or the muscles of the legs. Tackling and collisions can also cause dislocation of the shoulder joint or fracture of the acromioclavicular joint.

Injury to the forwards may arise due to foul play in the scrum and rucks, facial and head injuries being more common in this group. Collapsing of the scrum can lead to neck and spinal injuries.

7.2.5 Injuries relating to the game of Rugby League

The injuries occurring in Rugby League are similar to those in Rugby Union since both are aggressive contact sports. However the two games differ in style, Rugby League not having rucks, mauls and line-outs. Instead, once a player with the ball is tackled and stopped, play is resumed by a simple tap back to a team mate who stands behind ready to receive the ball. Therefore, the injuries that occur in Rugby League tend to be associated with tackling rather than the other phases of play discussed in section 7.2.3.

7.2.6 Factors increasing the risk of injury in rugby football

Factors that increase the risk and/or severity of injury in rugby include the incidence of foul play, ground conditions, failure to wear protective mouthguards, lack of fitness and fatigue.

Perhaps the most unnecessary cause of injury in rugby is violent and/or reckless play, which is against the rules. Indeed many pieces of research attribute a substantial proportion of injuries to such incidents. It is therefore important for the rules to protect the participants, for referees to enforce the rules and for coaches to encourage fair play.

The condition of the pitch is also believed to have a significant influence on the incidence of injuries since a hard playing surface will result in a greater force of impact when a player strikes the ground and the number of upper limb and shoulder injuries is greater on hard surfaces than on soft muddy pitches. Similarly, a hard pitch may cause the studs to grip unyieldingly so that any impact or twisting movement experienced by the leg is more likely to result in knee or ankle damage than on soft muddy pitches, which tend to allow the foot to slide and provide less purchase for the studs, thereby reducing the risk of ankle and knee injuries.

Fitness is important in the game of rugby: a lack of strength may predispose the player to additional injury and a lack of stamina may cause premature fatigue, which results in an increased risk of injury in the later stages of a game. Physique may also be a consideration in minimizing the risk of injury; some authorities recommend that individuals with long necks should not play in the front row of the scrum, where neck injuries are more common. Skill is also a factor, as an unskilful player is more likely to injure both himself and his opponents. A lack of warm-up has also been suggested as a cause of injury since there is a tendency for some injuries such as pulled muscles to occur during the early stages of the game if the player is cold. This may be especially important for the kickers, who are prone to pull hamstring muscles.

Because of the contact nature of rugby the rules often need to be modified for use by children, but even with such modifications it is still important for opposing players to be equally matched as oversized opposition or teams of unequal ability can cause injury.

7.2.7   Injury prevention in rugby football

Injury prevention in rugby requires adherence to all the standard approaches of warming up, fitness, skill, appropriate opposition, adherence to the rules, appropriate clothing and protective equipment. In rugby the amount of protection permitted is minimal, with some quilting permitted in the shirts, taping to protect the forwards' ears from damage, shin pads and mouthguards. The last of these is a topic of much debate but in general the wearing of a well-fitting mouthguard is believed to reduce the incidence of orofacial injuries, including general dental damage, and to reduce the incidence of concussion, as it cushions any blow to the jaw.

Various changes in the rules have also been associated with a reduction in certain injuries, most notable being those related to the collapsing of the scrum, rucks and mauls, where the frequency of serious cervical spinal injuries has declined.

7.2.8   The background to American football

American football is an aggressive contact sport in which the objective of the game is for the offence of one team to carry the ball into the opposition's 'end zone' while the defence of the opposition attempts to stop them. It is also possible for teams to score points by kicking the ball over the bar between the goal posts. The ball may be moved forwards by throwing (restricted to one forward pass per 'play'), players running with the ball or, in some circumstances, kicking it (usually just before the team gives up possession of the ball to their opponents and hence wishes to place the ball as deep into the opponents' half as possible). In general terms each team in American football is divided into an offence (which attempts to score points) and a defence (which attempts to prevent the opposing team from scoring points); these two components of any team are not on the pitch at the same time. Instead the offence of a team is on the pitch when the team is in possession of the ball, at which time it will confront the defence of the opposing team. When the ball changes possession the offence and defence of each team swap. In addition to this general set-up of offence and defence, there are a number of specific situations where a team may use a 'special team', consisting of specialist players; examples occur when returning a kick-off or when trying to block an opponent's kick at goal.

The rules of American football are complex but in general terms each 'play' during the game involves members of opposing teams facing each other across the pitch. The ball is placed between the two lines of players, which form the offensive line and defensive line. The team in possession of the ball then passes it back to their quarterback, who either throws the ball to one of his team, hands it to one of them or runs with it himself. In all cases the player with the ball attempts to run as far down the field as possible before being stopped by the opposition. In the initial stages of each 'play' members of the defence will try to tackle the quarterback with the ball while the members of the offence try to protect him. This therefore involves a considerable number of collisions and vigorous contact. In the later stages of a 'play' the player with the ball is liable to be tackled by the defence and is also therefore prone to aggressive collisions with the opposition.

In simplistic terms the offence of a team includes:

- **the quarterback**, whose function is to receive the ball each play and then pass it to other members of the offence;
- **offensive linemen**, who try to protect the quarterback, enabling him to pass the ball; these individuals therefore need to be large and strong to fend off the attempts of the defensive linesmen to tackle the quarterback;
- **wide receivers**, who run downfield and catch the ball thrown by the quarterback; these are therefore fast, agile individuals capable of great speed;
- **running backs**, who receive the ball from the quarterback and then try to charge through the defensive line; these individuals are therefore fast, powerful and agile but, because of the need to resist the tackles of the defensive line, they tend to be larger than the wide receivers.

The players of the defence include:

- **defensive linemen**, who try to tackle the quarterback and/or stop the progress of the offensive running back should they receive the ball; these individuals must be large and fast in order to beat the offensive linemen and catch the quarterback or running back;
- **safeties, corners** and other defensive players; these form the secondary and last line of defence – they will try to tackle the wide receivers should they receive the ball or alternatively they will try to catch the ball themselves or knock it away from the receivers if this is not possible. If a running back should break through the defensive line, defenders in

the secondary area of defence will attempt to tackle him.

In an attempt to minimize the risk of injury in American football a considerable amount of protective clothing has been developed. This includes padding, taping, mouthguards and the compulsory use of helmets. However the use of such clothing has enabled the players to be more aggressive in their contact which can result in additional injury. Another factor relating to injury in American football is the use of artificial surfaces by some teams. These permit the studs or cleats to grip the surface firmly, enabling the players to accelerate rapidly and make sudden changes in direction. However, this means that, when a player changes direction or is struck, his foot may remain locked in position on the pitch and hence any lateral or rotational forces may be transferred to the knee or ankle, causing injury.

7.2.9 The occurrence of injuries in American football

Injuries in American football include sprains, strains, fractures, dislocations, concussion, contusions and others, such as damage to the eyes. As with rugby football the injuries of most concern are the life-threatening and disabling injuries to the head, neck and spine. The sites of injury are similar to those in rugby, almost any area of the body being vulnerable.

Ankle and knee injuries may occur either in contact or non-contact situations. As mentioned previously the playing surface is sometimes implicated, artificial surfaces that do not permit the foot to slide or rotate being blamed for a number of such injuries. Non-contact ankle and knee injuries may occur when the player rapidly changes direction, such as when attempting to avoid a tackle. This situation may be made worse when the player is struck by an opponent; in such cases, if the foot is unable to move, the force of the tackle may injure the ankle or knee. Damage to the joints can include torn ligaments and cartilages. To reduce the risk of such injuries some authorities advocate the use of shoes with shorter cleats.

Upper-body injuries can occur through collisions with other players or the ground and can include contusions, fractures and dislocations. Additional injuries may occur if the player receives a finger in the eye; some players use eye guards or shields to prevent this. The kicker is a very specialist player who must be very flexible, especially in terms of hip flexion, because of the demands of kicking. Tight or cold hamstrings in these players will therefore predispose them to injury.

In addition to the injuries received through contact with other players the quarterback may also develop overuse injuries of the elbow and shoulder due to repeated throwing of the ball.

7.2.10   The prevention of injuries in American football

In addition to the protective clothing worn by American footballers there are strict rules concerning the tackling of opponents. These are devised to minimize the risk of serious neck and spinal injuries. Warming up and fitness are key issues, as is the compatibility of the opposition. Due to its aggressive nature, injuries in American football are common; fortunately most of these are minor and the player can return to full participation within a few weeks. However, despite the use of helmets, mouthguards and the rules associated with contact, serious injuries do occur, including a number of fatalities each year. It is therefore important that all those associated with the game take the utmost precautions to minimize the risk of such occurrences.

7.3   INJURIES IN BASKETBALL

Basketball is theoretically a non-contact sport, but incidental contact between players does

sometimes occur and can result in injury. Another common cause of injury is mistimed catches, causing stubbed fingers. Additionally, the rapid changes in direction that are required in the game predispose players to sprained ankles and damaged knee ligaments. Furthermore, the repeated explosive move-

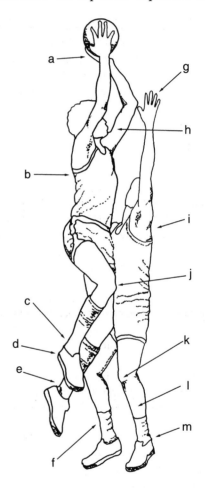

Figure 7.2   Common injuries occurring in basketball. (a) Fractures to arm and wrist. (b) Bruising to torso and cracked ribs. (c) Achilles tendinitis. (d) Bruised heels. (e) Sprained ankles. (f) Periostitis of the tibia. (g) Stubbed fingers. (h) Dental injuries. (i) Dislocations of shoulder. (j) Patellar tendinitis (jumper's knee). (k) Meniscal and ligament injuries to the knee. (l) Stress fractures of the tibia. (m) Ruptured Achilles tendons.

ments associated with jumping in basketball can also cause overuse injuries of the Achilles tendon and knee. Falls on to the hard ground can result in abrasions and knee pads are commonly used to minimize such injuries (Figure 7.2).

7.3.1 Background to the game of basketball

Basketball is a game involving two teams, each of up to 10 players but with only five players from each team on the court at any time. Substitutions are permitted throughout the game and are used to provide players with a chance to recover from the exertions of the game as well as for tactical reasons. The objective of the game is for players to score points by shooting the ball through the basket (a netted hoop suspended 3.15 m above the ground). Positioned behind the basket is a backboard, which may be used to rebound the ball off when shooting. In order to achieve a good shooting position the players may pass the ball to one another or dribble with it. The rules do not permit players to move into a space that is already occupied by another player, which should effectively prevent any body contact; however, in reality collisions do occur quite frequently.

Typical basketball injuries include stubbed fingers from misjudging the flight of the ball, contusions caused by collisions (often due to elbows when contesting a rebounding ball), abrasions caused by falls, strained Achilles tendons from repetitive jumping, and sprained ankles and damaged knees due to rapid turns and changes of direction.

The five players on a basketball team are typically made up of two guards, two forwards and one centre. Each of these positions fulfils a slightly different role during a game and their roles vary depending upon what kind of offence or defence the team is using. Essentially all players on the field will be involved in the offence when their team possess the ball and likewise all the players of a team will be involved in defence when the opposition has the ball. However, the general role of the guards is to defend under the basket and then pass or dribble the ball out from defence. The forwards attack the opponents' basket from the sides, often shooting from the corners and contesting rebounded balls when on the attack. The centre defends in a central position and attempts to get close to the opponents' basket when attacking; the centre must also contest rebounds. In reality the specific role of each player varies depending upon the kind of offence and defence being used by both teams, any difference in the emphasis of these roles making a particular player more or less vulnerable to particular types of injury.

The game of basketball can be divided into two key phases: offence and defence. The type of offence and defence used by a team dictates the types of offence and defence used by the opponents, each team altering its style of offence and defence throughout the game. The purpose of defence is to prevent the opposing team from scoring and to obtain possession of the ball. This may be achieved by the defenders forming a defensive zone around their basket or marking their opponents on an individual basis (man-to-man defence). The object of offence is to manoeuvre into a good shooting position from which to score a basket. This may be achieved by players attacking rapidly as soon as they have obtained possession of the ball or alternatively a more controlled and deliberate attacking move may be developed using practised manoeuvres.

7.3.2 The causes of injuries in basketball

In basketball, injuries may be caused in a variety of situations, including:

- falling;
- contact with another player;
- jumping or landing;
- contact with the ball;
- rapid movement or changes in direction.

Often a number of these circumstances occur together, as when players collide while jumping for a ball. This causes considerable overlap in the discussion of how injuries occur and the topic is covered accordingly.

(a) Injuries caused by falling

Since basketball is played on a hard surface any fall has the potential to cause injury. Falls may occur as a result of collisions or tripping. Most of the injuries that occur in this situation are minor, in the form of abrasions and contusions, the elbows and knees being particularly vulnerable. However if players strike their heads then concussion is possible or, alternatively, if they attempt to break their fall with their arms then fractures and dislocations can occasionally result.

Some of the most serious injuries of this kind occur if a player collides with another while airborne. This may cause the player to fall in an uncontrolled manner from a considerable height, with spinal and head injuries being possible. These injuries are discussed further in section 7.3.2(c). Occasionally, an injury may occur when two players both have possession of the ball and both have a strong grip on it. This should be resolved with a 'jump ball' but vigorous attempts to wrest the ball from the opponent's grasp may result in one player falling or may even causing damage to the fingers as the ball is forced from the player's grip.

(b) Injuries caused by contact with another player

Injuries caused by contact with other players can occur in numerous situations, including collisions both in general play, where players run into one another, and in specific phases of the game such as a rebounding ball. This latter phase of the game can be particularly hazardous, as airborne players may be knocked off balance and land awkwardly. The accidental or deliberate use of the knees and elbows can also contribute to injury when contesting a rebounding ball. Injuries from such contact vary from minor bruising to fractured ribs and broken teeth. Fortunately, more serious injuries such as fractures to the wrist and arm, dislocations of the shoulder and injuries to the head and spine, which can occur on landing, are relatively rare. Other injuries that occur include stubbed or dislocated fingers from contact with another player and eye injuries when players receive a finger in the eye.

(c) Injuries caused by jumping or landing

When players jump for the basket, as in the case of attempting a 'dunk' or lay-up shot, any contact in the air may cause them to fall awkwardly. Indeed, one of the potentially most dangerous situations in the game is when the lower part of an airborne player's body is struck, as this will cause the player to rotate in the air. In such situations the player may be spun into a horizontal position several feet up in the air, from which they will fall in an uncontrolled manner. The most serious injuries occurring in such situations are to the head and spine, with injuries to the wrist, hand, arm and shoulder also being possible on landing. If such fouls occur while a player is in the act of shooting it is commonly referred to as 'bridging'.

Contests for a rebounding ball also provide the potential for injury, with the accidental or deliberate use of the elbows being the cause of facial injuries and contusions to the upper body, including broken ribs and teeth. Raising the knee while jumping can also injure opponents, causing contusions and/or cracked ribs.

During a game players will repeatedly produce explosive movements such as jumping and also experience the subsequent forceful impact of landing on a hard surface, both of which put considerable stress on the ankles, knees, feet and lower leg. Common overuse injuries in basketball include Achilles tendinitis, patellar tendinitis (jumper's knee), bruised heels, periostitis and stress fractures to the tibia. A rupture of the Achilles tendon may also occur during jumping, especially if there are underlying factors of overuse and degeneration. Periostitis of the medial margin of the tibia (commonly referred to as 'shin splints') may be caused by the stress of repeatedly jumping off a hard surface while stress fractures of the tibia can be caused by the repeated stress of impact on landing. In any jumping situation, if the player's foot lands at an awkward angle it can result in ankle sprains or even fractures.

(d) Injuries caused by contact with the ball

Due to the speed at which the basketball may be passed and its weight (0.62 kg) it has the potential to cause injuries to the fingers and face should a catch be misjudged. 'Stubbed' fingers are a common result of this, joint dislocation being another possibility. This type of incident can occur either when receiving a pass or when jumping for a ball. Traumatic joint compression may cause synovitis (inflammation with swelling and stiffness) in the phalangeal or metacarpophalangeal joints. These tend to be the most common hand injuries, with ruptures of the ligaments of the finger and thumb accounting for most of the remainder. Hand injuries are considered to account for between 10% and 15% of basketball injuries.

(e) Injuries caused by rapid movement or changes in direction

In basketball the rapid acceleration and changes of direction that are required can cause injuries to the ankle and knee; a number of studies report the ankle as being the site of 20–30% and the knee of 14–40% of all injuries occurring in basketball. The risk of injury to the ankles and knees may be increased if the friction between the shoe and floor is too great. While this may permit more abrupt stopping, it exposes the lower leg to greater stress; this may be increased by the use of resin on the shoes. In the case of a sprained ankle it is usually the lateral ligament complex that is damaged and in an attempt to reduce the incidence of such injuries some individuals prefer to use 'high-top boots', which provide the ankle with more support. However it is argued by some authorities that on occasions, while this style of basketball boot may protect the ankle, any rotational forces that would normally be experienced by the ankle are transferred to the knee, causing more serious injury to that joint. The types of knee injury that can occur through excessive rotation or collision include damage to the meniscus and torn ligaments (cruciate, lateral and medial).

7.3.3 Injuries related to playing position

Because of the overall similarity in their roles, all players are susceptible to all the different forms of injury discussed, but a number of studies have indicated that forwards receive the most injuries to the upper body, possibly because of their role in rebounding.

7.3.4 Factors for consideration in injury prevention

The explosive nature of basketball makes it essential for all players to warm up adequately; failure to do so risks injury to cold muscles and tendons, which tear more easily. Keeping warm and flexible is also a consideration for players who are on the substitutes' bench waiting to return to the game. Coaches should therefore ensure that the team arrives in plenty of time for a warm-up and that those on the bench are kept in an adequate state of physical readiness to return to the game.

Collisions with the equipment around the court represents an unnecessary source of injury. It should therefore be ensured that all surplus equipment is removed and that there is adequate space around the edge of the court for the game to be played safely, the distance between the edge of the court and the wall being a major consideration. Courts must be kept in good condition: dusty and slippery floors may cause injury and in this respect any wet patches caused by sweat should be dried immediately.

Protective clothing such as knee and elbow pads may be recommended, while the use of high-top boots, which are advocated to reduce the incidence of ankle injuries but are reported at the same time to increase the incidence of knee injuries, should be considered carefully. The taping of the ankle and other joints may also be advocated by some to prevent sprains and in some cases injured fingers may be taped to adjacent digits to prevent further injury. The wearing of inappropriate clothing and jewellery such as rings, bracelets and earrings should not be permitted because of the additional injury risk it represents.

The strict enforcement of the rules should reduce the risk of injury from both accidental and deliberate fouls. A responsible attitude to play must always be enforced by referees, coaches and players, since deliberate fouls and aggressive or violent play can have serious consequences. The development of appropriate skills is also a consideration, as many players claim to receive more injuries in matches against unskilful and clumsy players than in those against players of a higher skill level.

The possession of a previous injury and a lack of appropriate fitness are also considered to be contributing factors, for which both the coach and physiotherapist must take some responsibility in deciding whether an individual is fit to play.

7.4   INJURIES IN NETBALL

7.4.1   Background to the game of netball

In many respects the physical demands of netball are similar to those of basketball and

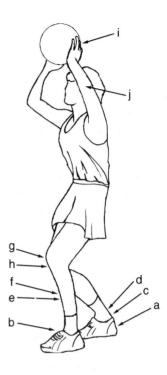

Figure 7.3 Common injuries occurring in netball. (a) Bruised heels. (b) Sprained ankles. (c) Ruptured Achilles tendon. (d) Achilles tendonitis. (e) Periostitis of the tibia (shin splints). (f) Stress fracture of the tibia. (g) Knee injury damage to the meniscus and torn ligaments. (h) Patellar tendinitis (jumper's knee). (i) Stubbed fingers. (j) Fractures to the arm and wrist.

therefore result in a similar injury profile (Figure 7.3).

Netball is a non-contact sport and injurious contact is uncommon; however, as in basketball, injuries may be caused by the rapid changes in direction required in the game, with sprained ankles and damaged knee ligaments occurring along with stubbed fingers from mistimed contact with the ball or another player. Points are scored in netball when players shoot the ball through a netted hoop 15 inches (38 cm) in diameter and positioned 10 feet (2 m) above the ground on a vertical post. Players are not permitted to run with the ball but must pass it in order to move it down the court. A netball team consists of seven players, each of whom has a specific role and whose range of movement is restricted to specific areas of the court.

The physical nature of the game requires the players to move quickly in order either to get in a position where they can receive the ball or, when the opposition has the ball, to try to stay close to their opponent in order to prevent them from receiving the ball. Hence the game requires rapid acceleration, changes of direction, abrupt stopping, fast passing and an ability to catch the ball, which may be thrown in a number of ways. The netball court is divided into thirds by two lines extending across the pitch and within the two end thirds are semicircles called the goal circles. During the game each player wears a top on which are letters that identify her playing position. The playing positions in netball are as follows: goal shooter (GS), goal attack (GA), wing attack (WA), centre (C), wing defence (WD), goal defence (GD) and goalkeeper (GK). The nature of the game is such that each playing position has an opposing player who will spend virtually the entire match with her. These playing positions are therefore discussed in pairs. While the descriptions given below briefly outline the roles of each player, they are of course a simplification since, when defenders such as the wing defence or goal defence receive the ball they will have to assume an attacking role and pass the ball to their team-mates and conversely those players who fulfil an attacking role while in possession of the ball will have to defend when the opposition has possession, for example by trying to prevent the opposition from passing the ball out of defence and by trying to regain possession by intercepting a pass.

(a)   The goal shooter and goalkeeper

The goal shooter's function is to score goals. Her movements are restricted to the third of the court in which the opponent's goal is situated and she will spend almost the entire match within the goal circle in close proximity to the goal. The role of the goalkeeper is to mark the goal shooter; she therefore has to prevent the goal shooter from receiving the ball and to prevent her from scoring. Her movements are also restricted to this third of the pitch, including the goal circle that contains the goal she is defending.

(b)   Goal attack and goal defence

Like the goal shooter the main role of the goal attack is to score goals. However she has a wider range of movement, which includes the centre third of the court as well as the third containing the opponent's goal. She is also permitted into the goal circle, within which she may shoot or pass the ball. Often she will 'feed' the ball to the goal shooter during an attack and may sometimes act as a decoy in order to free the goal shooter for a pass. The goal defence marks the goal attack, her function being to prevent the goal attack from receiving the ball and shooting. Her areas of movement therefore enable her to shadow the goal attack, as she is permitted in both the centre third and the third containing her team's goal (including the goal circle).

(c)   Wing attack and wing defence

The wing attack is permitted in the centre third of the court and the third containing the opponents' goal, but not within the goal circle. In order to fulfil her role the wing defence has a similar range of movement, which includes the centre third and the third containing the goal she is defending (again excluding the goal circle). The role of the wing attack is to pass the ball upfield, often linking with the defenders, centre and attackers of her team, one of her most important roles being to pass the ball to the goal shooter when she is in a good shooting position. The role of the wing defence is therefore to prevent such passing through close marking of the wing attack.

(d) Centre

The centres from each team have the greatest range of movement since they are permitted in all areas of the court except the goal circles. When her team is attacking the centre will tend to receive passes from the defenders and pass the ball on to the attackers, the goal shooter and goal attack. She therefore provides the link between the team's defenders and attackers; however when the opposition possess the ball she will assume a defensive role in marking the opposing centre.

7.4.2   Injuries occurring in netball and their prevention

In netball, injuries occur primarily in the same way as they do in basketball, i.e. through:

- falling;
- contact with another player;
- jumping or landing;
- contact with the ball;
- rapid movement or changes in direction.

Therefore, while certain aspects of the game may differ, it is possible to refer to the section on basketball injuries for details on typical netball injuries. For example, falling on a hard surface through loss of balance and tripping can cause abrasions; the rapid twisting, turning, jumping, landing and abrupt stopping can cause similar injuries in terms of the ankle and knee (both traumatic and overuse); mistimed catches can cause damage to the fingers and contact with another player may lead to contusions. However, because of the restrictions limiting the movement of players around the court, many of the injuries are less frequent as a result of the reduced opportunity for collisions and crowding. This may be particularly significant around the goal where the number of players is limited to four; this reduces the likelihood of injurious contact when contesting a high pass or missed shot. Furthermore, while players may jump for a high ball the fact that they are not permitted to jump while shooting may be a major factor in the reduced frequency of injury.

7.5   INJURIES IN SOCCER

7.5.1   Background to the game of soccer (association football) and the causes of injury

In soccer most injuries occur through contact with another player; others are caused by contact with the ball or ground, and the remainder result from excessive strain being placed upon a body part, e.g. when straining a muscle or twisting a joint beyond its normal range of movement. The relative incidence of soccer injuries, excluding minor injuries such as bruising and abrasions, is between 10 and 20 per 1000 playing hours (Figure 7.4).

The game itself involves two teams of 11 players who attempt to score goals by getting the ball into the opponents' goal, primarily by heading or kicking it. The ball is moved towards the opponents' goal by dribbling (running with the ball while controlling it with the feet) and passing (kicking or heading the ball towards a team-mate). Only the goalkeeper of each team, who normally provides the last line of defence, is permitted to touch the ball with the hands and in the process of defending the goal will punch, catch and 'handle' the ball within a specified area around it. For the remaining players, touching the ball with the hands or arms constitutes an offence. Opposing players attempt to dispossess players of the ball by tackling them. When tackling or challenging for the ball a player must 'go for the ball' and not the opposing player. Deliberately pushing or kicking an opponent constitutes foul play, as does an unintentional but unskilful challenge or tackle that risks injury to the opponent.

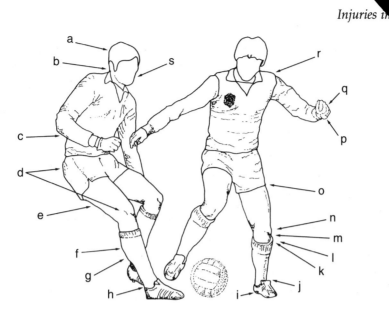

Figure 7.4 Common injuries occurring in soccer. (a) Concussion. (b) Orofacial injuries. (c) Fractures to the lower arm. (d) Avulsion fractures, Osgood–Schlatter's disease. (e) Strained hamstrings, quadriceps and adductors. (f) Bruised and strained calf muscles. (g) Bruising and fractures of the fibula. (h) Achilles tendon injury. (i) Fractures to bones of the foot. (j) Ankle sprains. (k) Dislocated patella. (l) Knee cartilage damage. (m) Knee ligament damage. (n) Myositis ossificans. (o) Bruising to thigh muscles. (p) Damage to hand and wrist. (q) Dislocation and fracture of fingers. (r) Dislocations of the shoulder. (s) Dental injuries.

Incidental contact frequently occurs in soccer, but provided that it is not violent and does not deliberately impede the opponent it may or may not be penalized by the referee depending upon the circumstances. Incidental and deliberate contact between players is the single most common cause of injury in soccer.

Within each team players are given specific roles, being designated attackers, midfield players, defenders and the goalkeeper. The goalkeeper fulfils a specialized role and is distinguished from the other players on the team by wearing a different-coloured top. Although the goalkeepers are permitted access to the entire pitch their role tends to require them to remain in close proximity to their own goal. Conversely, while the remaining players may be allocated specific roles within the team, they can all play as defenders, midfield players or attackers depending upon the circumstances of the game and the current phase of play. For example all players may fulfil a defensive role when the team is defending although some players may remain nearer to the opponents' goal ready for a quick attack once their team regains possession of the ball. Likewise, any player may attempt to score a goal, although specific players within the team will have that specialized role and train specifically for that purpose. The exception to these interchanging roles is the goalkeeper: only one is permitted on each team at any one time. The specialized role of the goalkeeper can make him/her more vulnerable to certain types of injury as s/he defends the goal, the details of which are discussed later.

The methods of tackling an opponent and physically contesting possession of the ball are restricted by rules that aim to ensure the safety of the players. However, these contests

urce of injury and ref-
o punish 'dangerous'
umber of sources the
injury are the ankles,
Injuries to the feet,
head do occur, but
e sites of injury are
th reference to the
, iry and their preven-
tion.

(a) Injuries to the head and neck

These injuries are most frequently due to contact with another player's head, elbow, fist or foot. Contact with the ball or goal posts may also be the cause in some cases. Injuries to this region of the body include cuts, abrasions, nose bleeds, dental injuries, concussion, ocular injuries and fractures of the bones of the face. Most of these will require immediate first aid, or hospitalization in the case of the more severe injuries. Head injuries commonly occur in crowded 'goalmouth' situations where several players contest for the ball. For example, as players jump for a high ball they may collide with their heads or in some cases a goalkeeper attempting to punch the ball away may make contact with another player. When jumping, players will often raise their elbows and in doing so may make contact with another player, intentionally or unintentionally. A further common cause of head injury is when the ball is travelling at chest height or bounces to that height. This may result in one player attempting to kick the ball as another attempts to head it thereby causing injury to the latter.

Goalkeepers tend to be more vulnerable to head injuries than other players as they will often have to dive at players' feet in order to retrieve the ball. Injuries to the neck occasionally occur when a player falls awkwardly, often as a result of a midair collision. Neck injuries resulting from the ball striking the head are also possible. Fortunately, these severe injuries are relatively rare.

(b) Injuries to the hands, arms and torso

Injuries to the hands are more frequent in goalkeepers because of their unique role in being able to handle the ball. A mistimed catch, parry or punch of the ball can cause a dislocation or fracture of the fingers. Likewise, the wrist is vulnerable if an attempted punch is mistimed. If a player falls awkwardly or from some height s/he may damage the wrist, lower arm or shoulder as s/he extends the arm to cushion the impact of the fall. Injuries occurring through such incidents include dislocations of the shoulder and fractures to the lower arm.

Injury to the torso can occur if a player is kicked while challenging for a ball a few feet off the ground; this can cause bruising or in extreme cases damage to the internal organs such as the kidneys. Another cause of torso injury is when the goalkeeper raises the knee while jumping to catch the ball. This represents a risk of injury to other players around him/her and may be penalized as 'dangerous play' by the referee.

An additional source of injury to the torso, head and neck is when players are struck by a rapidly moving ball. This can occur when they attempt to block a shot at goal. The most frequent situation in which this occurs is when one side are awarded a 'free kick'. The attacking team will often use this opportunity to take a shot at the goal if it is in range and a number of defenders from the opposing team will therefore line up 10 yards (9 m) away, forming 'a wall', in an attempt to block the direct line between the ball and goal. In such situations the defenders will protect their genitals with their hands. However all parts of their bodies will still be vulnerable to the violently struck ball which may be kicked at them with as much force as possible by an attacking player.

(c) Injuries to the upper leg

Injuries to the upper leg are commonly caused by kicks, which result in bruising to the thigh muscles, sometimes referred to as a 'dead leg'. If the blow is severe and the muscle is compressed against the underlying bone with sufficient force, bone cells may flake off into the damaged muscle. These may later develop and cause the condition of myositis ossificans.

Other common injuries to the upper leg include strained muscles of the hamstrings, quadriceps and adductors, which are commonly caused by overstretching when attempting to reach a ball or tackling an opponent. Another cause of pulled muscles is when sprinting, especially if it is cold and/or the player has not warmed up sufficiently.

(d) Injuries to the knee

In soccer the knee is often reported as the most common site for serious injury. Most injuries to the knees are caused by collisions, violent twisting movements or a blow to the side, all of which can violently overstretch the ligaments and damage the cartilages. These types of injury are more likely to occur if the victim's foot is fixed to the ground by his/her studs, thereby preventing any movement of the foot upon collision. Such injuries are therefore not surprisingly reported to be more common when playing on artificial surfaces, which provide a greater degree of traction. Likewise, if a player's foot remains fixed as s/he attempts to turn rapidly it will result in a violent twisting movement at the knee, which can cause damage to the cruciate ligaments and knee cartilages. Muddy pitches permit a degree of slippage and may therefore reduce the risk of these types of injury, although they may increase the risk of others. Another knee injury that occurs occasionally is dislocation of the patella, which may be dislodged if kicked.

(e) Injuries to the lower leg, ankle and foot

The most common injuries to the lower leg are caused by kicks during tackles. To protect the front of the leg players wear shin-pads although, despite this, on occasions severe bruising and fractures to the lower leg may occur, particularly to the fibula. Other injuries to the lower leg include pulled calf muscles when jumping or accelerating and bruised calf muscles if kicked from behind. The Achilles tendon is also vulnerable to injury from kicks or from tearing when jumping.

Other ankle injuries that are relatively common in soccer include sprained ankles due to a player 'going over' on the ankle when landing or changing direction. Such injuries are liable to damage the lateral ligaments of the ankle and can also cause compression damage on the medial side.

Fractures to the bones of the feet may occur from violent kicks or repeated overuse; the latter causes stress fractures. The repeated hyperextension and/or hyperflexion of the ankle can cause damage at the site where the joint capsule joins the bone and result in small bony growths. Severe traumatic fractures occasionally occur when a player falls upon an opponent's leg.

7.5.2 Soccer injuries in children

The smaller body mass of children makes them less vulnerable to certain forms of collision injury. However, their immature bodies can make them more vulnerable to others. For example, blows to the long bones may cause epiphyseal fractures, which will require surgery, and too much kicking of the ball can place excessive stress on the region below the knee where the quadriceps tendon inserts with the tibia, resulting in Osgood–Schlatter's disease. Avulsion fractures are also reported more commonly in children than in adults.

7.5.3 The prevention of soccer injuries

The prevention of injuries in soccer requires good refereeing, which ensures adherence to the rules and the prevention of dangerous play. Violent challenges and reckless tackling are the main causes of severe preventable injuries. The pitch conditions are also a factor, with hard pitches that are either frozen in winter or baked hard in summer increasing the risk of injury when players hit the ground. Conversely, if the pitch is too wet and muddy, players may not be able to stop and change direction effectively, hence increasing the risk of collisions. Ensuring that the pitch is fit to use and free of debris and faeces is also a consideration, and this can be a significant problem on public pitches, especially if dogs are exercised on them.

A player's fitness is also a major factor in injury prevention, since tight, unfit muscles are more prone to damage, as are players who are not fully recovered from a previous injury. In the professional game this is of particular concern: cortisone injections may enable players to play in the short term but can result in long-term permanent damage that prematurely finishes their playing careers. The reason for this is that the injection can temporarily mask the sensation of pain, enabling players to play without realizing that they are sustaining further injury. Under normal conditions the sensation of pain would inform them of the worsening injury and cause them to stop, preventing further damage.

Warming up prior to a game is also of key importance in the prevention of injury, with many teams failing to observe this requirement and considering that a 5-minute pre-match 'kick about' is sufficient, which it is not.

A limited amount of protective clothing is permitted in soccer. The use of shin pads should be encouraged and in some cases is compulsory. Quilted tops may also be used by the goalkeeper, to reduce the risk of impact injuries and abrasions when striking the ground. Specific goalkeeper's gloves are also available and are used by players to cushion the impact of the ball as well as to provide greater adhesion when catching.

Finally, while most of the reported injuries occur in matches, all the above factors should be considered in training as well.

7.6 INJURIES IN FIELD HOCKEY

7.6.1 Background to the game of field hockey

Hockey is an invasion game played by two teams of 11 players. It is played by both males and females at all levels from school to international standard. Typically, teams are made up of members of the same sex and play against members of the same sex, although mixed teams do occur, albeit usually at a somewhat more social level of play. The aim of the game is to score goals by hitting the ball into the opponents' goal using the hockey stick. To do this the ball is passed between players (again using the stick) while opponents may attempt to intercept a pass or tackle the player with the ball, using the stick. The rules governing the game are complex but in general prevent dangerous use of the stick and only the goalkeeper is permitted to kick the ball or use his/her hands to parry a shot. The players on each team have specific roles, such as attackers, midfield players, defenders and goalkeeper. They therefore tend to be allocated to particular areas of the pitch in order to fulfil these roles, although they are not restricted to them and will move around the pitch as dictated by the phase of the game, the obvious exception to this being the goalkeeper, who tends to remain close to his/her own goal as the last line of defence and whose mobility is largely restricted by protective equipment, which includes 'kickers' over the shoes and leg pads, as well as gloves, a helmet, body padding and often a face mask with neck protection.

Various pieces of research have indicated that over 75% of injuries sustained in field hockey are caused by a player being struck by either the ball or a stick (Figure 7.5).

As hockey is a fast game that requires the players to accelerate quickly and execute rapid changes in direction most of the remaining injuries can be attributed to these movements, with relatively few occurring through

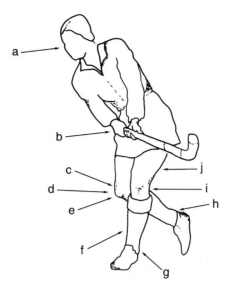

Figure 7.5   Common injuries occurring in field hockey. (a) Orofacial, dental and head injuries.
(b) Damage to fingers, abrasions, dislocations, bruising and fractures. (c) Knee dislocations. (d) Deep
abrasions to lower limbs, particularly the knee. (e) Knee ligament injuries. (f) Sore shins and stress
fractures. (g) Sprained ankles. (h) Achilles tendinitis. (i) Damage to knee cartilages. (j) Strained hamstring
and groin muscles.

contact with another player. An additional
factor of concern is the playing conditions
which, if uneven, can make the ball's movements unpredictable. Alternatively, in the
case of artificial surfaces an increase in the frequency of serious abrasions to the legs, particularly the knees, has been noted, along with
abrasions to the fingers, which also occur in
the indoor game. There is also a general feeling among many participants that joint injuries, particularly those to the knee and ankle,
are more common on artificial surfaces. This
may be related to the unrelenting nature of
the surface and the inability of the foot to
slide when turning or when the leg is struck.
Therefore, as with American football, another
game commonly played on both grass and
artificial surfaces, the extra traction provided
by the artificial surface may possibly increase
the incidence of knee and ankle injuries, particularly ligament sprains and cartilage
damage, while reducing the risk of others.
Some players have stated that they believe
the increased stresses caused by playing on

an artificial surface can shorten a playing
career by a number of years. Another reported
cause of injury relates to the stooped position
that players need to assume when dribbling
with the ball; this is believed to contribute to
the number of back complaints in hockey
players.

7.6.2   Common injuries in field hockey

(a)   *Injuries caused by a stick or ball*

In hockey the ball can reach velocities of up to
80 mph (130 kmh^{-1}), which if it strikes a
player, can cause serious injury. Of greatest
concern in this context are ocular, facial, dental and general head injuries, many of which
may have permanent consequences. With the
exception of the goalkeeper, most hockey
players wear relatively little protection and
are therefore vulnerable to blows to any part
of the body. Typically, the type of protection
worn by players includes shin-pads, groin
protectors and, in some cases, mouthguards,

although these are optional. Female players may wear padding to protect the breasts but this is again optional.

The 'short corner' is generally considered to be the phase of play in which injuries are most likely to occur, as it involves defenders rushing out of the goalmouth towards an attacker, who is likely to hit the ball as hard as possible in the direction of the goal. This can result in the oncoming defenders being struck by the ball on any part of their body, causing bruising or fractures. Since the goal-keeper is the most likely player to be struck by a fast-moving ball s/he must wear addi-tional protective clothing, including a helmet with face mask, leg pads, gloves, 'kickers' over the shoes and padding for the torso, which should make him/her adequately pro-tected and in reality less vulnerable than his/her team-mates.

In addition to the risk of being hit by the ball, players may also be struck by a stick to which they are in close proximity. With refer-ence to this, there are rules that penalize 'dan-gerous play', although in crowded conditions it can still occur.

(b) Traumatic injuries to muscles and joints

As with any fast-moving game that requires rapid acceleration and changes in direction, hockey results in a variety of injuries to the muscles and joints. Typical among them are:

- pulled hamstrings and groin muscles which occur when rapidly accelerating;
- sprained ankles and knee ligament injuries when rapidly changing direction.

Dislocations of the knee are also reported and can occur if the knee is struck when in a flexed position. A number of researchers have reported an increased incidence of mus-cle and joint injuries when playing on artifi-cial surfaces, which, while providing a greater degree of traction, place far more strain on the joints.

(c) Injuries caused by the playing surface

As stated above, the playing surface may con-tribute to the incidence of traumatic muscle and joint injuries. If it is uneven it can cause the ball's movements to be unpredictable and the ball to fly up when hitting a bump, increasing the risk of this form of injury. Uneven surfaces also increase the risk of sprained joints, particularly to the knee and ankle, with associated damage to ligaments and cartilages in the case of the knee.

Of additional concern are the seriousness of the deep abrasions that occur when players slide on artificial surfaces, the most vulner-able site being the knee, although abrasion injuries can occur almost anywhere.

7.6.3 Rules, protective clothing and footwear

While rules exist to ensure that players wear a minimum amount of protective clothing, many researchers would argue that most players do not wear enough. The goalkeeper is the most vulnerable player on the pitch but is usually adequately protected by his/her compulsory clothing. Other players, espe-cially defenders at short corners, should also consider wearing protective garments. Appropriate taping of the fingers can prevent serious abrasions of the knuckle joints and suitable pads on the knees can protect this vulnerable area. The choice of footwear is important and should be appropriate for the playing surface, permitting adequate cushion-ing and traction. Sore shins and even stress fractures can occur from the repeated stress of playing on a hard surface.

7.7 INJURIES IN ICE HOCKEY

7.7.1 Background to injuries in ice hockey

Ice hockey is a fast-moving game that includes an accepted level of 'violence' in the form of body contact. The aim of the game is to score goals by hitting the 'puck' into the opponents' goal; the team is composed of many players but only six are allowed on the ice at any one time. Typically this would include three attackers, two defenders and a goalminder (goalkeeper). However, the constant use of substitutions can alter this combination in accordance with the state of the game and in some situations a team may temporarily have less than six players on the ice because of individuals being penalized for foul play and having to spend a designated period of time in the penalty box, commonly called the 'cooler' or 'sin-bin'. Collisions are part of the game and include the technique of 'checking', which involves forcing an opponent against the rigid boarding that surrounds the playing area. However, in addition to the permitted level of contact and collisions, ice hockey at some levels also has a reputation for deliberate foul play. This includes the illegal use of the stick to hit players, and fighting. Indeed some players are reputed to deliberately foul opponents or provoke them into fighting as part of their game. Unfortunately these incidents can result in further injury and their occurrence is being reviewed by many ice hockey authorities, not only in the context of unnecessary injuries but also in the context of how it affects the reputation of the sport among spectators and sponsors.

The speed with which the 'puck' can be hit, up to 120 mph (200 kmh^{-1}), makes it a hazard to players, as are the sticks, skates and goal posts. The ice playing surface is also a factor in the incidence of injuries, since slipping is common and can result in muscle, tendon or joint injuries if they are forced beyond their normal range of movement during a fall. Injury rates in ice hockey are generally calculated to be between 40 and 80 per 1000 player hours, the vast majority occurring in matches rather than in practice. The difference in injury rate between practice and matches (a three- to sixfold difference) is likely to be related to the increase in forceful contact that occurs during matches.

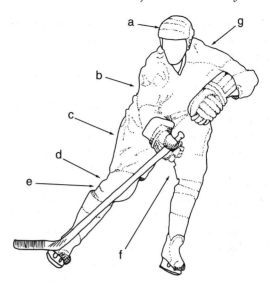

Figure 7.6 Common injuries occurring in ice hockey. (a) Concussion, contusions, lacerations and general orofacial damage. (b) Cervical, spinal injury. (c) Bruised thighs. (d) Patellar tendinitis. (e) Knee cartilage damage. (f) Adductor muscular-tendon injuries. (g) Shoulder dislocations.

7.7.2   Causes of injury, site of injury and prevention

In ice hockey the majority of injuries are caused by trauma, less than 20% being attributed to overuse (Figure 7.6).

The most common causes of injury are blows from a stick and collisions with other players, including tackling and checking. Collisions with the goal posts, being hit by the puck and accidental falls are reported to account for most of the remaining traumatic injuries. The head and face are often reported as the most common site of injury in ice hockey, with the knee being the most vulnerable joint. When combined these account for over half the reported injuries. The extensive amount of protective equipment worn by ice hockey players may help to explain this distribution of injuries since most of the body is well protected, only the face being exposed. In general, facial injuries are caused by being struck by the puck or stick although illegal punches from opponents also contribute to the number of injuries. Head and facial injuries include concussion, contusions, lacerations to the face, and eye and dental damage. In ice hockey, helmets are generally compulsory, the use of visors and mouth guards also being recommended by most authorities to reduce the incidence of eye and dental injuries. Injuries to the knee tend to include ligament damage and occur in all players, some researchers reporting the goalkeeper to be the most vulnerable. Some authorities therefore recommend the use of knee protectors that contain a means of preventing excessive rotation or lateral movement at this joint.

The relatively violent nature of the game means that foul play is considered to be a factor in about 15% of reported injuries, foul play involving the stick being the most significant. The commonly reported overuse injuries in ice hockey include: patellar tendinitis and adductor muscular–tendon injuries, which can be related to the biomechanics of skating.

The prevention of ice hockey injuries therefore depends upon good refereeing that prevents unnecessary foul play and the fitness of the players, which will help to ensure that they are physically capable of withstanding the stresses of the game.

7.8   INJURIES IN VOLLEYBALL

7.8.1   Background to the game of volleyball and the causes of injury

Volleyball is played by both males and females, with a team consisting of six players. The court is 18 m × 9 m and divided in half by a net set at 2.43 m for the men's game and 2.24 cm for the women's game or for junior boys. The aim of the game is to get the ball to land in the opponents' court. The two teams are separated by the net and players are not permitted to enter the opponents' side of the court or even to touch the net. However this may occur accidentally and

can be a cause of injury as players trip over or land on an opponent while playing at the net (Figure 7.7).

During the game points are only scored by the team who is serving and if the serving team loses the rally the opposing team are then given service. Each time a team gains service they rotate in a clockwise direction; thus, although some players may be employed for specialist skills, all players will have the opportunity to play at the front of the court,

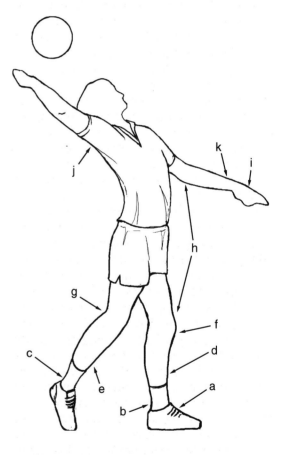

Figure 7.7   Common injuries occurring in volleyball. (a) Sprained ankle. (b) Achilles tendinitis. (c) Achilles tendon rupture. (d) Shin soreness. (e) Stress fracture of the lower leg. (f) Knee ligament and cartilage damage. (g) Patellar tendon injury (jumper's knee). (h) Abrasions to elbows and knees. (i) Injuries to hands and fingers. (j) Shoulder injuries. (k) Bruising of the arms.

play at the back of the court and serve. After serving each team is allowed to touch the ball three times (an attempted block at the net not counting as a touch) with no player being permitted to touch the ball twice in succession (again an attempted block would not count as the first touch).

Typically when a team receives the ball it will be coming over the net from either a serve or an attacking shot such as a smash (spike). Therefore, the team's first touch of the ball will usually be a 'dig' (bump pass), which is played on both forearms at about waist height, although one-handed digs and other defensive shots are used if the former is not possible. This may involve diving to try and reach the ball. In playing this first shot the player will attempt to prevent the ball hitting the ground and thus winning the rally; it is therefore a defensive pass. It is also the first phase of setting up the team's own attack, so when playing the dig the player will also attempt to hit the ball high in the air in order to give his/her teammates the maximum amount of time to position and prepare themselves for the next phase of the attack. If possible the dig pass will be directed to a specialist player at the front of the court called the 'setter'. If the dig has been well played the setter will receive the ball from a height that will enable him/her to position him/herself for the next pass, which is usually a 'set' or volley pass. If the team initially received the ball at a speed and height that permitted it, the volley pass may be used as an alternative to the dig. The volley or set pass is played with two hands from just above head height and is directed towards another member of the team, who will attempt to smash (spike) the ball down into the opponents' court. A variation on this attacking shot would be to volley the ball into a space in the opponents' defences.

As the spiker jumps to spike the ball one, two or even three defenders may oppose him/her on the other side of the net. These defenders will jump and raise their hands as high as possible in an attempt to 'block' the spike, preventing it from landing on their side of the court and possibly causing it to fall into the opponents' court, giving them the rally. This is the phase of the game that results in most traumatic injuries, as players are in close proximity. As players land they can step on each other, resulting in sprained ankles; other injuries are caused by falls. Furthermore, even though players of opposing teams are separated by the net it is not uncommon for one to land with his/her feet on the opponents' side of the net, increasing the risk of injury to themselves and the opponents should s/he land on them. The other cause of injury during this phase of the game is the ball, which, if hit hard by the attacking player, may injure the opponents' fingers or faces if they are struck by it.

Volleyball is a fast, explosive game that requires rapid movement around the court, hitting the ball with a large amount of force and blocking or retrieving a fast-moving ball before it hits the ground. The injury profile of the game of volleyball reflects this, with injuries to the hands and fingers, knees and ankles. Shoulder injuries are caused by hitting the ball. Traumatic hand and finger injuries are caused by hitting and blocking the ball, while sprained ankles and traumatic knee injuries are caused by landing awkwardly. These may also occur if a player lands or steps upon a member of the opposition who has accidentally intruded on to the wrong side of the net, usually as a result of a fall that has caused his/her feet to protrude across to the wrong side of the court. Knee injuries can include both ligament and cartilage damage. Jumper's knee is a common overuse injury among volleyball players and reflects the demands of the game.

The phases of play most likely to result in injury are blocking and spiking. When taking off to block the ball the player may pull muscles and place a considerable amount of strain upon the Achilles and patellar tendons. Hence, players are susceptible to injuries of the Achilles tendon and patellar tendon (jumper's knee) in much the same way as those involved in the athletic jumping events. Upon landing the player may step on the feet of a team member, who will often be in close proximity through the use of two or three blockers. This can result in ankle sprains and knee damage. Landing on the feet of an opponent is also a possibility if either have crossed the line of the net through too much forward momentum while jumping. While in the air the fingers, hand and wrist are used to block the ball hit by the opposing attacking player, who has usually attempted to spike (smash) it into the opposite court. Fingers are obviously vulnerable in this phase. Diving to dig a ball (hit it up before it hits the ground, usually from an opponent's spike) can result in abrasions and knee pads should be worn by all players. Bruising of the arms from repetitive 'digging' of the ball is common among novices. The incidence of overuse injuries such as stress fractures to the lower leg is increased if the playing surface is very hard and/or the player's footwear lacks adequate cushioning.

7.9   INJURIES IN CRICKET

7.9.1   Background to the common injuries occurring in cricket

The game of cricket involves two teams of 11 players and, while the rules are complex, the object of the game are to score more 'runs' than the opposing team. The game is divided into two key phases: fielding and batting. When a team is batting they will attempt to score as many runs as possible while the fielding team try to keep the number of runs scored down to a minimum. The pitch consists of a large roughly circular area, towards the centre of which is the batting square. In this area two sets of stumps are erected (three stumps in each set) with a pair of bails laid across each set of stumps. Only two members of the batting team are on the pitch at any

time while they attempt to score runs against the entire fielding team. The fielding team consists of a number of specialist positions, including the bowler, who 'bowls' the ball at the stumps using a particular style or technique in an attempt to knock the stumps over. 'Fast bowlers' are recognized for the speed with which they bowl the ball while 'spin bowlers' obviously try to hit the stumps using various techniques of spin. Positioned behind the stumps is the wicket keeper, who stops the ball if it reaches him/her and prevents it travelling further as this could result in the batting team gaining runs. The batsman defends the stumps from the ball using a cricket bat, with which s/he hits the ball. If the ball hits the stumps the batsman is out and will be replaced by another member of the team. This continues until the allocated time is completed or until ten of the batting team are out. Runs are achieved by either hitting the ball over the boundary of the pitch (six runs if the ball crosses the boundary without bouncing and four if it bounces before crossing) or by the batsmen running between the two sets of stumps. The batsmen run after hitting the ball if they believe that they can get to the other set of stumps before a fielder can hit the stumps with the ball. A batsman can also be 'out' if s/he hits the ball and it is caught by a fielder before it hits the ground. When a side completes its turn of batting (its innings) the teams change round.

The above description is obviously a very superficial description of the game of cricket, which is extremely complex, with many other rules that govern play and how batsmen may be out. It should, however, give those unfamiliar with the game a brief insight into its demands and therefore the potential causes of injury.

The most likely cause of injury in cricket (Figure 7.8) is being hit by a fast ball while either batting or fielding.

This can result in bruising or fractures to almost any part of the body that is not adequately protected. Head and eye injuries are

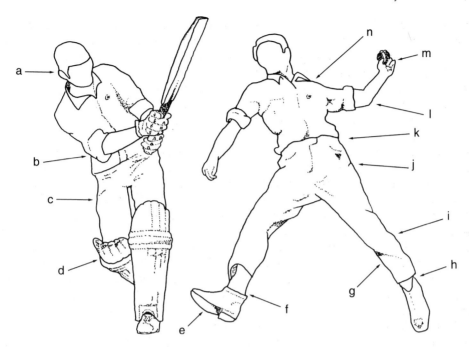

Figure 7.8 Common injuries occurring in cricket. (a) Orofacial injuries, head injury. (b) Elbow injuries. (c) Hamstring muscle strain. (d) Knee ligament and meniscal cartilage injury. (e) Stress fractures of feet. (f) Achilles tendinitis. (g) Stress fractures. (h) Sprained ankle. (i) Calf muscle strain. (j) Hip joint injuries. (k) Stress factures of the vertebrae, spondylolysis. (l) Medial epicondylitis (thrower's elbow). (m) Stubbed fingers. (n) Shoulder injuries.

usually of greatest concern at all levels of the game and the use of appropriate protective equipment should therefore be strongly advocated. The feet are also vulnerable, especially when batting, and the use of cricket boots that offer some degree of protection is to be recommended.

Muscular and tendon injuries such as pulled hamstring muscles and damaged Achilles tendons can occur when bowling, chasing after the ball when fielding or when attempting to run between the stumps. As a group, fast bowlers also suffer from a range of back injuries, including stress fractures of the vertebrae (spondylolysis), intervertebral disc damage and strained muscles. The repeated pounding of the legs experienced by this group also makes them vulnerable to knee and foot injuries such as stress fractures and cartilage damage. Shoulder injuries are also possible because of the repetitive action of fast bowling. Stubbed fingers from mistiming the ball occurs in fielders, the wicket keeper being particularly vulnerable despite his/her protective gloves.

Repeatedly throwing the ball can cause medial epicondylitis (thrower's elbow), an inflammation at the site of muscular attachment of the medial epicondyle of the humerus caused by the pronatory action of throwing. This may be more prevalent among juniors because of the relative weakness of the immature skeleton in this region.

7.9.2 The prevention of injuries in cricket

In cricket the incidence of many injuries can be minimized by adhering to the general recommendations made in Chapter 1. The use of a hard ball, which can be thrown or bowled at speed, makes it a potentially dangerous game and a number of specific points relating to the prevention of cricket injuries are as follows.

(a)   Protective clothing

The batsman is potentially the most vulnerable player and should be adequately protected. Leg pads, gloves and a 'cricket box' to protect the genitals are used by batsmen at all levels. In addition to this a helmet with protective visor, and additional padding to protect the thighs and body, are used in games of a standard where the speed of bowling can make batting particularly hazardous.

The wicket keeper wears specific protective clothing such as wicket keeper's gloves because of the necessity for him/her to repeatedly catch a hard ball travelling at great speed. Other fielders who may be positioned close to the batsman may also wear protective helmets in case they are struck by a ball hit by the batsman.

(b)   Inappropriate opposition

This is particularly pertinent when considering the case of a inexperienced batsman facing a fast bowler. A lack of skill may make him/her unable to avoid a ball bowled at them at speed and result in serious injury. This must therefore be a consideration in the attitude of players, especially at the recreational level, where players of a great range of abilities may take part in the same match.

(c)   Dangerous pitches

An uneven cricket square that results in an unpredictable bounce of the ball is an unnecessary hazard for batsmen as it provides them with virtually no time in which to protect themselves. An uneven pitch can also present a hazard to bowlers and fielders, who can sprain ankles on it. These occurrences are more likely at the lower levels of the game where the pitch may have several uses throughout the year, including pastureland for grazing animals.

(d)   Bad light and poor weather conditions

The speed of the ball gives the batsman little time to react. In conditions of bad light this problem is heightened and is a consideration for the umpires, who may terminate the game if they consider it to be dangerous. Rain can make the pitches slippery, causing individuals to slip, fall and pull muscles even if wearing the correct footwear. Inappropriate footwear will make slipping more likely.

(e)   Poor technique and overuse among bowlers

During a match a bowler may be asked to bowl a large number of overs. Throughout a season these demands can build to the level where overuse injuries are almost inevitable. Therefore the demands being placed upon a bowler must be carefully considered if s/he is not to suffer from the common cricketing injuries to the back, knees, ankles and Achilles tendons. The likelihood of any overuse injury among this group of players may be greatly affected by their bowling technique. In general the front-on bowling technique is more likely to cause injury than the side-on technique because the former requires the bowler to hyperextend the back with a laterally flexed spine and rotate the shoulder more than the side-on technique.

(f)   Warming up and fitness

All players, but in particular fast bowlers, must possess a high level of fitness and gradually increase the amount of bowling they undertake. Specific fitness training programmes for this group are therefore essential to ensure that they can cope with the physical demands of each match. Within such programmes a gradual build-up of the number of balls bowled each day must be a factor.

As with all sports a level of sport-specific fitness is essential. The fit squash player may be surprised by stiff joints and aching muscles the day after a social game of cricket. In this context, warming up is also very important. Cricket can involve sudden exertion, such as sprinting for a ball, and while most sportspeople will warm up for their own sport they tend not to bother if they are playing another game as a one-off just for fun. In cricket it is not uncommon for a tea or lunch interval to separate the two phases of the match and warming up again after the interval is just as important as before the commencement of the match.

7.10 FURTHER READING

7.10.1 Rugby injuries

Addley, K. and Farren, J. (1988) Irish rugby injury survey. *British Journal of Sports Medicine*, **22**(1), 22–24.

Blignaut, J.B., Carstens, I.L. and Lombard, C.J. (1987) Injuries sustained in rugby by wearers and non-wearers of mouthguards. *British Journal of Sports Medicine*, **21**(2), 5–7.

Burry, H.C. and Calcinai, C.J. (1988) The need to make rugby safer. *British Medical Journal (Clinical Research edn)*, **296**(6616), 149–150.

Chapman, P.J. (1985) Orofacial injuries and mouthguards: a study of the 1984 Wallabies. *British Journal of Sports Medicine*, **19**(2), 93–95.

Duda, M. (1988) Reducing catastrophic injuries in rugby. *Physician and Sportsmedicine*, **16**(10), 29.

Durkin, T.E. (1977) Survey of injuries in a 1st class Rugby Union Football Club from 1972–1976. *British Journal of Sports Medicine*, **11**(1), 7–11.

Fairclough, J.A. and Farquhar, G.A. (1986) Mechanisms of injury: a pictorial record. *British Journal of Sports Medicine*, **20**(3), 107–108.

Gallagher, J. E. and Dineen, P. F. (1981) Survey of rugby injuries. *Irish Medical Journal*, **74**(5), 137.

Gonzales, A. (1975) Rugby: a game for hooligans played by gentlemen. *Physician and Sportsmedicine*, **3**(3), 109–113.

Harrison, D.H., Walkden, L., Moffat, R. *et al.* (1980) Rugby injuries in schools. *British Journal of Sports Medicine*, **14**(4), 234–235.

Hawkins, S.B. (1986) Head, neck, face, and shoulder injuries in female and male rugby players. *Physician and Sportsmedicine*, **14**(7), 111–118.

Jennings, D.C. (1990) Injuries sustained by users and non-users of gum shields in local rugby union. *British Journal of Sports Medicine*, **24**(3), 159–165.

Kay, E.J., Kakarla, P., Macleod, D.A.D. and McGlashan, T.P.L. (1990) Orofacial and dental injuries in club rugby union players. *British Journal of Sports Medicine*, **24**(4), 271–273.

McLean, D.A. (1990) Role of the team physiotherapist in rugby union football. *British Journal of Sports Medicine*, **24**(1), 19– 24.

O'Brien, C. (1992) Retrospective study of rugby injuries in the Leinster province of Ireland 1987–1989. *British Journal of Sports Medicine*, **26**(4) 243–244.

Pearson, J. (1979) Sports injuries. *British Journal of Physical Education*, **10**(6), 166–184.

Reilly, T. and Hardiker, R. (1981) Somatotype and injuries in adult student rugby football. *Journal of Sports Medicine and Physical Fitness*, **21**(2), 186–191.

Scher, A.T. (1987) Rugby injuries of the spine and spinal cord. *Clinics in Sports Medicine*, **6**(1), 87–99.

Silver, J.R. (1984) Injuries of the spine sustained in rugby. *British Medical Journal (Clinical Research edn)*, **288**(6410), 37–43.

Sparks, J.P. (1985) Rugby football injuries 1980–1983. *British Journal of Sports Medicine*, **19**(2), 71–75.

Stokes, A.M. and Chapman, P.J. (1991) Mouthguards, dental trauma and the 1990 All Blacks. *New Zealand Journal of Sports Medicine*, **19**(4), 66–67.

Tomasin, J.D., Martin, D.F. and Curl, W.W. (1989) Recognition and prevention of rugby injuries. *Physician and Sportsmedicine*, **17**(6), 114–126.

Tscher, A.T. (1991) Catastrophic rugby injuries of the spinal cord: changing patterns of injury. *British Journal of Sports Medicine*, **25**(1), 57–60.

Turl, S. (1992) Rugby injuries: are the clubs medically prepared? *Physiotherapy in Sport*, **14**(1), 7–8.

Walker, R.D. (1985) Sports injuries: rugby league may be less dangerous than union. *Practitioner*, **229**(1401), 205–206.

Webb, J. and Bannister G. (1992) Acromioclavicular disruption in first class rugby players. *British Journal of Sports Medicine*, **26**(4) 247–248.

Whytehead, C. (1982) Examining rugby injuries. *Action: British Journal of Physical Education*, **13**(5), 145.

7.10.2 American football injuries

Canale, S.T., Cantler, E.D., Sisk, T.D. and Freeman, B.L. (1981) Chronicle of injuries of an American intercollegiate football team. *American Journal of Sports Medicine*, **9**(6), 384– 389.

Halpern, B., Thompson, N., Walton, W. *et al.* (1987) High school football injuries: Identifying the risk factors. *American Journal of Sports Medicine*, **15**(4), 316–320.

Karpakka, J. (1993) American Football injuries in Finland. *British Journal of Sports Medicine*, **27**(2) 135–137.

Prager, B.I., Fitton, W.L., Cahill, B.R. and Olson, G.H. (1989) High school football injuries: a prospective study and pitfalls of data collection. *American Journal of Sports Medicine*, **17**(5), 681–685.

Thompson, N., Halpern, B., Walton, W. *et al.* (1987) High school football injuries: evaluation. *American Journal of Sports Medicine*, **15**(2), 117–124.

7.10.3 Basketball injuries

Apple, D.F. (1988) Basketball injuries: an overview. *Physician and Sportsmedicine*, **16**(12), 64–76.

Apple, D.F., O'Toole, J. and Annis, C. (1982) Professional basketball injuries. *Physician and Sportsmedicine*, **10**(11), 81– 86.

Blazina, M.E., Fox, J. M. and Carlson, G.J. (1975) Certain basketball injuries. *Physician and Sportsmedicine*, **3**(1), 68–71.

Henry, J.H., Lareau, B. and Neigut, D. (1982) Injury rate in professional basketball. *American Journal of Sports Medicine*, **10**(1), 16–18.

Moretz, A. and Grana, W.A. (1978) High school basketball injuries. *Physician and Sportsmedicine*, **6**(10), 92–96.

Purdam, C. (1987) A survey of netball and basketball injuries. *Excel*, **3**(3), 9–11.

7.10.4 Netball injuries

Hopper, D. (1986) A survey of netball injuries and conditions related to these injuries. *Australian Journal of Physiotherapy*, **32**(4), 231–239.

Purdam, C. (1987) A survey of netball and basketball injuries. *Excel*, **3**(3), 9–11.

Steele, J. and Milburn, P. (1988) Reducing the risk of injury in netball: changing rules or changing techniques? *New Zealand Journal of Health, Physical Education and Recreation*, **21**(1), 17–21.

7.10.5 Association football injuries

Ekstrand, J. and Gillquist, J. (1983) Avoidability of soccer injuries. *International Journal of Sports Medicine*, **4**(2), 124– 128.

Ekstrand, J. and Gillquist, J. (1983) Soccer injuries and their mechanisms: a prospective study. *Medicine and Science in Sports and Exercise*, **15**(3), 267–270.

Ekstand, J. and Gillquist, J. (1984) Prevention of sport injuries in football players. *International Journal of Sports Medicine*, **Suppl. 5**, 140–144.

Ekstrand, J., Gillquist, J. and Liljedahl, S.O. (1983) Prevention of soccer injuries. *American Journal of Sports Medicine*, **11**(3), 116–120.

Fried, T. and Lloyd, G.J. (1992) An overview of common soccer injuries. Management and prevention. *Sports Medicine*, **14**(4), 269–275.

Hoy, K., Lindblad, B.E., Helleland, H.E. and Terkelsen, C.J. (1992) European soccer injuries. A prospective epidemiologic and socioeconomic study. *American Journal of Sports Medicine*, **20**(3), 318–322.

Hunt, M. and Fulford, S. (1990) Amateur soccer: injuries in relation to field position. *British Journal of Sports Medicine*, **24**(4), 265.

Klasen, H.J. (1984) Acute soccer injuries. *International Journal of Sports Medicine*, **Suppl. 5**, 156–158.

McCarroll, J.R., Meaney, C. and Sieber, J.M. (1984) Profile of youth soccer injuries. *Physician and Sportsmedicine*, **12**(2), 113–117.

Maehlum, S. and Daljord, O.A. (1984) Football injuries in Olso: a one-year study. *British Journal of Sports Medicine*, **18**(3), 186–190.

Mozes, M., Papa, M.Z., Zweig, A. *et al.* (1985) Iliopsoas injuries in soccer players. *British Journal of Sports Medicine*, **19**(3), 168–170.

Muckle, D.S. (1981) Injuries in professional footballers. *British Journal of Sports Medicine*, **15**(1), 77–79.

Nielsen, A.B. and Yde, J. (1989) Epidemiology and traumatology of injuries in soccer. *American Journal of Sports Medicine*, **17**(6), 803–807.

Poulsen, T.D., Freund, K.G., Madsen, F. and Sandvej, K. (1991) Injuries in high-skilled and low-skilled soccer: a prospective study. *British Journal of Sports Medicine*, **25**(3), 151–153.

Sadat-Ali, M. and Sankaran-Kutty, M. (1987) Soccer injuries in Saudi Arabia. *American Journal of Sports Medicine*, **15**(5), 500– 502.

Sandelin, J., Santavirta, S. and Kiviluoto, O. (1985) Acute soccer injuries in Finland in 1980. *British Journal of Sports Medicine*, **19**(1), 30–33.

Schmidt-Olsen, S., Buenemann, L.K.H., Lade, V. and Brassoe, J.O.K. (1985) Soccer injuries of youth. *British Journal of Sports Medicine*, **19**(3), 161–164.

Schmidt-Olsen, S., Jorgensen, U., Kaalund, S. and Sorensen, J. (1991) Injuries among young soccer players. *American Journal of Sports Medicine*, **19**(3), 273–275.

7.10.6 Injuries in field hockey

Bolhuis, J.H.A., Leurs, J.M.M. and Flogel, G.E. (1987) Dental and facial injuries in international field hockey. *British Journal of Sports Medicine*, **21**(4) 174–177.

Jamison, S. and Lee, C. (1989) The incidence of female injuries on grass and synthetic playing surfaces. *Australian Journal of Science and Medicine in Sport*, **21**(2), 15–17.

Lindgren, S. and Maguire, K. (1985) Survey of field hockey injuries. *Sports Science and Medicine quarterly*, **1**(3), 7–12.

7.10.7 Ice hockey injuries

Daly, P.J., Sim, F.H. and Simonet, W.T. (1990) Ice hockey injuries: a review. *Sports Medicine*, **10**(2), 122–131.

Hayes, D. (1975) Hockey injuries: how, why, where and when? *Physician and Sportsmedicine*, **3**(1), 61–65.

Hayes, D. (1978) Reducing risks in hockey: analysis of equipment and injuries. *Physician and Sportsmedicine*, **6**(1), 67– 70.

Jorgenson, U and Schmidt-Olsen, S. (1986) The epidemiology of ice hockey injuries. *British Journal of Sports Medicine*, **20**(2), 7–9.

Ryan, A.J. (1985) Study: hockey eye injuries preventable. *Physician and Sportsmedicine*, **13**(2), 32.

Sim, F.H. and Simonet, W.T. (1988) Ice hockey injuries. *Physician and Sportsmedicine*, **16**(3), 92–105.

Sim, F.H., Simonet, W.T., Melton, L.J. and Lehn, T.A. (1987) Ice hockey injuries. *American Journal of Sports Medicine*, **15**(1), 30–40.

Tegner, Y. and Lorentzon, R. (1991) Ice hockey injuries: incidence, nature and causes. *British Journal of Sports Medicine*, **25**(2), 87–89.

7.10.8 Volleyball injuries

Bracker, M.D., Cohen, M. and Blasingame, J. (1990) Chronic shoulder pain in a volleyball player. *Physician and Sportsmedicine*, **18**(10), 85–88.

Ferretti, A., Puddu, G., Mariani, P.P. and Neri, M. (1984) Jumper's knee: an epidemiological study of volleyball players. *Physician and Sportsmedicine*, **12**(10), 97–106.

Ferretti, A., Papandrea, P. and Conteduca, F. (1990) Knee injuries in volleyball. *Sports Medicine*, **10**(2), 132–138.

Ferretti, A., Papandrea, P., Conteduca, F. and Mariani, P. P. (1992) Knee ligament injuries in volleyball players. *American Journal of Sports Medicine*, **20**(2), 203–207.

Lo, Y.P.C., Hsu, Y.C.S. and Chan, K.M. (1990) Epidemiology of shoulder impingement in upper arm sports events. *British Journal of Sports Medicine*, **24**(3), 173–177.

Schafle, M.D., Requa, R.K., Patton, W. L. and Garrick, J.G. (1990) Injuries in the 1987 national amateur volleyball tournament. *American Journal of Sports Medicine*, **18**(6), 624–631.

Watkins, J. and Green, B.N. (1992) Volleyball injuries: a survey of injuries of Scottish National League male players. *British Journal of Sports Medicine*, **26**(2), 135–137.

7.10.9 Cricket injuries

Bell, P.A. (1992) Spondylolysis in fast bowlers: principles of prevention and a survey of awareness among cricket coaches. *British Journal of Sports Medicine*, **26**(4) 273–275.

Foster, D., John, D., Elliott, B. *et al.* (1989) Back injuries to fast bowlers in cricket: a prospective study. *British Journal of Sports Medicine*, **23**(3), 150–154.

Jones, N.P and Tullo, A.B. (1986) Severe eye injuries in cricket. *British Journal of Sports Medicine*, **20**(4), 178–179.

Temple. R. (1982) Cricket injuries: fast pitches change the gentleman's sport. *Physician and Sportsmedicine*, **10**(6), 186–192.

Weightman, D. and Browne, R.C. (1975) Injuries in eleven selected sports. *British Journal of Sports Medicine*, **9**(3), 136–141.

8. Injuries in individual sports and racquet sports

8.1 RUNNING INJURIES – SPRINTING, ENDURANCE EVENTS, CROSS-COUNTRY AND ORIENTEERING

8.1.1 Introduction to running injuries

The injuries most commonly seen in runners are inevitably those to the lower limbs, although a number of back complaints also occur (Figure 8.1).

While any runner may acquire almost any of the following running injuries, the distance and terrain over which they compete will have some influence over the likelihood of their suffering from a particular type of injury. For example, sprained ankles are more common among those who run over rough

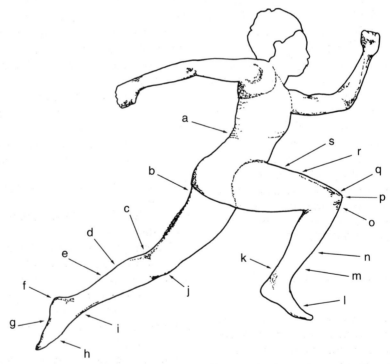

Figure 8.1 Common running injuries. (a) Sciatica. (b) Strained hamstrings and adductor muscles. (c) Damage to lateral and medial ligaments. (d) Strained gastrocnemius. (e) Compartment syndrome. (f) Server's disease. (g) Plantar fasciitis. (h) Tenosynovitis. (i) Sprained ankle. (j) Osgood–Schlatter's disease. (k) Achilles tendon injury (rupture and overuse). (l) Stress fractures of metatarsals. (m) Sore shins. (n) Fractures to lower leg. (o) Knee cruciate ligament damage. (p) Knee meniscal damage. (q) Chondromalacia patella. (r) Iliotibial band syndrome. (s) Strained quadriceps.

ground while torn hamstring muscles occur more frequently in sprinters. Likewise, runners of particular ages or gender are more susceptible to certain injuries, with older runners reporting a greater incidence of Achilles tendon soreness and female runners being more prone to chondromalacia patellae. The repetitive nature of endurance running can cause a number of overuse injuries the occurrence of which may be partially attributed to factors such as running gait, biomechanical imbalances and anatomical factors. If these are not considered by the practitioner when dealing with the injured athlete and steps are not taken to address them, the injury is quite likely to recur. Therefore a thorough analysis of potential problems such as heel–forefoot alignment, knee configuration – including genu varum, valgum and recurvatum, hip alignment, relative bone length and the pattern of shoe wear is essential; examples and details are given in Chapter 4.

Running injuries are perhaps the most extensively documented area of all sports injuries; indeed, whole books have been devoted to the subject. This chapter will not therefore attempt to cover all the vast number of possible injuries in detail but will attempt to briefly review the most frequent, as well as providing the practitioner with guidelines on how to approach their treatment and rehabilitation.

In this section running injuries are classified according to the site of injury. Further details of these injuries are found in Chapters 2–6.

8.1.2 Injuries to the foot, ankle and Achilles tendon

A sprained ankle – damage to the lateral ligaments with the additional possibility of compression damage to the medial side of the ankle – most commonly occurs when running across rough terrain. It is therefore relatively common among orienteers and cross-country runners, especially when the ground is very hard, for example when rutted and frozen in the winter. In orienteering the additional hazards of brashings and rough undergrowth further increases the incidence of this injury and can occasionally result in fractures to the lower leg and ankle. The other commonly reported cause of sprained ankles in runners is accidentally stepping off a kerb during a momentary lapse of concentration or when running in poorly lit areas at night.

A partially or fully ruptured Achilles tendon can occur when the tendon is overstretched and/or a forceful contraction of the calf muscles (plantarflexors) exceeds the tensile strength of the tendon. This can happen when sprinting, jumping, hurdling or landing and is therefore an injury to which all runners are prone, although fortunately it occurs relatively infrequently.

The excessive mileage attempted by many long-distance runners in their endeavour to reach a peak of fitness is the cause of many overuse injuries, including inflammation of the Achilles tendon (Achilles tendinitis) and its surrounding tissues (Achilles peritendinitis). Another related injury in this region is Achilles bursitis – inflammation of the bursae in the region of the Achilles tendon's insertion on the calcaneum bone of the heel (Chapter 2). Factors that are reported to contribute to overuse injuries of the Achilles tendon include:

- a rapid increase in the mileage run in training;
- a switch from steady running to speed work;
- changing to a new running surface (artificial track surfaces are often a factor);
- running on one side of the road, which, because of the camber, puts additional stress on the tendon;
- wearing old shoes that lack the necessary cushioning;
- wearing shoes with high heel-tabs;
- a running gait with excessive pronation.

Focal degeneration of the Achilles tendon may occur if it is repeatedly overstressed by forceful contractions, such as when sprinting uphill. This damage will not only make the tendon sore but will increase the risk of rupture if training is continued at the same intensity without permitting it to heal.

Plantar fasciitis is another overuse injury found in distance runners. It is inflammation of the fascia, connective tissue, under the foot and is found to occur more frequently in runners who pronate excessively. Attempting to run during icy conditions, which can cause the runner to alter gait to accommodate the loss of traction, may also be a factor in causing this injury and similar injuries to the ligaments under the foot.

Another consequence of running too many miles can be stress fractures in the metatarsal bones of the feet, especially if running on hard surfaces. Here again, footwear and running gait can also be a factor. This injury is sometimes referred to as a 'march fracture' because of its occurrence in army recruits, where it is caused by marching long distances in rigid boots. Bruising of the heel may occur in all runners, including hurdlers and sprinters. In young athletes this may be complicated and any heel pain could be due to damage to the growing region of the calcaneum heel bone (Sever's disease).

Tenderness and inflammation of the tendons on the top of the foot (tenosynovitis) is sometimes caused by tight lacing, tight footwear or tight strapping. All of these can prevent the tendons from moving freely, as they are pressed against their sheaths and the surrounding tissues, which causes them to rub against each other as the tendon moves, resulting in inflammation.

8.1.3   Injuries to the lower leg

Sore shins and 'shin splints' are general terms commonly used by athletes to describe pain in this region, although in reality the terms are somewhat imprecise and therefore cover a number of possible injuries. These range from inflammation of the muscle's attachment to the bone (periostitis) to stress fractures. They may be caused by:

- running too many miles on a hard surfaces;
- a change in the training surface or type of training;
- running in old worn out shoes or even a change in footwear.

Another group of injuries that occur in the lower leg are the 'compartment syndromes'. These can be caused by overuse or trauma such as a pulled muscle. In the case of the former, number of different compartment syndromes may be caused by large amounts of training, which can cause the muscle to enlarge beyond the capacity of its surrounding sheath. This will inhibit the flow of blood to the exercising muscle fibres, resulting in a build-up of lactic acid and the development of oedema, which will cause additional swelling. This will further inhibit the flow of blood and result in the development of a fatiguing cramp in the muscle. In some cases the condition can be attributed to a rapid increase in training volume resulting in either posterior or anterior compartment syndrome. Compartment syndromes may also arise from internal bleeding within the muscle caused by a blow or tear (Chapter 2). The build-up of fluid within the muscle increases the pressure, thereby inhibiting the flow of oxygenated blood into the muscle and resulting in a cramp-like pain.

Tears to the muscles of the lower leg, particularly the gastrocnemius, can occur during powerful contractions of the plantarflexors, as when accelerating, jumping or running fast uphill. Here the excessive stress placed on the lower leg may cause the muscle to tear rather than the Achilles tendon (as discussed previously).

8.1.4   Injuries to the knee

Traumatic damage to the knee most commonly occurs when it is twisted. The structures of the knee that can be damaged by this rotatory movement are the cruciate ligaments and the meniscus cartilages within the knee;

damage to the lateral and medial ligaments are also possible. A forced lateral flexion of the knee may also damage these ligaments and cartilages. This is fortunately a relatively infrequent occurrence in most runners, but can occur when running over rough terrain.

Chondromalacia patellae is a roughening of the back of the kneecap. It occurs in many endurance runners but is found to be more common among female runners with relatively wide pelvises. The suggested reason for this is the increased angle of pull of the rectus femoris at the knee (Q angle), which causes the articular surface of the patella to rub against the femur, usually the lateral condyle.

Osgood–Schlatter's disease is the condition of inflammation at the point where the patellar tendon joins the tibia, just below the knee. It occurs in running and other sports where there is excessive and/or repeated knee extension, which causes the patellar tendon to pull on its insertion on the periosteum of the tibia, resulting in inflammation. It more frequently occurs in the junior age groups below the age of 18, and upon healing a permanent lump often forms.

Iliotibial band syndrome is characterized by pain down the lateral side of the knee and is caused by inflammation of the iliotibial band tendon. This tendon connects the ilium to the tibia and therefore has to move across the lateral side of the femur when the knee is flexed and extended. In long-distance runners, where training involves a high mileage, repeating this movement an excessive number of times can cause inflammation. Other contributing factors include excessive pronation and running on roads with a steep camber.

8.1.5 Injuries to the upper leg

Strained quadriceps and hamstring muscles tend to occur when there is a slight miscoordination in the contraction and relaxation sequence of these two muscle groups.

For example, if one group is forced to lengthen (by the contraction of the opposing group) before it has started to relax, it will still be tense and hence vulnerable to being torn as the fibres are forced to lengthen. This is most commonly seen in sprinters as they accelerate, or in the later stages of a race when fatigue may affect the runner's coordination. Hurdlers are also prone to hamstring injuries, especially if they overstretch when attempting to clear a hurdle. In both cases, tight inflexible hamstrings and/or a lack of warm-up can contribute to the risk of injury.

Hamstring tears also occur in endurance runners, often as they attempt to sprint or when they slip in muddy or icy conditions. This latter cause occurs because when the runner slips the hamstrings are stretched rapidly while at the same time a reflex reaction causes the muscles to contract in order to restore the individual's balance. A similar scenario can cause strains in the adductor muscles. Adductor strains also occur in sprinters, where they are associated with the rapid acceleration phase of a sprint, and in poorly conditioned hurdlers, where the hurdling technique requires good adductor flexibility.

While most sprinters and hurdlers will spend a considerable amount of time developing their flexibility (although some don't), many endurance runners possess very poor flexibility, especially in the hamstrings, and should therefore be encouraged to undertake a regular stretching routine which will promote their range of movement and reduce the risk of injury to this muscle group.

8.1.6 Injuries to the back

Sciatica is a back complaint that occasionally affects runners. Typically, its symptoms include pain in the hamstrings, which may be mistaken for a pulled muscle. It is caused by pressure on the sciatic nerve in the region of the back, often caused by a slipped disc.

8.1.7 Epiphyseal plate injuries

Young runners can suffer from epiphyseal plate damage due to the repeated stresses placed upon this area of growth cartilage within the bone. In extreme cases this can cause the premature cessation of bone growth in this region and a resultant asymmetry in the developing skeleton.

8.1.8 Factors that contribute to running injuries

The most commonly reported factors include:

- **a lack of flexibility**, which is extremely common in distance runners;
- **training on hard surfaces and/or running on one side of the road**, which can mean that because of the camber certain anatomical structures experience additional stress;
- **running in old shoes or inappropriate shoes**, which in some cases may promote injuries rather than prevent them; this is clearly illustrated by the current concerns over high heel tabs, which are reported to aggravate the Achilles tendon;
- **running gait** – runners with particular running styles or gaits, such as extreme pronators or supinators, may be predisposed to particular types of injury;
- **biomechanical imbalances**, such as a discrepancy in bone length, muscle flexibility between certain muscles, the relative strength of related muscle groups and anatomical factors (Chapter 4).

Injuries are also caused by external factors such as falling while running. The severity of the injury resulting from such incidents can vary considerably, from slight abrasions to fractures. Stepping out into the path of a cyclist is also a potential cause of injury and all runners should be careful about this, especially when running in a group and stepping into the road to overtake. At night, additional reflective clothing should be worn to make the runner more visible to other road users. Lightweight headlamps, which are designed for runners and night orienteering, may be advocated in poorly lit areas to illuminate the running surface and make the runner more visible to oncoming traffic.

8.2 INJURIES IN THE THROWING EVENTS – DISCUS, JAVELIN, SHOT PUT AND HAMMER

8.2.1 Introduction to injuries in the throwing events

The athletic throwing events require explosive power to project the implement as far as possible. To do this the participants must use the permissible technique(s) that are laid down in the rules of the governing body. During athletic training and competition strict rules must be enforced to ensure the safety of the participants, spectators, judges and other users of the athletic arena. The throwers must ensure that the projectile lands within a designated sector and in events such as the discus and hammer the projectile is thrown from within a protective cage designed to prevent the implement from being thrown in an unpredicted direction and injuring any persons in that direction. Because of the need for maximum power and strength in the throwing events most throwers will spend a considerable amount of time training with weights. This is the cause of many injuries in this group of athletes. Other injuries are caused by the specific strains associated with the throwing techniques used in each event (Figure 8.2).

At most levels of athletics it is usual for a 'thrower' to participate in more than one of the throwing events and any injury may therefore be the result of a mixture of stresses placed upon his/her body by each event. Furthermore, it is not uncommon in club competitions for non-specialist throwers to participate in these events just to gain points for their club. Since these events require a consid-

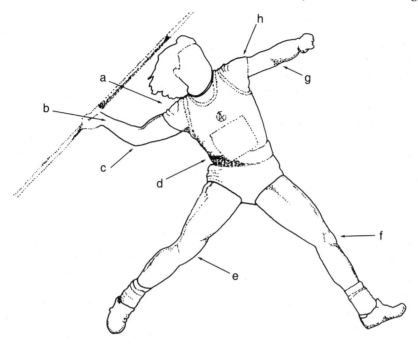

Figure 8.2 Common injuries occurring in the athletic throwing events. (a) Shoulder injuries. (b) Wrist injuries. (c) Elbow injuries (medial epicondylitis). (d) Spondylolysis. (e) Knee ligament injury. (f) Knee injuries to the meniscal cartilages. (g) Avulsion fractures. (h) Injuries to the rotator cuff.

erable amount of strength and the execution of the correct technique if they are to be performed safely 'non-throwers' are often injured when attempting the events. A common back injury among throwers is spondylolysis.

For each of the throwing events the exact competition weight of the implement will depend upon the age and gender of the participant. If young or novice throwers attempt to use a weight that is too heavy for them, this can lead to injury, especially if they lack the necessary strength to cope with it. The use of lighter implements is therefore often advocated with novices and those who have not yet developed the necessary strength and skill to safely throw the designated weight of implement.

In all the throwing events it is important for the throwing area to have sufficient traction, since a slippery surface is likely to cause injury and inappropriate footwear is likely to increase this risk. The explosive nature of the throwing events means that a thorough

warm-up is essential. The latter stages of the warm-up should include throwing specific activities such as practising the technique with submaximal effort before gradually progressing up to full throws with maximum effort.

8.2.2 The shot put

There are a number of established shot putting techniques all of which ultimately involve extending the knee and hip before finally extending the arm and pushing the shot out as fast as possible. This requires the explosive and coordinated use of legs, trunk and arms to attain the maximum speed of the shot and the optimum angle of release. While novice throwers may attempt this from a stationary position, established shot putters will employ a variety of techniques to increase the speed with which the shot is moving when it is released. These primarily involve commencing the throw from the far side of the throwing circle and then moving rapidly across it either in a direct line (as a glide or shift) or rotating in a similar manner to the discus technique. The rules of the shot put require that the shot is kept close to the neck in the initial stages of the throw, prior to the stage when the arm is extended, thereby ensuring that the event primarily requires a pushing action.

The wrist is perhaps the most vulnerable site of injury in shot putters, sprains being quite common. This is because it carries the weight of the shot and applies a final 'flick' before the shot is released. The elbow and shoulder are also prone to injuries, avulsion fractures being a possibility. Knee injuries are also quite common among shot putters because of the strain that is placed upon the knee. This occurs when landing just after the shot has been released and the participant tries to prevent him/herself from overbalancing and stepping out of the front of the throwing circle, which would constitute a foul.

8.2.3   The javelin

The rules of the javelin do not permit any 'unorthodox' throwing techniques, although some were tried prior to the introduction of this ruling. The javelin throw is preceded by a run-up, which is used to increase the final release speed of the implement. The two joints most prone to injury when throwing the javelin are the elbow and knee, with back and shoulder injuries also being quite common. Elbow injuries tend to result from the forceful extension, and in some cases hyperextension, of the elbow as the javelin is released. A common injury to this region is medial epicondylitis (thrower's elbow) at the site of muscular attachment to the medial epicondyle of the humerus. This may be more prevalent in junior throwers due to the presence of the epiphyseal growth plates and relative weakness of the bone in this region. The knee is prone

to injury because of the strain placed upon it as the thrower attempts to stop before the throwing line. In attempting to stop in the shortest possible distance the thrower plants his/her foot firmly in the ground and the knee then experiences a considerable amount of strain as s/he attempts to decelerate as quickly as possible. To facilitate this rapid deceleration javelin boots have spikes in the heel of the shoe as well as the forefoot. The explosive movements used in the javelin throw can also strain the muscles of the back, as the javelin is pulled through in the process of throwing, and the shoulder, which needs to rapidly move through a large range of movement as the thrower attempts to convey the maximum amount of force to the implement.

8.2.4   The discus

The normal technique for throwing the discus involves the thrower moving across the throwing circle in a rotatory motion, at the end of which s/he flings the discus out into the designated sector. The rotation technique can cause knee injuries if the knee is twisted as the upper body rotates while the foot remains fixed to the floor. These knee injuries tend to involve the meniscus cartilages and occasionally the ligaments. Inappropriate footwear, which prevents the foot from rotating across the circle, can be a contributing factor, as can an inappropriate throwing surface. Injuries to the elbow and rotator cuff of the shoulder are prevalent among this group of throwers because of the stresses placed upon these areas by the explosive movements used in the throwing action.

8.2.5   The hammer

Like the discus, the established technique for the hammer involves the athlete rotating rapidly across the throwing circle before releasing the implement. This can cause similar knee injuries to those reported in the discus, including damage to the meniscus cartilages and knee ligaments. Again, inappropriate footwear may be a contributing factor. The 'hammer' itself consists of a weighted ball attached to a wire (up to 4 feet/1.2 m) and handle. While rotating across the circle the wire is extended horizontally, enabling the ball to rotate with a maximum radius and angular acceleration. This places considerable strain upon the thrower and can cause back injuries, especially if the thrower is not properly conditioned for the event.

8.3 INJURIES IN THE ATHLETIC JUMPING EVENTS – LONG JUMP, TRIPLE JUMP, HIGH JUMP AND POLE VAULT

8.3.1 Introduction to injuries in the athletic jumping events

The long jump, triple jump and pole vault all require good sprinting speed. The training for these events is therefore similar to that of sprinters and the physiological stresses placed upon the body are reflected in the common injuries reported in these activities (Figure 8.3).

Training for the high jump often involves bounding exercises (plyometrics), which are also used by the other jumping events and can results in overuse injuries such as stress fractures and 'jumper's knee'. Pole vaulters often use weight training to develop the additional upper body strength they require in their event and weight training is also sometimes employed by other jumpers. Therefore, injuries resulting from this form of training may occur in these athletes.

The explosive power needed on take-off for all the jumping events places considerable strain upon the Achilles tendon, calf muscles and patellar tendon. This can result in repetitive overuse injuries and focal degeneration of the Achilles tendon and patellar tendon, making them vulnerable to partial rupture; complete ruptures of the Achilles tendon are also possible. The calf muscles are also prone to strains, as are the hamstring muscles during the take-off phase. Furthermore, the stresses placed upon the foot and heel during take-off can result in stress fractures and bruised heels.

During both training and competitions it is important for coaches and officials to ensure that the jumping and landing areas are safe. Excess water on any of the take-off areas can cause the athletes to slip, resulting in various

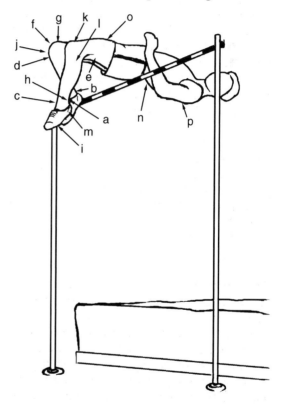

Figure 8.3 Common injuries occurring in the athletic jumping events. (a) Achilles tendinitis. (b) Achilles tendon rupture. (c) Sprained ankle. (d) Damage to the patellar tendon. (e) Hamstring strains. (f) Knee injuries. (g) Osgood–Schlatter's disease. (h) Sever's disease (i) Stress fracture to the metatarsal bones of the foot. (j) Sprained knee ligaments. (k) Knee meniscal cartilage damage. (l) Strains to the gastrocnemius. (m) Bruised heel. (n) Back injuries. (o) Adductor strains. (p) Rotator cuff tendinitis.

injuries. The landing pit in the long and triple jumps must be checked for debris that might cause injury and the sand should be dug properly to the correct depth. This involves digging and loosening the sand to a depth of at least 45 cm rather than just the surface, as this will leave hard, compacted sand just below the surface and will not provide adequate cushioning. The use of landing beds that fulfil the required safety standards are essential in the high jump and pole vault, where they must be of the correct size and be correctly positioned.

Competitions in the jumping events can last for over an hour, with the competitors having to wait between their attempts. During this time it is important for them to remain fully warmed up and flexible, since cold, tight muscles are more easily damaged.

8.3.2   The long and triple jump

The sprinting and explosive take-off aspects of the long and triple jump can result in damage to the Achilles tendon and patellar tendon. The repeated stresses can cause focal degeneration of these tendons and predispose the Achilles tendon to rupture. Hamstring injuries are another common injury in this group.

During the hop phase of the triple jump considerable strain is placed on the leg, which has to absorb the shock of landing and then generate the explosive force needed to propel the body forward for the next phase. This makes triple jumpers particularly vulnerable to knee injuries and concern has been expressed about the stresses experienced by juniors who participate in the event. Osgood–Schlatter's disease is not uncommonly found among junior jumpers. Other injuries found in young triple jumpers include Sever's disease (damage to the heel bone), caused by the impact of landing during the various phases of the triple jump, and stress fractures to the metatarsal bones of the foot.

Landing in the pit can cause injuries in any of the jumping events if joints are forced beyond their permissible range of movement. Knee and ankle injuries are most commonly reported in the long and triple jump, along with minor abrasions.

8.3.3.   The high jump

Like the other jumping events the stresses experienced by the foot, heel, Achilles tendon, calf muscles and hamstrings upon take-off in the high jump can cause injuries, which include stress fracture of the foot, bruised heel, various degree of traumatic and/or overuse damage to the Achilles tendon and strained muscles. Other injuries occurring in the high jump tend to reflect the technique used: the commonly used Fosbury flop can result in back injuries from poor landings and the repeated hyperextension of the back. The now less commonly used straddle technique can cause injury to the hamstrings and adductors if they are overstretched.

8.3.4   The pole vault

The injuries associated with the pole vault are usually related to accidents occurring during a vault. These include snapped poles or missing the landing bed. The latter of these is more likely with novice vaulters, who may swing out sideways with the pole rather than pulling themselves up in a direct vertical line. This can cause them to collide with the upright stands and risk missing the landing area. An awkward landing can also result in sprained ankles and a variety of other injuries, including back injuries. The need for upper body strength when executing the pole vault technique requires these athletes to pursue additional strengthening programmes and the strains of such training can cause injuries to the shoulder, most notably to the rotator cuff, which can suffer from tendinitis.

8.4 INJURIES IN GYMNASTICS

8.4.1 Introduction to injuries in gymnastics

A number of studies have indicated that gymnastics is one of the major sources of sports injuries in women. This is reflective of the relatively high levels of participation and the age group involved, as well as the physical demands of the sport. Both traumatic and overuse injuries occur in gymnastics with approximately equal frequency, although some studies would suggest that traumatic injuries are slightly more common (Figure 8.4).

The lower extremities appear to be most vulnerable followed by the elbow, wrist, back and spine. Sprains and strains account for most of these injuries, although a number of fractures also occur. Mild overuse injuries such as blisters to the hands commonly occur and will need to be treated using standard first aid procedures. To reduce the incidence of these problems handguards and chalk are often advocated, as these will reduce the amount of friction between the hands and apparatus. Traumatic injuries in gymnastics are most commonly caused by falling from the apparatus or mistakes when executing a movement such as a somersault. Some of these can be extremely serious, such as back and neck injuries, the treatment of which will usually be the concern of specialized medical practitioners rather than the general sports injury therapist. Consequently, the type of gymnastic injuries the practitioner is most likely to encounter are the more significant overuse injuries and any damage caused to the tendons, ligaments, muscles and joints during training or competition.

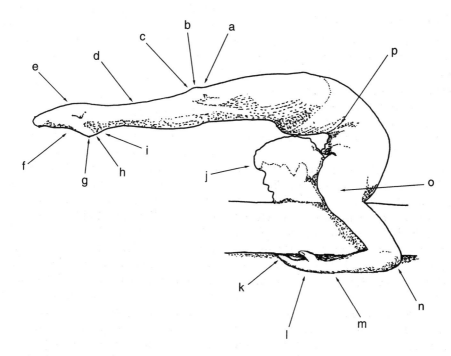

Figure 8.4 Common injuries occurring in gymnastics. (a) Knee ligament and meniscal cartilage injuries. (b) Osgood-Schlatter's disease. (c) Partial rupture of patellar tendon. (d) Stress fractures of tibia. (e) Ankle sprains. (f) Plantar fasciitis. (g) Bruised heel. (h) Sever's disease. (i) Achilles tendon injuries. (j) Traumatic injuries to head and spine. (k) Blisters. (l) Fractures to wrist and hand. (m) Epiphyseal plate injuries. (n) Elbow hyperextension. (o) Shoulder injuries. (p) Spondylolysis, spondylolisthesis.

A number of studies have indicated that the incidence of injuries in gymnastics increases with the standard of the performer. This is probably related to:

- the number of hours spent training and thus exposure to the risk of traumatic injury;
- the increased likelihood of overuse injury from repeating movements a larger number of times;
- the tendency for higher level performers to attempt more complex movements.

The vast majority of gymnastic injuries have been shown to occur in training. Here a number of factors may contribute, including:

- loss of concentration when attempting to execute a movement;
- fatigue;
- failure to use protective equipment such as foam landing areas, belts and padding;
- the absence of spotters;
- attempting new movements or sequences;
- the obvious difference in the amount of time spent training versus competing.

Another factor that may contribute to the risk of injury in some gymnasts is their stage of development. Prepubescent female gymnasts appear to be far less prone to injury than older, pubescent gymnasts. It has been suggested that the reasons for this are:

- a change in the relative lengths of muscle and bones, causing muscle–tendon tightness;
- a change in muscle strength relative to bone length;
- an increase in moments of inertia with increasing limb length;
- the vulnerability of the growth cartilage at this stage.

In women's gymnastics the discipline most likely to cause injury is floor work. In this activity incorrectly executed somersaults, handsprings and flips often result in the per-former injuring herself on landing. Injuries also occur when working on the balance beam and asymmetric bars, where poorly executed dismounts, falling and colliding with the apparatus are the most commonly reported causes. Somewhat surprisingly, the vault appears to be the discipline in which the smallest number of injuries occur, although the causes of injury are similar – poor landings or colliding with the apparatus. Colliding with any piece of apparatus can cause bruising and is a common occurrence at all levels of gymnastics.

Gymnastics requires extreme levels of flexibility, and therefore a comprehensive warm-up that includes a relatively large amount of stretching is vital before training and competition. It should also be remembered that in competitions there may be some time between individual components of the competition and that gymnasts will need to keep warm and flexible if they are not to risk pulling muscles. They may therefore need to repeat their warm-up routine, or part of it, at regular intervals during the competition.

8.4.2 Injuries to the foot and ankle

The joint most commonly damaged during gymnastics is the ankle. Ankle sprains occur when landing awkwardly, either when dismounting from a piece of apparatus or when landing from a jump. Often in the process of landing the gymnast will execute a complex manoeuvre that involves twisting and rotating, both of which increase the chance of landing awkwardly. In gymnastics the apparatus must be checked for safety and there must be no gaps between landing mats, another cause of falls and ankle injuries. The most common overuse injuries to the feet and ankles include:

- fractures to the metatarsals and tarsals;
- plantar fasciitis;
- bruised and damaged heels, including Sever's disease;

- damage to the Achilles tendon and associated structures, including tendinitis, tenoperiostitis, focal degeneration of the tendon and bursitis. The Achilles tendon is also vulnerable to traumatic rupture (partial or complete) due to the stress placed upon it during take-off.

8.4.3 Injuries to the leg, including the knee

Sprains to the knee ligaments and meniscal cartilage damage can occur with poorly executed landings that cause violent twisting movements or hyperextension of the knee. Additional traumatic injuries include patellar tendon ruptures and epiphyseal fractures as a result of collisions. Repetitive stress can also cause epiphyseal plate damage, which has been reported in the long bones of the arms as well as the legs. Osgood–Schlatter's disease is a problem encountered by many young gymnasts. This overuse injury is caused by the repetitive strain placed on the insertion of the patellar tendon on the tibia by frequent of powerful extension and eccentric contractions of the knee extensors during jumping and landing movements. Stress fractures to the tibia can be caused by repeatedly landing on hard surfaces. Partial rupture of the patellar tendon (jumper's knee) may be caused by the excessive stresses placed upon it during take-off. Often these partial ruptures, and in a few cases complete ruptures, are a result of repetitive overuse causing an initial degeneration of the tendon, making it more vulnerable to rupture during explosive movements. Anterior compartment syndrome is also reported among gymnasts.

8.4.4 Injuries to the hand, wrist, arm and shoulder

The use of the upper limbs in movements such as flick-flacks and handsprings makes the wrist and elbow vulnerable to both traumatic and overuse injuries. Hyperextending the elbow or wrist is a common cause of injury to these joints and the repetitive stress of taking the weight of the body when landing on the hands can cause a number of overuse problems. Epiphyseal damage may occur from either a collision or repetitive overuse, with other fractures of both the wrist and elbow also possible. The most commonly reported shoulder injuries include supraspinatus tendinitis.

8.4.5 Injuries to the back and spine

In addition to the obvious traumatic injuries caused by poorly executed landings or falls a number of overuse injuries are also possible. Spondylolysis is the most commonly reported overuse injury to the back in female gymnastics, where the cause is reported to be repeated hyperextension of the spine and the repeated impact of landing. These stresses can result in a stress fracture to the vertebrae and may also cause the forward slippage of the vertebrae (spondylolisthesis). It usually occurs in the lumbar region of the spine. 'Back walkovers' and 'back flips', both of which require considerable hyperextension of the back, are considered to be contributing factors.

8.5 INJURIES IN SWIMMING

8.5.1 Background to swimming injuries

Swimming is a relatively injury-free sport with a very low incidence of traumatic injuries. However the large training volumes undertaken by most competitive swimmers almost inevitably makes them vulnerable to overuse injuries (Figure 8.5).

The most common sites of injury are the shoulders, back and knee. Shoulder injuries include supraspinatus tendinitis, bursitis of the subacromial bursae and damage to the tendon of the long head of the biceps. The front crawl and backstroke arm action are likely to be the main causes of this injury

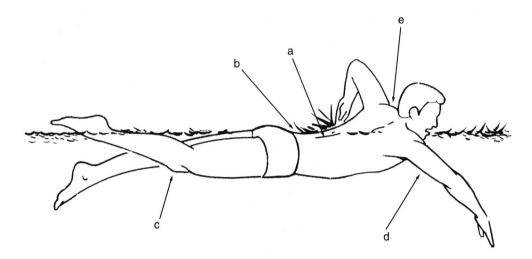

Figure 8.5   Common injuries occurring in swimming. (a) Spondylolysis, back injury (butterfly). (b) Lordosis of the back. (c) Knee ligament and cartilage injury (breast stroke). (d) Biceps tendinitis. (e) Swimmer's shoulder and supra spinatus tendinitis (front crawl) and Kyphosis.

because of the large range through which the shoulder moves. In the swimming events the arm action can cause the subacromial bursa and supraspinatus tendon to become pinched under the acromion process of the scapula and the coracoacromial ligament, resulting in tenderness and inflammation, commonly referred to as 'swimmer's shoulder' (subacromial impingement syndrome).

Overuse injuries of the knee are usually associated with the breast stroke, which can damage the medial ligaments. Hyperflexion of the spine during the dolphin kick in butterfly can cause back injuries including spondylolysis (stress fracture of the vertebrae) and kyphosis (a rounding of the back also called Scheuermann's disease).

8.6   INJURIES IN COMPETITIVE CYCLING

8.6.1   Background to injuries in competitive cycling

Competitive cycling events take place in a number of environments including velodrome stadiums, roads, paths, tracks and open country. The distance over which cyclists race also ranges considerably, from relatively short sprints to multiday events such as the Tour de France. The format of cycling races also varies, including time trials and team pursuit events as well as races in which all the competitors start together. The bicycles used in these events vary according to the terrain and the requirements of the event; the machines used in top-class velodrome, road and mountain bike events differ considerably. Cycling is also a component in events such as the triathlon, and hence competitors in these events can suffer from cycling injuries as well as those experienced by runners and swimmers.

Cycling injuries include both the traumatic and overuse types (Figure 8.6).

Most traumatic cycling injuries are caused by falls and result in abrasions to the thigh, hip and lower leg, with more serious injuries such as fractures occurring occasionally. The repetitive nature of cycling makes the participants also prone to overuse injuries, particularly to the knee. Maintaining one position for a prolonged period of time can cause back injuries and cyclist's palsy.

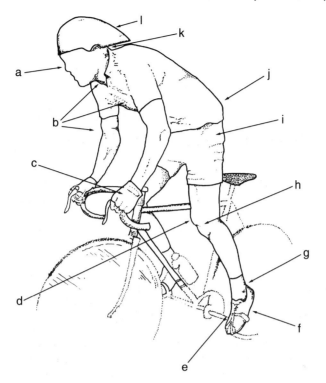

Figure 8.6 Common injuries occurring in competitive cycling. (a) Orofacial and eye injuries. (b) Fractures to elbows, ribs and collar bone. (c) Cyclist palsy (ulnar neuropathy). (d) Patellar tendinitis and bursitis. (e) Metatarsalgia. (f) Plantar fasciitis. (g) Achilles tendinitis. (h) Biker's knee, chondromalacia patellae. (i) Tronchenteric bursitis. (j) Lower back pain. (k) Neck pain. (l) Head injuries

8.6.2 Common causes of cycling injuries

(a) Traumatic injuries

The commonest cause of the traumatic type of cycling injury is a fall, sometimes resulting from collisions with other cyclists or motor vehicles. Attempting to corner too fast is also a problem, especially on wet, slippery roads. Obstructions or debris in the road are cited as causes in some cases, along with punctures. To minimize the risk of these injuries the bike should be well maintained and carefully checked before each ride. The wearing of helmets is advocated by governing bodies to reduce the risk of head injuries and their use is compulsory in some races. The wearing of glasses or visors will protect the eyes from stones, grit and flying insects. Cycling shorts and tops will reduce the severity of abrasions when falling. The development of a high level of skill and good tactics should minimize the risk of falling and collisions.

(b) Overuse injuries

In the course of training and competition cyclists will repeat the pedalling action many thousands of times. This makes them prone to overuse injuries, especially to the knee. The factors that may contribute to such injuries are an inappropriate pedalling action due to a poorly set-up bike, an inappropriate pedalling action due to anatomical factors, and anatomical weaknesses. Maintaining the same position during long rides can also contribute to injuries such as neck pain, ulnar neuropathy (cyclist's palsy) and lower back pain, all of which may again be partially attributed to the set-up of the bike. It is therefore essential that the bike is correctly set up for each individual rider. Numerous factors must be considered, including (1) the saddle height, (2) the distance between the saddle and the handlebars and (3) the height of the handlebars, along with numerous other variables, which make it an area of specialism but one which the practitioner should be aware of when considering the likely cause of any injury. Simple overuse problems such as blisters and saddle-soreness can be treated with the usual first aid procedures with, in some cases, a change of saddle being appropriate.

8.6.3   Common cycling injuries and their prevention

(a)   Knee injuries (biker's knee, patellofemoral pain syndrome, chondromalacia patellae, patellar tendinitis and patellar bursitis)

Knee pain is common in cyclists, especially early in the season when they may rapidly increase the amount of training. Indeed the term 'Easter knee' is often used to reflect its occurrence in the spring. A factor relating to this could be the weather at this time of year, which can be cold and wet. This can chill the exposed knee as it moves rapidly through the cold air decreasing the lubricating capacity of the knee fluids and contributing to the likelihood of overuse problems. Common causes of knee pain are:

- saddle set too high or too low;
- using too high a gear and hence pedalling against a high resistance at a relatively low cadence;
- rotation of the foot on the pedals/pronation of the rearfoot (rearfoot valgus);
- malalignment of the knee extensor mechanism, possibly related to a poorly fitting bike.

When pedalling, the patellofemoral joint is under considerable stress, which can be increased by the above factors; hence, by altering them, the problem may be alleviated. The patella tracks over the femur as the knee extends and if the amount of friction between the two is increased then chondromalacia-type pain is likely to result from the inflammation at the back of the kneecap. As with runners, a large Q angle of the quadriceps muscle group may be a contributing factor, as can dysplasia of the vastus medialis obliquus or a high/lateral position of the patella. Pronation of the rearfoot (rearfoot valgus) while pedalling can only be effectively diagnosed by video techniques that involve the cyclist using their own bike while pedalling on rollers. This may be resolved by realigning the saddle or the use of orthotics such as a medial heel wedge.

(b)   Foot and ankle injuries (Achilles tendinitis, plantar fasciitis, metatarsalgia)

Foot problems such as metatarsalgia are generally caused by using toe clips and straps that are too tight. Modifying these and pedalling in a lower gear that provides less resistance usually reduces the likelihood of recurrence. Achilles tendinitis and plantar fasciitis may occur if the saddle is too low, as this can cause excessive dorsiflexion while pedalling.

(c)   Neck and back pain

Neck pain can result from excessive hyperextension of the neck and usually involves the first three cervical vertebrae. Cycling with the handlebars set too low or with the hands in the dropped position for prolonged periods will cause the cyclist to hyperextend the neck in order to see ahead. Using a bike that is 'too long' will also cause this problem, as s/he will have to over-reach. Raising the torso while cycling or adjusting the set-up of the bike are therefore the usual remedies. Lower back pain may also result from an inappropriately set-up bike and prolonged periods of using the handlebars in the dropped position, so appropriate changes in the cycling position and/or adjustments to the set-up of the bike are likely to resolve the problem.

(d) Head and ocular injuries

Head injuries usually result from falls. To minimize their occurrence the cyclist should possess the necessary skills, ensure that s/he concentrate and wear a protective helmet. Eye injuries and more minor inconveniences can result from grit, small stones and flying insects. To prevent these the use of glasses or visors is advocated. In the case of sunglasses those with some form of UV protection are recommended to prevent damage to the eye, since the use of glasses may cause the pupil to be somewhat more dilated than usual, thereby exposing the eye to additional UV.

(e) Fractures and abrasions

Fractures and abrasions, like head injuries, are caused by falls. Possessing adequate levels of skill and concentration are the best means of minimizing their occurrence. The severity of abrasions may be reduced by wearing appropriate cycling clothing. When fractures do occur a number of sites are vulnerable, including the wrist, elbow, ribs and collarbone.

(f) Hand and wrist injuries

A common overuse injury experienced by cyclists is 'cyclist's palsy' (ulnar neuropathy). It is caused by compression of the ulnar nerve in the region of Guyon's canal. It causes a tingling and numbness in the areas served by the ulnar nerve and in particular the ring and little fingers. In more severe cases it causes pain, weakness of the intrinsic muscles of the hand and coordination problems which, if untreated, may have permanent effects. It is caused by cycling for prolonged periods

with the hands in the dropped position on the handlebars. In this position the hands are dorsiflexed and a significant amount of the cyclist's weight is over the hands, which results in the nerve being compressed.

To alleviate the problem cyclists should minimize the amount of time spent in the 'dropped position', pad the handlebars or use padded gloves and, where appropriate, adjust the bike so that in the normal cycling position they don't lean so far forward and hence place less weight on the hands.

(g) Hip injuries (trochanteric bursitis and iliopsoas tendinitis)

Trochanteric bursitis is caused by the repetitive movement of the fascia lata over the greater trochanter and, like tendinitis of the iliopsoas, may be caused by the saddle being too high.

8.7 INJURIES IN GOLF

8.7.1 General background to common golfing injuries, causes and prevention

The traumatic injuries reported in golf tend to relate to being hit by the ball, being hit by a club or falling over, while the overuse injuries are related to the repeated action of swinging the golf club (Figure 8.7).

In right-handed players the most common sites of injury are the left wrist, left hand, elbow, shoulder and back. Overuse injuries in golf are usually linked to a poor swing; some golfers compensate for poor technique with brute force. Holding the club too tightly is another common error which can cause tendinitis of the tendons in the hand. Sprained wrists usually occur on the radial (thumb) side and muscle strains of the wrist extensors (extensor carpi radialis brevis and extensor carpi radialis longus) are also fairly common.

One of the most common complaints of right-handed golfers is lateral epicondylitis,

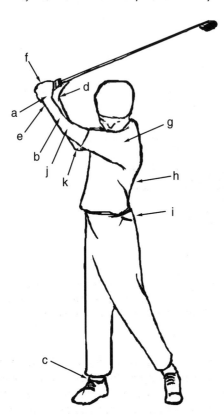

Figure 8.7 Common golfing injuries. (a) Carpal fractures. (b) Ulnar and median neuropathies. (c) Achilles tendonitis. (d) Sprained wrist. (e) Strains of the wrist extensor. (f) Tendinitis/tenosynovitis of the tendons of the hand. (g) Shoulder injuries (rotator cuff). (h) Back pain. (i) Hip pain. (j) Lateral epicondylitis of the leading elbow. (k) Medial epicondylitis of the following elbow.

consisting of a combination of tendinitis and periostitis of the extensor tendons in the left elbow. Holding the club too tightly is likely to increase the risk of this. Medial epicondylitis (golfer's elbow) can sometimes occur in the other elbow.

Injuries of the shoulder usually relate to the rotator cuff and range from tendinitis to full tears. Back injuries are often attributable to a lack of warm-up before playing and a poor technique. Other reported injuries include Achilles tendinitis and various causes of pain in the hips.

The prevention of golfing injuries can be assisted by ensuring the gradual resumption of the game and an adequate level of general fitness. Attempting to play several games on consecutive days after the winter break will almost certainly result in an aching back, sore shoulders and overused joints. A good level of fitness, perhaps through the use of a general weight training and conditioning programme, may help to ensure that the golfer's body can cope with the demands made on it while playing. Warming up before playing is also essential as many backs are strained on the first tee.

8.8 INJURIES IN ROWING, CANOEING AND KAYAKING

8.8.1 Background to common injuries in rowing canoeing and kayaking, causes and prevention

All water sports carry an element of risk associated with the environment. When canoeing or rafting in white water this is obviously increased and all the necessary safety precautions should therefore be adhered to.

Most injuries in these sports occur to the wrist and forearm due to the repetitive action of paddling or rowing (Figure 8.8).

In the Canadian canoeing events the canoeists kneel in the boat and use a paddle with a single blade. The paddling action involves holding the paddle with one hand on top of the shaft of the paddle and the other lower down the shaft nearer the blade. This paddling action can cause some asymmetry in paddlers. Kayakers, by contrast, use a double-bladed paddle on alternate sides of the boat. Competitive canoeing and kayaking include both single and doubles classes.

Competitive rowing also includes a number of classes and variations from singles to eights. The doubles may be coxed or coxless and depending upon the class a rower may use one or two oars. The use of one oar, as in

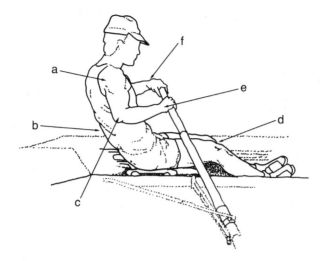

Figure 8.8   Common injuries occurring in rowing, canoeing and kayaking. (a) Shoulder injuries, subacromial impingement syndrome in Canadian-style canoeists. (b) Back pain. (c) Lateral and medial epicondylitis. (d) Chondromalacia patellae (rowing). (e) Wrist sprains and extensor tenosynovitis. (f) Median nerve entrapment.

the eights, can lead to asymmetrical development in participants.

In canoeists, kayakers and rowers one of the most common repetitive strain injuries is extensor tenosynovitis, with a similar overuse injury also occurring in the flexors in some participants. In general both of these injuries are likely to be attributed to gripping the paddle/oar too tightly. The paddling/rowing action can also cause both medial and lateral epicondylitis in the elbow.

In the Canadian-style canoeing events the paddling action can cause the subacromial bursa and supraspinatus tendon to become pinched under the acromion process of the scapula and the coracoacromial ligament, resulting in tenderness and inflammation (subacromial impingement syndrome).

Lower back pain occurs in canoeists, kayakers and rowers since much of the power used in the paddling/rowing action is generated here. Rowers can also suffer from chondromalacia patellae due to the leg movements involved as they slide forward and back in the rowing action.

The prevention of injuries in these events largely centres upon the participants possessing a good level of general fitness with appropriate muscle strength and flexibility. A lack of these will almost inevitably result in overuse injuries. Faulty paddling/or rowing technique is also a factor in the incidence of injuries and a good warm-up before any strenuous work is essential.

8.9   INJURIES IN WEIGHT LIFTING AND WEIGHT TRAINING

8.9.1   Introduction to weight-lifting and weight-training injuries

The competitive sports of Olympic weight lifting and power lifting obviously require the participants to undertake training with heavy weights. In addition to these individuals, weight training is also undertaken by a large number of sports performers from a variety of sports as a means of developing their muscular strength. Although some individuals and coaches prefer not to use weights, many do, especially those training for the athletic throwing events and team games such as rugby. Others who might incorporate weight training into a general conditioning programme include individuals who participate in the combat sports, sprinting, swimming and gymnastics. Many of these coaches and sports performers find that the increased strength gained from this form of training can enhance performance. However this form of training can also be a source of injury if it is not undertaken properly with the correct adherence to safe techniques and the principles of gradual progressive overload (Figure 8.9).

One of the adaptations of the body to weight training is to increase the strength of the muscles, initially through an enhanced neurological recruitment of the muscle fibres and then through hypertrophy of the muscle. Strength training will also cause adaptations in the tendons and their connection to the bone. However it is suggested that these adaptations occur more slowly and therefore, if an individual attempts to progress too rapidly with their training programme, while the muscles may be able to cope with the heavier weights, the tendons and tenoperiosteal junctions may not. This makes these structures vulnerable to overuse injury, rupture and even avulsion fractures.

Many authorities would recommend that preadolescents do not participate in weight training because of the risk of injury to their immature skeleton. In particular, concern is expressed about the incidence of injuries to the epiphyseal plates, which it is suggested can be damaged by the large stresses placed upon them resulting in their premature closure and hence stunting of the individual's growth. The relative weakness of these areas of growth cartilage also makes them vulner-

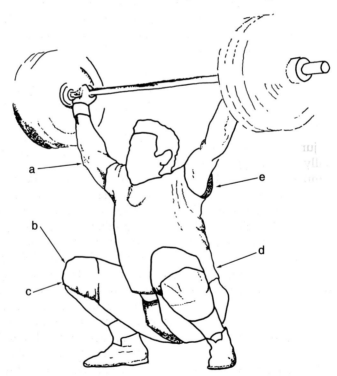

Figure 8.9 Common injuries occurring in weight training and weight lifting. (a) Biceps rupture. (b) Knee cartilage injuries. (c) Patellar tendon injuries including rupture. (d) Back injuries, spondylolysis, spondylosis, spondylolisthesis. (e) Shoulder injuries including of the rotator cuff.

able to fracture; documented reports of such injuries include those to the distal radial epiphyses.

Most of the traumatic injuries that occur when training with weights are as a result of the individual dropping the weight or the weights not being securely attached to the bar with the appropriate collars. This can make the use of exercise machines preferable as they may be safer in this respect, although it is argued by some that, since they restrict the range of movement and assist with its control, they are not as effective at training some of the muscle groups, especially those involved with controlling and stabilizing movement. When using any form of exercise machine or multi-gym it is essential that all the safety aspects are adhered to and that the correct lifting technique is used. Furthermore when using 'free weights', helpers and spotters must also be present and aware of their responsibilities. In addition to the traumatic injuries caused by dropping weights a number of other injuries occur to the back, knees and shoulder; these and their causes are highlighted below.

8.9.2 Back injuries

A common site of injury from weight training is the back, especially if it is hyperextended during the lift. Examples of this are the military press and bench press where a poor technique can result in hyperextension. These injuries may be associated with poor technique or the individual possessing inadequate strength to cope safely with the weight s/he is lifting and the effect of the repeated loads placed upon the spine. Common back injuries include:

- **spondylolysis** – a stress fracture of the vertebral arch;
- **spondylosis** – the degeneration of an intervertebral disc;
- **spondylolisthesis** – the forward movement of a vertebra, causing it to be out of align-

ment with the one below it; this most commonly occurs in the fifth lumbar vertebra.

8.9.3 Knee injuries

Exercises involving knee flexion and extension can cause knee damage, especially when using heavy weights or large resistances. Leg flexion and extension machines may be a source of injury here, as is deep squatting, where the individual supports a weight on the shoulders and then squats down beyond the point where the thigh is parallel to the floor. This can place excessively large strains upon the knee, causing overuse injury or even rupture of the patellar tendon.

8.9.4 Shoulder injuries

Shoulder injuries are common among weight lifters and typically involve strained muscles and tendons in this region, including the rotator cuff.

8.10 INJURIES IN THE COMBAT SPORTS AND MARTIAL ARTS

8.10.1 Introduction to injuries in the combat sports and martial arts

The nature of the combat sports and martial arts almost inevitably means that most of the injuries will occur as a result of contact during competitions (Figure 8.10).

The level of permissible contact and the amount of permissible protective clothing varies considerably among these sports and even among variations of the same sport, and will influence the frequency and severity of injury. Many of the injuries that occur during competitions will require immediate first aid and are therefore likely to be the concern of the medical staff at the venue rather than being presented to the practitioner at a later date. Safety within these sports is best ensured by close adherence to the rules, an

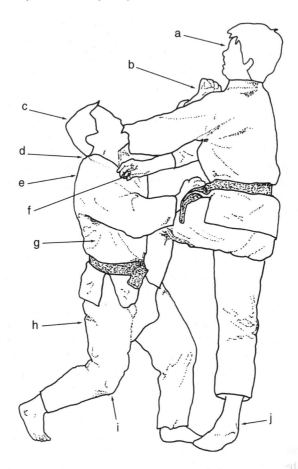

Figure 8.10 Common injuries occurring in the combat sports and martial arts. (a) Orofacial injuries. (b) Fractures, compression injuries and dislocations of the fingers. (c) Traumatic encephalopathy (boxing). (d) Neck injuries. (e) Shoulder dislocations. (f) Wrist and arm fractures from falls. (g) General bruising. (h) Strained hamstring and adductor muscles. (i) Damaged knee ligaments and meniscal cartilages. (j) Sprained ankles.

equal matching of the participants in terms of size and skill and an appropriate level of fitness of the participants.

8.10.2 Background to injuries in karate, tae kwon do and related martial arts

The competitive martial arts involve a variety of styles of combat that primarily use the hands and feet to punch and kick the opponent. The amount of violent contact that is permitted in competitive bouts varies considerably, depending upon the style of martial art. For example, most forms of karate permit no contact or minimal contact, which should be light. This therefore requires the participants to 'pull' punches and kicks before they make contact. However other forms of karate permit full contact, which therefore conveys a much greater risk of injury, making the risks of participation similar to those of other contact martial arts such as tae kwon do.

The head is a vulnerable and common target in the martial arts, which results in the head and neck region suffering from the greatest number of reported injuries. These include lacerations, fractures of the nose, dental damage, ocular injuries and concussion. Since the usual means of attack are the hands and feet these are also prone to damage in the form of fractures and dislocations. Bruising to the arms and legs is common since they are used to block an attack. Other injuries include shoulder dislocations and injuries to the trunk, the frequency and severity of which depend upon the style of combat and the amount of protection worn by the participants. Some of the most serious injuries to the body include damage to the spleen, liver, kidneys and lungs.

The extreme range of movement that is required in the sport can cause pulled muscles in those who lack the necessary flexibility, especially in the hamstrings and adductors. Damaged joints may result from a fall, loss of balance or a blow. Sprained ankles are relatively common and damaged knee ligaments may be caused by twisting, falling awkwardly or receiving a blow to the side of the knee.

8.10.3 Karate

The amount of physical contact that is permitted in karate contests varies considerably, depending upon which variation of the rules is being applied. The amount of contact varies from no permissible contact to full contact and this will obviously influence the likelihood of injury. Typically a kick or punch has to stop (be pulled) just prior to contact; often light contact is permitted but more forceful contact is usually penalized. Punches are the most common cause of injury, with most injurious punches being aimed at the head and causing lacerations, concussion and fractures (mainly nasal and teeth). Injuries to the fingers also occur in the form of fractures and dislocations, as a consequence of which the use of padded gloves has been advocated by some authorities as a means of protecting the hands when punching as well as the recipient of the punch by lessening the impact. Other

protective equipment such as gum shields, head protectors, groin protectors and padding for the arms, lower leg and feet have also be suggested but are not widely used. An argument against their use is that the additional protection would reduce the emphasis on not making contact with the opponent and would thereby increase the risk of contact and hence injury. Therefore it is the strict enforcement of the rules that currently provides the main assurance of preventing injury.

8.10.4 Tae kwon do

Tae kwon do, unlike most forms of karate, permits full contact in the form of kicks and punches. Punching is allowed to all parts of the body above the belt except the head and kicks to all parts of the body including the head. No head protection is worn but padding to the trunk and genitalia is permitted, as are mouthguards. As might be expected, most recorded injuries occur to the head and neck, with others to the hands, arms legs and feet, the causes of which are similar to those described in the section on karate.

Other martial arts, which may emphasize a slightly different technique or style of combat, produce similar injury profiles.

8.10.5 Boxing

Most boxing injuries are related to the combat aspect of the sport and most will require immediate first aid and medical treatment. Blows to the head can result in immediate injury either from the opponent's glove when punching or from the floor if a boxer falls and hits the back of his head. The cumulative effect of punches to the head can also result in traumatic encephalopathy, with the distinctive symptoms that give it its common name of 'punch drunk'. Facial injuries to the eyes, nose and mouth would all require appropriate first aid and are therefore unlikely to fall into the realm of most practitioners unless they were in attendance when they occurred. Injuries to the hand include thumb injuries (joint compression and dislocation) from poor punching technique. The wearing of appropriate protective equipment such as headgear, mouthguards and groin protectors is mandatory at most levels of the sport. Strict adherence to the rules and good refereeing that stops a fight once a participant is unable to defend himself will also prevent unnecessary injury. Skill is an obvious factor and a boxer must know how to protect himself as well as how to punch correctly. It is also important to ensure that the participants are appropriately matched. Weight divisions go some way towards ensuring this, although appropriate matching in accordance with ability is also essential.

8.10.6   Judo and wrestling

Compared with other combat sports, judo and wrestling are relatively low-risk. In these sports most injuries occur when falling and making contact with the ground. Often it is the elbow that is most vulnerable if the participant attempts to break his/her fall with an outstretched arm, which can also result in fractures. The wrist and shoulder are also prone to injury, shoulder dislocations also being caused by falls. Wrestling can result in a similar injury profile, with the addition of neck injuries if it is hyperextended in movements such as bridging.

8.11   INJURIES IN THE RACQUET SPORTS

8.11.1   Introduction to the racquet sports and common injuries

Since badminton, squash and tennis are the most widely played racquet games, most of the research into the incidence of racquet game injuries has focused upon these three.

In respect of the incidence, causes and prevention of injuries, while these racquet games obviously differ in some respects, they also possess a number of similarities, which means that the physical stresses placed upon the bodies of the participants are similar and hence they produce a similar injury profile (Figure 8.11). This would also be true of other racquet sports such as racquet ball and hence much of the content of this chapter can be applied to all racquet games.

In racquet sports most of the reported sports injuries occur to the lower limbs. This is due to the demands of the games, which involve rapid changes of direction, abrupt stopping, explosive jumping and lunging to reach the ball or shuttlecock. A second group of injuries occur to the upper limbs and are related to the stresses placed upon the racquet arm, with additional injuries occurring to the torso because of the movements involved in stroke play. A final group of injuries are caused by the projectile (ball or shuttlecock) and racquet (usually that of the partner or opponent). Of this latter group the most serious injuries are those to the face and eyes. While the practitioner may not be directly involved with the treatment of facial and ocular injuries s/he may be in a position to advise on their prevention and hence should be aware that they occur.

8.11.2   Injuries to the lower limb – causes and prevention

All racquet games require rapid movements and changes in direction, which can stress the muscles, tendons and joints. Strained adductor muscles are fairly common in all racquet sports and are primarily caused by overstretching the muscles when lunging for a shot or rapidly changing direction. Strained muscles of the quadriceps and hamstring groups are also caused in this manner, as are strains to the gastrocnemius. In all cases research has often highlighted an inadequate warm-up as a contributing factor and in

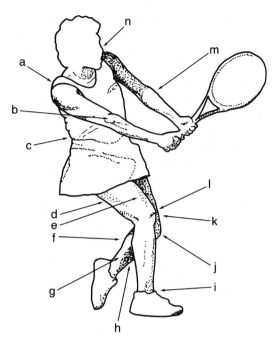

Figure 8.11 Common injuries occurring in the racquet sports. (a) Overuse of rotator cuff of shoulder. (b) Medial and lateral epicondylitis (tennis elbow). (c) Back injuries, muscular strains and disc prolapse. (d) Strained adductors, hamstrings. (e) Strained quadriceps. (f) Strained gastrocnemius. (g) Achilles tendon injuries, including rupture. (h) Shin soreness and stress fractures. (i) Sprained ankle. (j) Chondromalacia patellae. (k) Knee ligament injury: cruciate, medial and lateral ligaments. (l) Knee meniscal cartilage damage. (m) Overuse of forearm extensors. (n) Eye injuries (primarily squash and badminton)

some cases a previous injury that has predisposed the tissue to further damage. This is also the case with injuries to the Achilles tendon, with badminton being the most common cause of sports-related Achilles tendon rupture. Therefore, players should not attempt to continue to play with underlying injuries but should seek treatment and permit the injury to heal before resuming their sport.

Injuries to the knee and ankle joint are caused by the joint being forced beyond its permissible range of movement. In the case of the ankle the most common injury is a sprain of the lateral ligaments, which is caused by excessive inversion of the foot, often when changing direction. To reduce the risk of this injury appropriate footwear should be worn and in some cases strapping may be advocated although some authorities

would suggest caution with its use, as reliance upon the external support could reduce the effectiveness of the musculature around the joint, causing weakness and the risk of future instability leading to further injury. Injury to the knee is usually caused by over-rotation, often due to the foot remaining fixed to the ground as the upper leg rotates. This can damage the meniscal cartilage and cruciate ligaments. Other knee injuries include strains to the medial and lateral ligaments and chondromalacia patellae due to overuse.

The hard surface upon which racquet sports tend to be played can also result in sore shins or even stress fractures. The choice of footwear is therefore important in injury prevention since it must provide adequate traction (while not increasing the risk of knee injuries), stability and cushioning. In the case of the latter, additional insoles or extra socks may be worn. Some authorities have suggested additional heel inserts for badminton players to reduce the risk of overstretching the Achilles tendon and hence its rupture.

For most racquet games players, appropriate flexibility exercises for the leg muscles and Achilles tendon, coupled with an adequate warm-up routine, could reduce the number of injuries quite considerably. It is quite remarkable how many squash players expend a large amount of strenuous effort in warming up the ball for a match without first warming up themselves.

8.11.3 Injuries to the upper limb and torso – causes and prevention

The most widely reported upper limb injury is 'lateral epicondylitis', commonly called 'tennis elbow' although it occurs in all racquet sports. Essentially this is an overuse injury, which is frequently attributed to poor stroke technique, especially of the backhand, which places excessive strain on the elbow at the point of origin of wrist and finger extensor muscles where they attach to the humerus. Of the racquet sports it is most prominent in tennis because of the greater forces involved due to the weight of the racquet and ball. The impact of the racquet striking the ball causes these forces to be conveyed up the arm to the elbow. With good technique these will be distributed over the entire arm and shoulder rather than being focused on the elbow. Hence good stroke technique is often the key to preventing tennis elbow. The same is also true for medial epicondylitis, which may be caused by poor forehand technique. In both cases some authorities suggest that the use of racquets that are too tightly strung, are too heavy or have the wrong size of grip may also be contributing factors; however this has not yet been conclusively demonstrated in all cases. Although lateral and medial epicondylitis occur in all racquet sports they are less common in badminton

because of the lighter weight of the racquet and projectile, which results in less stress being placed upon the elbow.

An excessive use of the wrist in racquet games can result in overuse of the forearm extensors. In squash some players may deliberately use the wrist to conceal the type of shot being played, while others may possess a 'wristy' or poor overall technique that makes them susceptible to this form of injury. In badminton the use of the wrist is part of the stroke technique and is therefore used extensively, but because of the use of lighter implements the risk of injury to the forearm extensors is lessened.

Overuse injuries of the 'rotator cuff' of the shoulder of the racquet arm occur in all racquet games. However, they are most common in tennis, where the forceful overhead serve and overhead smash place the most amount of stress on this region. The excessive forces are again related to the use of a relatively heavy racquet and ball.

Back injuries in racquet sports are related to rapid movements of the torso and attempting to play shots while the back is in a vulnerable position. Playing shots while the spine is flexed, hyperextended, laterally flexed and rotated all place stress on the back. The forces placed upon the back in these positions can result in a number of injuries, including muscular strains and disc prolapse. A specific cause of back injury is reported to be the twist serve in tennis.

8.11.4 Head and eye injuries – causes and prevention

Racquet sports are the cause of over half the reported sports-related eye injuries. Of these, squash is the most common cause, followed by badminton and then tennis. In racquet games, head and eye injuries may be caused by a racquet or the projectile, most eye injuries being caused by the latter. Injuries caused by the racquet are more common in squash due to the two opponents being confined in a small area. When playing the game players must ensure that they do not get too close to each other and that good, safe stroke play is employed at all times. A player who swings wildly at the ball instead of using the orthodox squash stroke play, in which the racquet remains relatively close to the body, is an obvious danger to his/her opponent. In badminton and tennis, injuries caused by the racquet are less likely to occur because opponents are confined to separate areas of the court by the net. However injuries do occur in doubles when a player may be struck by his/her partner, or occasionally by an opponent if both are close to the net.

The predominant cause of eye injuries in racquet games is the ball or shuttlecock. In squash this tends to occur when a player turns to look behind them at his/her opponent, who is playing a shot from the back of the court. All players should be made aware of this danger and warned against it. In badminton and tennis it is players close to the net who are most at risk because of the short time in which they have to react to the projectile coming towards them, although turning to observe their partner's shot can convey the same risks as in squash.

The prevention of eye injuries is best ensured by the wearing of eye guards in the form of visors or toughened safety lenses. The wearing of contact lenses or glasses provides no protection and can complicate an injury. Therefore, most authorities would recommend that if a person normally wears glasses or contact lenses they should not wear them while playing but instead should wear toughened safety lenses, which provide protection as well as correcting their sight. For those who do not normally wear glasses, plain toughened safety lenses are readily available. An awareness of safe court procedures and the observance of safe play on the court will also reduce the incidence of such injuries.

8.11.5 Summary of racquet sports injuries

Injuries occur to racquet sports players of all ages and standards. The incidence among higher level players may be due to the frequency of play, while for those of a lesser standard a lack of specific fitness may be a factor, especially in those who play infrequently or who have just taken up the sport. The prevention of injury in racquet sports includes the use of protective eye guards, appropriate footwear, the development of good stroke technique, the adherence to good safe play while on court, ensuring an adequate warm-up is undertaken before all training and matches, an appropriate choice of racquet and an adequate level of fitness.

8.12 FURTHER READING

8.12.1 Running injuries

Caine, D.J. and Lindner, K.J. (1984) Growth plate injury: a threat to young distance runners? *Physician and Sportsmedicine*, **12**(4), 118–124.

Cibulka, M.T., Sinacore, D.R. and Mueller, M.J. (1994) Shin splints and forefoot contact running: a case report. *Journal of Orthopaedic and Sports Physical Therapy*, **20**(2), 98–102.

Clement, D.B., Taunton, J.E., Smart, G.W. and McNicol, K.L. (1981) A survey of overuse running injuries. *Physician and Sportsmedicine*, **9**(5), 47–58.

Cook, S.D., Brinker, M.R. and Poche, M. (1990) Running shoes: their relationship to running injuries. *Sports Medicine*, **10**(1), 1–8.

Falsetti, H.L., Burke, E.R., Feld, R.D., Frederick, E.C. and Ratering, C.R. (1983) Hematological variations after endurance running with hard- and soft-soled shoes. *Physician and Sportsmedicine*, **11**(8), 118–127.

Fick, D.S., Albright, J.P. and Murray, B.P. (1992) Relieving painful 'shin splints'. *Physician and Sports Medicine*, **20**(12), 105–110; 112–113.

Hintermann, B. and Hintermann, M. (1992) Ankle sprains in orienteering – a simple injury? *Scientific Journal of Orienteering*, **8**(2), 79–86.

Holmich, P., Darre, E., Jahnsen, F. and Hartvig-Jensen, T. (1988) The elite marathon runner: Problems during and after competition. *British Journal of Sports Medicine*, **22**(1) 19–21.

Houeberigs, J.H. (1992) Factors related to the incidence of running injuries: a review. *Sports Medicine*, **13**(6), 408–422.

Johnasson, C. (1986) Injuries in elite orienteers. *American Journal of Sports Medicine*, **14**(5), 410–415.

Korkia, P.K., Tunstall-Pedoe, D.S. and Maffulli, N. (1994) An epidemiological investigation of training and injury patterns in British triathletes. *British Journal of Sports Medicine*, 28(3), 191–196.

Linde, F. (1986) Injuries in orienteering. *British Journal of Sports Medicine*, **20**(3), 125–127.

Lucas, C.A. (1992) Iliotibial band friction syndrome as exhibited in athletes. *Journal of Athletic Training*, **27**(3), 250–252.

McCaw, S.T. (1992) Leg length inequality. Implications for running injury prevention. *Sports Medicine*, **14**(6), 422–429.

Messier, S.P., Edwards, D.G., Lowery, R.B. et al. (1995) Etiology of iliotibial band friction syndrome in distance runners. *Medicine and Science in Sport and Exercise*, **27**(7), 951–960.

Nike Sport Research Laboratory (1989) Common running injuries. *Physician and Sportsmedicine*, **17**(3), 143–146.

Powell, K.E., Kohl, H.W., Caspersen, C.J. and Blair, S.N. (1986) An epidemiological perspective on the causes of running injuries. *Physician and Sportsmedicine*, **14**(6), 100–114.

Rolf, C. (1995) Overuse injuries of the lower extremity in runners. *Scandinavian Journal of Medicine and Science in Sports*, **5**(4), 181–190.

Stacoff, A., Denoth, J., Kaelin, X. and Stuessi, E. (1988) Running injuries and shoe construction: some possible relationships. *International Journal of Sports Biomechanics*, **4**, 342–357.

Van Mechelen, W. (1992) Running injuries. A review of the epidemiological literature. *Sports Medicine*, **14**(5), 320–335.

Van Mechelen, W. (1995) Can running injuries be effectively prevented (guest editorial)? *Sports Medicine*, **19**(3), 161–165.

Warren, B.L. (1990) Plantar fasciitis in runners: treatment and prevention. *Sports Medicine*, **10**(5), 338–345.

8.12.2   Injuries in athletic throwing and jumping events

Falster, O. and Hasselbalch, H. (1992) Avulsion fracture of the tibial tuberosity with combined ligament and meniscal tear. *American Journal of Sports Medicine*, **20**(1) 82–83.

Haw, D.W.M. (1981) Avulsion fracture of the medical epicondyle of the elbow in a young javelin thrower. Case report. *British Journal of Sports Medicine*, **15**(1), 47.

Hogan, P. and Ryan, A.J. (1975) Pain of the high jumper. *Physician and Sportsmedicine*, **3**(3), 25.

Hughes, A. W. (1985) Case report: avusion fracture involving the body of the patella. *British Journal of Sports Medicine*, **19**(2), 119–120.

Hulkko, A., Orava, S. and Nikula, P. (1986) Stress fractures of the olecranon in javelin throwers. *International Journal of Sports Medicine*, **7**(4), 210–213.

Paley, D. and Gillespie, K. (1986) Chronic repetitive unrecognized flexion injury of the cervical spine (high jumper's neck). *American Journal of Sports Medicine*, **14**(1), 92–95.

Payton, J. (1981) Australian pole vault injuries. *Modern Athlete and Coach*, **19**(3), 33–35.

Sing, R.F. (1984) Shoulder injuries in the javelin thrower. *Journal of the American Osteopathic Association*, **83**(9), 680–684.

8.12.3   Injuries in gymnastics

Andrish, J.T. (1985) Knee injuries in gymnastics. *Clinics in Sports Medicine*, **4**(1), 111–121.

Bak, K., Kalms, S.B., Olesen, S. and Jorgensen, U. (1994) Epidemiology of injuries in gymnastics. *Scandinavian Journal of Medicine and Science in Sports*, **4**(2), 148–154.

Caine, D.J. and Lindner, K.J. (1985) Overuse injuries of growing bones: the young female gymnast at risk? *Physician and Sportsmedicine*, **13**(12), 51–64.

Dixon, M. and Fricker, P. (1993) Injuries to elite gymnasts over 10 yr. *Medicine and Science in Sports and Exercise*, **25**(12), 1322–1329.

Goldstein, J.D., Berger, P.E., Windler, G.E. and Jackson, D.W. (1991) Spine injuries in gymnasts and swimmers: an epidemiologic investigation. *American Journal of Sports Medicine*, **19**(5), 463–468.

Kerr, G. (1990) Preventing gymnastic injuries. *Canadian Journal of Sport Sciences/Journal Canadien des Sciences du Sport*, **15**(4), 227.

Lindner, K.J. and Caine, D.J. (1990) Injury patterns of female competitive club gymnasts. *Canadian Journal of Sport Sciences/Journal Canadien des Sciences du Sport*, **15**(4), 254–261.

Mackie, S.J. and Taunton, J.E. (1994) Injuries in female gymnasts: trends suggest prevention tactics. *Physician and Sportsmedicine*, **22**(8), 40–45.

McAuley, E., Hudash, G., Shields, K. et al. (1987) Injuries in women's gymnastics: the state of the art. *American Journal of Sports Medicine*, **15**(6), 558–565.

Meeusen, R. and Borms, J. (1992) Gymnastic injuries. *Sports Medicine*, **13**(5), 337–356.

Micheli, L.J. (1985) Back injuries in gymnastics. *Clinics in Sports Medicine*, **4**(1), 85–93.

Nattiv, A. and Mandelbaum, B.R. (1993) Injuries and special concerns in female gymnasts. Detecting, treating and preventing common problems. *Physician and Sportsmedicine*, **21**(7), 66–67; 70; 73–74; 79–82.

Priest, J.D. (1985) Elbow injuries in gymnastics. *Clinics in Sports Medicine*, **4**(1), 73–83.

Ruggles, D.L., Peterson, H.A. and Scott, S.G. (1991) Radial growth plate injury in a female gymnast. *Medicine and Science in Sports and Exercise*, **23**(4), 393–396.

Sands, W.A., Shultz, B.B. and Newman, A.P. (1993) Women's gymnastics injuries. A five-year study. *American Journal of Sports Medicine*, **21**(2), 271–276.

Silver, J.R., Silver, D.D. and Godfrey, J.J. (1986) Injuries of the spine sustained during gymnastic activities. *British Medical Journal (Clinical Research Edn)*, **293**(6551), 861–863.

Steele, V.A. and White, J.A. (1986) Injury prediction in female gymnasts. *British Journal of Sports Medicine*, **20**(1), 31–33.

Weiker, G.G. (1992) Hand and wrist problems in the gymnast. *Clinics in Sports Medicine*, **11**(1), 189–202.

8.12.4 Swimming injuries

Becker, T. (1982) Competitive swimming injuries: their cause and prevention, in *American Swimming Coaches Association World Clinic Yearbook*, American Swimming Coaches Association, Fort Lauderdale, FL, pp. 9–38.

Ciullo, J.V. and Stevens, G.G. (1989) The prevention and treatment of injuries to the shoulder in swimming. *Sports Medicine*, **7**(3), 182–204.

Fowler, P.J. and Regan, W.D. (1986) Swimming injuries of the knee, foot and ankle, elbow, and back. *Clinics in Sports Medicine*, **5**(1), 139–148.

Goldstein, J.D., Berger, P.E., Windler, G.E. and Jackson, D.W. (1991) Spine injuries in gymnasts and swimmers: an epidemiologic investigation. *American Journal of Sports Medicine*, **19**(5), 463–468.

Greipp, J.F. (1985) Swimmer's shoulder: the influence of flexibility and weight training. *Physician and Sportsmedicine*, **13**(8), 92–105.

Korkia, P.K., Tunstall-Pedoe, D.S. and Maffulli, N. (1994) An epidemiological investigation of training and injury patterns in British triathletes. *British Journal of Sports Medicine*, **28**(3), 191–196.

Lo, Y.P.C., Hsu, Y.C.S. and Chan, K.M. (1990) Epidemiology of shoulder impingement in upper arm sports events. *British Journal of Sports Medicine*, **24**(3), 173–177.

McMaster, E.C. and Troup, J. (1993) A survey of interfering shoulder pain in United States competitive swimmers. *American Journal of Sports Medicine*, **21**(1), 67–70.

Vizsolyi, P., Taunton, J., Robertson, G. et al. (1987) Breastroker's knee: an analysis of epidemiological and biomechanical factors. *American Journal of Sports Medicine*, **15**(1), 63–71.

8.12.5 Injuries in competitive cycling

Bohlmann, J.T. (1981) Injuries in competitive cycling. *Physician and Sportsmedicine*, **9**(5), 116–126.

Braithwaite, I.J. (1992) Bilateral median nerve palsy in a cyclist. *British Journal of Sports Medicine*, **26**(1), 27–28.

Brogger-Jensen, T., Hvass, I. and Bugge, S. (1990) Injuries at the BMX cycling European Championships 1989. *British Journal of Sports Medicine*, **24**(4) 269–270.

Dickson, T. B (1985) Preventing overuse cycling injuries. *Physician and Sportsmedicine*, **13**(10), 116–123.

Frontera, W.R. (1983) Cyclist's palsy: clinical and electrodiagnostic findings. Case report. *British Journal of Sports Medicine*, **17**(2), 91–93.

Hannaford, D.R., Moran, G.T. and Hlavac, H.F. (1986) Video analysis and treatment of overuse knee injury in cycling: a limited clinical study. *Clinics in Podiatric Medicine and Surgery*, **3**(4), 671–678.

Harvey, J. and Schonning, J. (1987) Cycling injuries. *Sports Medicine Digest*, **9**(7), 13.

Holmes J.C., Pruitt, A.L. and Whalen, N.J. (1991) Cycling knee injuries. Common mistakes that cause injuries and how to avoid them. *Cycling Science*, **3**(2), 11–15.

Holmes, J.C., Pruitt, A.L. and Whalen, N.J. (1993) Iliotibial band syndrome in cyclists. *American Journal of Sports Medicine*, **21**(3), 419–424.

Holmes, J.C., Pruitt, A.L. and Whalen, N.J. (1994) Lower extremity overuse in bicycling. *Clinics in Sports Medicine*, **13**(1), 187–203.

Ireland, M.L. (1987) Patellofemoral disorders in runners and bicyclists. *Annals of Sports Medicine*, **3**(2), 77–84.

Korkia, P.K., Tunstall-Pedoe, D.S. and Maffulli, N. (1994) An epidemiological investigation of training and injury patterns in British triathletes. *British Journal of Sports Medicine*, **28**(3), 191–196.

Kronisch, R.L. and Rubin, A.L. (1994) Traumatic injuries in off-road bicycling. *Clinical Journal of Sport Medicine*, **4**(4), 240–244.

Maimaris, C. and Zedeh, H.G. (1990) Ulnar nerve compression in the cyclist's hand; two case reports and a literature review. *British Journal of Sports Medicine*, **24**(4), 245–246.

McLennan, J.G., McLennan, J.C. and Ungersma, J. (1988) Accident prevention in competitive cycling. *American Journal of Sports Medicine*, **16**(3), 266–268.

Mellion, M.B. (1991) Common cycling injuries. Management and prevention. *Sports Medicine*, **11**(1), 52–70.

Munnings, F. (1991) Cyclist's palsy: making changes brings relief. *Physician and Sportsmedicine*, **19**(9), 112–119.

Pleffer, R.P. and Kronisch, R.L. (1995) Off-road cycling injuries. An overview. *Sports Medicine*, **19**(5), 311–325.

Pfeiffer, R.P. (1994) Off road bicycle racing injuries – the NORBA Pro/Elite category. *Clinics in Sports Medicine*, **13**(1), 207–218.

Rogak, L. (1987) How to avoid cyclist's knee. *Women's Sports and Fitness*, **9**(6), 11–12.

Roos, R. (1987) Medical coverage of endurance events: part 1. *Physician and Sportsmedicine*, **15**(11), 140–146.

8.12.6　Injuries in golf

Batt, M.E. (1992) A survey of golf injuries in amateur golfers. *British Journal of Sports Medicine*, **26**(1), 63–65.

Batt, M.E. (1993) Golfing injuries: an overview. *Sports Medicine*, **16**(1), 64–71.

Brendecke, P. (1990) Golf injuries. *Sports Medicine Digest*, **12**(4), 1–2.

Duda, M. (1987) Golf injuries: they really do happen. *Physician and Sportsmedicine*, **15**(7), 190–196.

Hannafin, J.A. (1996) Home exercises for tennis and golfer's elbow. *Physician and Sportsmedicine*, **24**(2), 71.

Jobe, F.W., Moynes, D.R. and Antonelli, D.J. (1986) Rotator cuff function during a golf swing. *American Journal of Sports Medicine*, **14**(5), 388–392.

McCarroll, J.R. and Gioe, T.J. (1982) Professional golfers and the price they pay. *Physician and Sportsmedicine*, **10**(7), 64–70.

McCarroll, J.R., Rettig, A.C. and Shelbourne, R.D. (1990) Injuries in the amateur golfer. *Physician and Sportsmedicine*, **18**(3), 122–126.

Voss, M.W. (1982) Medical support system for a professional golf tournament. *Physician and Sportsmedicine*, **10**(8), 63–70.

Voss, M.W. (1983) Golf injuries. *Sportsmedicine Digest*, **5**(7), 1–2.

8.12.7　Injuries in rowing, canoeing and kayaking

Brosh, S. and Jenner, J.R. (1988) Injuries to rowers. *British Journal of Sports Medicine*, **22**(4), 169.

Burrell, C.L. and Burrell, R. (1982) Injuries in white-water paddling. *Physician and Sportsmedicine*, **10**(8), 118–124.

MacAuley, D. (1992) Medical aspects of rowing. *Physiotherapy in Sport*, **14**(1), 8–9.

Edwards, A. (1993) Injuries in kayaking. *Sport Health*, **11**(1), 8–11.

Jones, R.T. (1979) Rowing injuries. *Rowing*, **23**(268), 23–24.

Kizer, K.W. (1987) Medical aspects of white-water kayaking. *Physician and Sportsmedicine*, **15**(7), 128–137.

Lo, Y.P.C., Hsu, Y.C.S. and Chan, K.M. (1990) Epidemiology of shoulder impingement in upper arm sports events. *British Journal of Sports Medicine*, **24**(3), 173–177.

Pelham, T.W., Holt, L.E. and Stalker, R.E. (1995) The etiology of paddler's shoulder. *Australian Journal of Science and Medicine in Sport*, **27**(2) 43–47.

Raymond, P. (1977) Care of the hands. *Oarsman*, **9**(2), 40–41.

Walsh, M. (1989) Sports medicine for paddlers: the cause, care and treatment of paddler's injuries. *Canoe*, **17**(2), 36–38.

Walsh, M. (1985) Preventing injury in competitive canoeists. *Physician and Sportsmedicine*, **13**(9), 120–128.

Weightman, D. and Browne, R.C. (1975) Injuries in eleven selected sports. *British Journal of Sports Medicine*, **9**(3), 136–141.

8.12.8　Weight lifting and weight training injuries

Albright, J.P., Saterbak, A. and Stokes, J. (1995) Use of knee braces in sport: current recommendations. *Sports Medicine*, **20**(5), 281–301.

Basford, J.R. (1985) Weightlifting, weight training and injuries. *Orthopedics*, **8**(8), 1051–1056.

Blimkie, C.J.R. (1993) Resistance training during preadolescence. Issues and controversies. *Sports Medicine*, **5**(6), 389–407.

Brady, T.A., Cahill, B.R. and Bodmar, L.M. (1982) Weight training-related injuries in the high school athlete. *American Journal of Sports Medicine*, **10**(1), 1–5.

Carmichael, D. (1986) What every adult should know about children and sport. *Sports Coach*, **10**(3):41–45.

Gray, M. and Young, J. (1986) Weight training and the prepubescent athlete. *Journal of Applied Research in Coaching and Athletics*, **1**(3), 201–211.

Jenkins. N.H. and Mintowt-Czyz, W.J. (1986) Bilateral fracture separations of the distal radial epiphysis during weight lifting. *British Journal of Sports Medicine*, **20**(2), 72–73.

Kulund, D.N., Dewey, J.B., Brubaker, C.E. and Roberts, J.R. (1978) Olympic weightlifting injuries. *Physician and Sportsmedicine*, **6**(11), 111–119.

Mazur, L.J., Yetman, R.J. and Risser, W.L. (1993) Weight training injuries: common injuries and preventative methods. *Sports Medicine*, **16**(1), 57–63.

Reilly, T. (1978) Some observations on weight-training. *British Journal of Sports Medicine*, **12**(1), 45–47.

Risser, W.L., Risser, J.M.H. and Preston, D. (1990) Weight-training injuries in adolescents. *American Journal of Diseases of Children*, **144**, 1015–1017.

Wilson, R.W. (1993) Entrapment neuropathy of the inferior suprascapular nerve in a weight lifter. *Journal of Sport Rehabilitation*, **2**(3), 208–210.

8.12.9 Injuries in combat sports and martial arts

Birrer, R., Birrer, C., Son, D.S. and Stone, D. (1981) Injuries in taekwondo. *Physician and Sportsmedicine*, **9**(2), 97–103.

Burns, R.J. (1986) Boxing and the brain. *Australian and New Zealand Journal of Medicine*, **16**(3), 439–440.

Butler, R.J. (1994) Neuropsychological investigation of amateur boxers. *British Journal of Sports Medicine*, **28**(3), 187–190.

Estwanik, J.J. and Rovere, G.D. (1983) Wrestling injuries in North Carolina high schools. *Physician and Sportsmedicine*, **11**(1), 100–108.

Harvey, J., Magsamen, B. and Strauss, R.H. (1987) Medical problems of wrestlers. *Physician and Sportsmedicine*, **15**(1), 136–148.

Haugegaard, M., Rasmussen, S.W. and Jensen, P. (1993) Avulsion fracture of the medial humerus epicondyle in young wrestlers. *Scandinavian Journal of Medicine and Science in Sports*, **3**(3), 178–181.

Hillman, S., Dicker, G. and Sali, A. (1993) Non contact karate injuries. *Australian Journal of Science and Medicine in Sport*, **25**(4), 73–75.

Johannsen, H.V. and Noerregaard, F.O.H. (1988) Prevention of injury in karate. *British Journal of Sports Medicine*, **22**(3), 113–115.

Jordan, B.D. and Campbell, E.A. (1988) Acute injuries among professional boxers in New York State: a two-year survey. *Physician and Sportsmedicine*, **16**(1), 87–91.

Jordan, B.D., Voy, R.O. and Stone, J. (1990) Amateur boxing injuries at the US Olympic Training Center. *Physician and Sportsmedicine*, **18**(2), 80–90.

Kort, H.D. and Hendriks, H.A. (1992) A comparison of selected isokinetic trunk strength parameters of elite male judo competitors and cyclists. *Journal of Orthopaedic and Sports Physical Therapy*, **16**(2), 92–96.

Kurland, H.L. (1980) Injuries in karate. Protective equipment and enlightened attitudes could help prevent most karate injuries. *Physician and Sportsmedicine*, **8**(10), 80–85.

Lennox, S. (1991) A study of amateur boxing injuries. *Physiotherapy in Sport*, **13**(1), 89.

Lorish, T.R., Rizzo, T.D., Ilstrup, D.M. and Scott, S.G. (1992) Injuries in adolescent and preadolescent boys at two large wrestling tournaments. *American Journal of Sports Medicine*, **20**(2), 199–202.

Lubell, A. (1989) Chronic brain injury in boxers: is it avoidable? *Physician and Sportsmedicine*, **17**(11), 126–132.

Ludwig, R. (1986) Making boxing safer. The Swedish model. *Journal of the American Medical Association*, **255**(18), 2482.

Marsh, C. (1990) Injuries in amateur wrestling. *Sports Coach*, **13**(3), 37–40.

Mbubaegbu, C.E. and Percy, A.J. (1994) Femoral osteochondral fracture – a non contact injury in martial arts? A case report. *British Journal of Sports Medicine*, **28**(3) 203–205.

McLatchie, G. (1981) Karate and karate injuries. *British Journal of Sports Medicine*, **15**(1), 84–86.

McLatchie, G. and Jennett, B. (1994) Head injury. *Sports Exercise and Injury*, **1**(3), 118–123.

Morris, E.W. and McLatchie, G.R. (1977) Prevention of karate injuries a progress report. *British Journal of Sports Medicine*, **11**(2), 78–82.

Nobel, C. (1987) Hand injuries in boxing. *American Journal of Sports Medicine*, **15**(4), 342–346.

Pieter, W. and Lufting, R. (1994) Injuries at the 1991 Taekwondo World Championships. Traumi nei Campionati del Mondo di Taekwondo del 1991. *Journal of Sports Traumatology and Related Research*, **16**(1), 49–57.

Ransom, S.B. and Ransom, E.R. (1989) The epidemiology of judo injuries. *Journal of Osteopathic Sports Medicine*, **3**(1), 12–14.

Ross, R.J., Casson, I.R., Siegel, O. and Cole, M. (1987) Boxing injuries: neurologic, radiologic, and neuropsychologic evaluation. *Clinics in Sports Medicine*, **6**(1), 41–51.

Siana, J.E., Borum, P. and Kryger, H. (1986) Injuries in taekwondo. *British Journal of Sports Medicine*, **20**(4),165–166.

Snook, G.A. (1980) Survey of wrestling injuries. *American Journal of Sports Medicine*, **8**(6), 450–453.

Strauss, R.H. and Lanese, R.R. (1982) Injuries among wrestlers in school and college tournaments. *Journal of the American Medical Association*, **248**(16), 2016–2019.

Tuominen, R. (1995) Injuries in national karate competitions in Finland. *Scandinavian Journal of Medicine and Science in Sports*, **5**(1), 44–48.

Wroble, R.R., Mysnyk, M.C., Foster, D.T. and Albright, J.P. (1986) Patterns of knee injuries in wrestling: a six year study. *American Journal of Sports Medicine*, **14**(1), 55–66.

Uzych, L. and Ryan, A.J. (1992) Banning boxing. *Physician and Sportsmedicine*, **20**(2), 29.

Zemper, E.D. and Pieter, W. (1989) Injury rates during the 1988 US Olympic Team Trials for taekwondo. *British Journal of Sports Medicine*, **23**(3), 161–164.

The medical aspects of boxing: a round table. (1985) *Physician and Sportsmedicine*, **13**(9), 56–72.

8.12.10 Injuries in racquet sports

Berson, B.L., Rolnick, A.M., Ramos, C.G. and Thornton, J. (1981) Epidemiologic study of squash injuries. *American Journal of Sports Medicine*, **9**(2), 103–106.

Bigiliani, L.U., Kimmel, J., McCann, P.D. and Wolfe, I. (1992) Repair of rotator cuff tears in tennis players. *American Journal of Sports Medicine*, **20**(2), 112–117.

Brown, M. (1995) The older athlete with tennis elbow: rehabilitation considerations. *Clinics in Sports Medicine*, **14**(1), 267–275.

Chard M.D. and Lachmann, S.M. (1987) Racquet sports patterns of injury presenting to a sports injury clinic. *British Journal of Sports Medicine*, **21**(4), 150–153.

Ellenbecker, T.S. (1995) Rehabilitation of shoulder and elbow injuries in tennis players. *Clinics in Sports Medicine*, **14**(1), 87–110.

Feit, E.M. and Berenter, R. (1993) Lower extremity tennis injuries: prevalence, etiology and mechanism. *Journal of American Podiatric Medical Association*, **83**(9), 509–514.

Field, L.D. and Altchek, D.W. (1995) Elbow injuries. *Clinics in Sports Medicine*, **14**(1), 59–78.

Gecha, S.R. and Torg, E. (1988) Knee injuries in tennis. *Clinics in Sports Medicine*, 7(2)435–452.

Hannafin, J.A. (1996) Home exercises for tennis and golfer's elbow. *Physician and Sportsmedicine*, **24**(2), 71.

Hardlng, W.G. (1992) Use and misuse of the tennis elbow strap. *Physician and Sportsmedicine*, **20**(8), 65–74.

Hensley, L.D. and Paup, D.C. (1979) Survey of badminton injuries. *British Journal of Sports Medicine*, **13**(4), 156–160.

Hoy, K., Lindblad, B.E., Terkelsen, C.J. et al. (1994) Badminton injuries - a prospective epidemiological and socioeconomic study. *British Journal of Sports Medicine*, **28**(4), 276–279.

Ishikawa, H., Ueba, Y., Yonezawa, T. et al. (1988) Osteochondritis dissecans of the shoulder in a tennis player. *American Journal of Sports Medicine*, **16**(5), 547–550.

Jorgensen, U. and Winge, S. (1987) Epidemiology of badminton injuries. *International Journal of Sports Medicine*, **6**(8), 379–382.

Jorgensen, U. and Winge, S. (1990) Injuries in badminton. *Sports Medicine*, **10**(1), 59–64.

Kaalund, S., Lass, P., Hogsaa, B. and Nohr, M. (1989) Achilles tendon rupture in badminton. *British Journal of Sports Medicine*, **23**(2), 102–104.

Kamien, M. (1989) The incidence of tennis elbow and other injuries in tennis players at the Royal Kings Park Tennis Club of Western Australia from October 1983 to September 1984. *Australian Journal of Science and Medicine in Sport*, **21**(2), 18–22.

Kelly, S.P. (1987) Serious eye injury in badminton players. *British Journal of Ophthalmology*, **71**(10), 746–747.

Kennerley-Bankes, J.L. (1985) Squash rackets: a survey of eye injuries in England. *British Medical Journal (Clinical Research edn)*, **291**(6508), 1539.

Kroner, K., Schmidt, S.A., Nielsen, A.B. et al. (1990) Badminton injuries. *British Journal of Sports Medicine*, **24**(3), 169–172.

Kuhn, J.E. and Hawkins, R.J. (1995) Surgical treatment of shoulder injuries in tennis players. *Clinics in Sports Medicine*, **14**(1), 139–161.

Kulund, D.M., McCue, F.C., Rockwell, D.A. and Gieck, J.H. (1979) Tennis injuries: prevention and treatment. A review *American Journal of Sports Medicine*, **7**(4), 249–253.

Legwold G. (1984) The pros face the cons of constant play. *Physician and Sportsmedicine*, **12**(6), 187–189.

Lehman, R.C. (1988) Surface and equipment variables in tennis injuries. *Clinics in Sports Medicine*, **7**(2), 229–232.

Lee, H.W. (1995) Mechanisms of neck and shoulder injuries in tennis players. *Journal of Orthopaedic and Sports Physical Therapy*, **21**(1), 28–37.

Maffulli, N., Regine, R., Carrillo, F. et al. (1990) Tennis elbow: an ultrasonographic study in tennis players. *British Journal of Sports Medicine*, **24**(3), 151–155.

Medhurst, D. and McNaughton, L. (1984) Badminton injuries in Australia. *Sports Coach*, **8**(2), 10–11.

Nirschl, R.P. (1988) Prevention and treatment of elbow and shoulder injuries in the tennis player. *Clinics in Sports Medicine*, **7**(2), 289–308.

Northcote, R.J., Evanst, A.D. and Ballantyne D. (1984) Sudden death in squash players. *Lancet*, i(8369), 148–150.

Pintore, E. and Maffulli, N. (1991) Osteochondritis dissecans of the lateral humeral condyle in a table tennis player. *Medicine and Science in Sports and Exercise*, **23**(8), 889–891.

Renstrom, A.F.H. (1995) Knee pain in tennis players. *Clinics in Sports Medicine*, **14**(1), 163–175.

Zecher, S.B. and Leach, R.E. (1995) Lower leg and foot injuries in tennis and other racquet sports. *Clinics in Sports Medicine*, **14**(1), 223–239.

9. Children and sports injuries

9.1 INTRODUCTION

Children can suffer from all of the sports injuries that are seen in adults. Furthermore, they can also suffer from a number of additional injuries related to their stage of development. This means that some injuries are only seen in children and the relative frequency of many other injuries differs between children and adults (Figure 9.1).

Many children participate in serious competitive sport from a very young age and in order to achieve success at a young age they are being given very strenuous and demanding training schedules that are more suited to adults. Indeed, many authorities would emphasize that children are not miniature adults since their growing bodies are unable to take the physical stresses that an adult body can endure. Training programmes for children should therefore be designed accordingly. However, despite these recommendations the incidence of overuse injuries in children is on the increase and it is evident from a number of sports that children are attaining high levels of performance from a very young age; examples being swimming, female gymnastics and tennis. It is quite likely, therefore, that the practitioner will encounter such injuries not infrequently. A number of the sports injuries observed in children are related to: (1) their immature skeleton, which can be more vulnerable to injury, and (2) the anatomical imbalances that can occur during the growth spurt. The key areas of most concern are the injuries that occur to the growth plates and the back, since these can have permanent consequences for the growth and physical development of the child. The incidence of certain injuries may be related to the rapid increase in bone length which occurs early in the growth spurt without an accompanying increase in muscle length, which occurs later. A consequence of this disproportionate growth is often a loss of flexibility, much of which may be regained as the muscles lengthen in the later stages of the growth spurt. However, the possession of tight muscles during the early phase of the growth spurt has obvious implications for the risk of musculoskeletal injury.

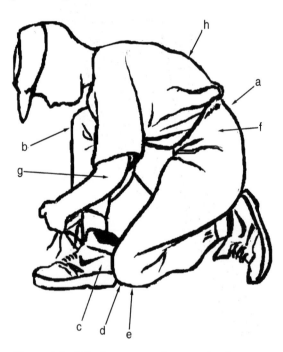

Figure 9.1 Injuries commonly occurring in children. (a) Spondylolysis and spondylolisthesis. (b) Chondromalacia patellae. (c) Sever's disease. (d) Sinding-Larson–Johansson disease. (e) Osgood–Schlatter's disease. (f) Avulsion fractures. (g) Thrower's elbow. (h) Sheuermann's disease (roundback)

The child also has relatively weak bones compared to the strength of their muscles and ligamentous tissue. This means that if a part of the body is subjected to tension or torsion the site of damage is often somewhat different to that of an adult. For example avulsion fractures (where the tendon pulls away from the bone, taking a small piece of bone with it) are far more common in children because of the different relative strengths of the tendons and bone. Similarly, overuse injuries such as Osgood–Schlatter's disease and Sever's disease also occur in children because of the relative weakness of the skeleton and the presence of the growth cartilages. The causes of such injuries are discussed in section 9.3.

The risk of injury to the epiphyseal growth plates (Figure 9.2) is a topic of great concern among practitioners, since the cartilage and bone of which they are composed is relatively weak and is therefore vulnerable to both traumatic fractures upon impact and overuse.

The main significance of such injuries is the possibility of stunted growth, since the growth plates are the sites at which the

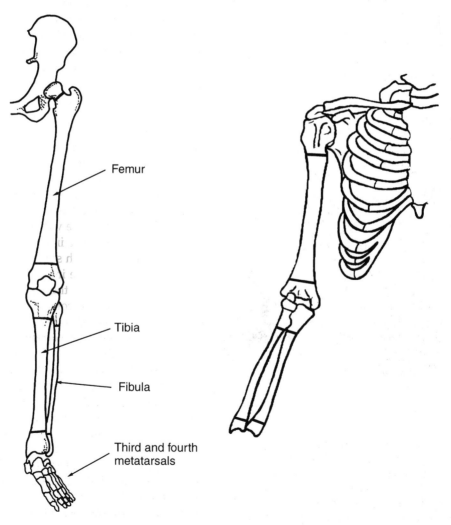

Femur

Tibia

Fibula

Third and fourth metatarsals

Figure 9.2 Position of the growth plates.

bones increase in length. In adults these areas have ossified and are therefore no longer of concern. The cause of such injuries is discussed in more detail later.

In young females the increase in bodyweight and the deposition of gender-related fat at puberty can cause the individual to be unable to perform at the levels she was previously attaining; furthermore the relative increase in hip width in females at puberty can also increase the risk of chondromalacia patellae in runners if they continue with the training volumes they were attempting prior to the growth spurt.

In summary, coaches should be made aware of the vulnerability of children at this age and should be prepared to adjust their training schedules accordingly. Once the individual has attained full physical maturity the training loads can then be increased again to match those of other adult performers. In this respect the sports injury practitioner has an important role to play as an adviser and educator.

9.2 THE PREVENTION OF SPORTS INJURIES IN CHILDREN

To minimize the risk of sports injuries in children all the usual factors need to be considered (Chapter 1) plus a number of specific issues which relate primarily to children.

(a) Warming up before sport and strenuous exercise

Like adults, children should be encouraged to warm up before strenuous physical activity. This should also help to establish the habit, ensuring that it will be continued into their adult sporting life.

(b) Sport-specific fitness and physique

If the child does not possess the necessary levels of fitness for a particular sport or activity, then the physical stresses that they experience during it may cause injury. A lack of strength, speed, flexibility or endurance can all contribute towards injury. Furthermore, the physique of some children makes them unsuited to certain sports. Of particular concern here are the contact sports such as rugby for the slightly built young boy or gymnastics for the girl who lacks the necessary flexibility to execute a particular movement.

(c) Attempting to pursue adult training programmes

The correct training and level of fitness will reduce the risk of the child suffering from a sports injury and there is a large body of evidence to support the notion that in terms of benefiting their general health most children are at risk of doing too little exercise rather than too much. However, as with adults, inappropriate or too much training can cause injury. When considering what training a child should do a number of factors need to be reviewed. These include their physical condition, stage of physical development and current level of participation as well as the intended type of training, duration, intensity and frequency. If a child attempts to do too much, too often, at too high an intensity, then s/he is likely to suffer from overuse injuries, especially to the skeleton (such as spondylolysis), and overuse injuries of the epiphyseal growth plates. Their training must therefore be modified and should not be the same as that undertaken by adults, whose skeletons are fully matured. For example, running too many miles on a hard surface can injure the growth plates through the repeated compressional strain and in soccer the tension exerted on the tenoperiosteal junction between the patellar tendon and tibia when kicking a ball is a common cause of Osgood–Schlatter's disease. Furthermore, it must also be remembered that what is appropriate for one child is not necessarily so for another, since it depends upon their physical capacity to train, their level of fitness and their stage of physical development. Commencing a training programme at a relatively easy level with gradual progression is also important and should be remembered especially if a child joins a club and is put into a group with his/her friends who because they have been training for some time will possess bodies that are therefore likely to be more adapted to the training loads placed upon them.

Undertaking the wrong type of exercise or using a poor technique can also cause injury. This is most obvious in activities such as gymnastics where a poor technique can cause strain to areas such as the back. Spondylolysis is a common problem in young gymnasts and butterfly swimmers who repeatedly hyperextend the back. Other back problems such as spondylolisthesis can also occur in these sports and from weight training if back hyperextension occurs. Indeed, the whole topic of prepubescent weight training is a controversial topic among coaches, exercise physiologists and medical practitioners. The concern about this form of training once again centres upon the child's immature skeleton and the presence of the growth plates, which are vulnerable to compression injuries. A large increase in muscle strength can also increase the likelihood of skeletal damage if the strong muscles exert too much tension on the tenoperiosteal junction with the bone.

(d)   Recovery between exercise sessions

As with adults, children need time to recover between training and competition. The physical and mental stresses imposed upon children by competitive sport can cause staleness and burnout as well as overuse injuries if they are not given time to recover from the exertions of the activity. In this context it should also be remembered that, unlike most adults, children will often be involved in many additional activities outside their specialist sport, e.g. playing for school teams and participating in PE lessons, all of which can place additional stresses on the body and require the training programmes to be modified accordingly to prevent excessive fatigue and overuse. It is unrealistic to expect a child to complete a full training session on the track if s/he has just played football for the school team.

(e)   Biomechanical imbalances and anatomical factors associated with the child's growth

During the growth spurt the bones lengthen in advance of the skeletal muscles. This results in the child losing much of his/her flexibility and developing tight muscles. As a consequence of this, additional strain is placed upon the skeleton as the tight muscles pull on the relatively weak bone. The loss of flexibility is also likely to prevent the child from performing certain movements that s/he could easily execute a few months before. Those involved in gymnastics and other activities should be particularly aware of this, although it can affect all sports.

The relatively weak immature skeleton is vulnerable to injury, including avulsion fractures, apophysitis and epiphyseal plate damage. The incidence of chondromalacia patellae in female runners has been previously discussed, along with the effects of weight gain in this group of female performers.

(f)   Skill

Children are introduced to many new sporting activities and, as discussed previously, all of these convey an element of risk. Therefore, in order to minimize this risk it is important that the child is taught the correct techniques and attains the necessary levels of skill required to participate in the sport safely. Clumsy tackles in games such as rugby, hockey and soccer can injure both the tackler and the tackled. Likewise, correct codes of conduct and levels of skill in racquet games also reduce the risk of injury.

(g) Equipment, environment and rules

The guidelines relating to footwear, clothing and protective equipment are the same for children as for adults. However, because of their smaller stature and levels of strength, additional consideration needs to be given to the use of sports equipment. It is not unusual to see a child struggling with a tennis racket that is too big for him/her or trying to throw a shot that is too heavy. Sports equipment should be scaled down to suit the child's capabilities and, where necessary, the rules of the game should be modified, along with the size of the pitch and the duration of the event. Full-sized pitches are usually far too large for the child and the duration of an event suitable for the physical capabilities of adults is likely to far exceed those of a child. Many governing bodies have rules that determine these factors, such as what distances a child can compete in when running or the duration of a match.

(h) Inappropriate opposition

In the case of children, the issue of competing against inappropriate opposition is even more significant than it is with adults. This is especially so in contact sports, where playing against opponents who are significantly larger can cause an increase in injury, although the risk can also extend to other sports such as cricket, hockey and the racquet games, where larger children may be able to hit or throw the ball much harder. The problems in this area lie in the fact that children are usually asked to compete against other children of their own age. However there are often vast differences in the stages of physical maturity of children of the same age. To try and overcome these discrepancies an alternative form of categorization based upon anthropometric matching is sometimes used and should result in individuals of the same level of physical maturity competing against one another, thereby reducing the risk of injury to those who are less well developed.

(i) Prior injury

A child will often participate in a sport to impress their parents, coach or other adults. However whereas adults may be in a position to make a decision about a niggling injury and if necessary stop playing, a child may continue regardless. Therefore all adults involved with children's sport should be sensitive to the comments of a child who complains of pain or who appears to have an injury.

(j) The need to make sport enjoyable

A child should participate in sport for the fun and enjoyment s/he gains from it in both training and competition. It is therefore the responsibility of adults to ensure that the child can get the most from sport in terms of the physical, mental and social benefits it conveys, while at the same time minimizing the risk of injury to the child. In this context, the practitioner has an important role to play as an informed and qualified expert who may occasionally have to temper the overenthusiasm of parents and coaches who may attempt to push the child beyond their capabilities. A child should participate in sport for his/her own benefit and not that of parents and other associated adults.

9.3 KEY INJURIES RELATING TO THE CHILD

9.3.1 Overuse and traumatic injuries to the epiphyseal plates

The epiphyseal plates (Figure 9.2) are the sites of bone growth in the child. They are made of cartilage, which ossifies as the child reaches physical maturity. Since they are made of cartilage rather than bone they are vulnerable to fracture and overuse. Fractures may occur as a

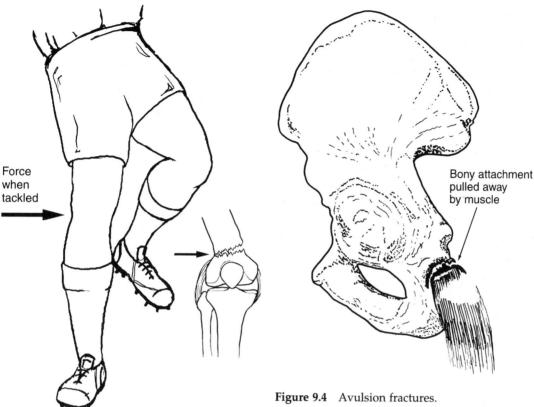

Force
when
tackled

Bony attachment
pulled away
by muscle

Figure 9.4 Avulsion fractures.

Figure 9.3 Epiphyseal fractures.

result of a collision, for example when tackled in rugby, or a fall in gymnastics (Figure 9.3).

Furthermore, a number of epiphyseal fractures, particularly to the distal radial epiphyses, have been caused by weight-training activities. Epiphyseal fractures require immediate surgery to realign the bones and minimize the consequences.

The relatively soft cartilage is also vulnerable to overuse injuries such as are caused by the compressional forces experienced from running an excessively high mileage on hard surfaces. This kind of repetitive trauma can cause the growth plates to ossify prematurely (premature epiphyseal closure), thereby preventing any further lengthening of the bone and hence stunting the growth of the child. The administration of anabolic ster-

oids to children in the context of sport can also cause closure of the growth plates with the same consequences.

9.3.2 Avulsion fractures

The relative weakness of children's bones compared to their muscles and ligamentous tissues can mean that if excessive stress is experienced in the region of the tenoperiosteal junction it is the bone that fractures rather than the tendon rupturing. As with other fractures, these require immediate surgery. Avulsion fractures to the proximal tibial epiphysis are reported in jumping activities and sports such as basketball that involve a lot of jumping (Figure 9.4). Other common sites are the front of the pelvis and the ischium at the origin of the posterior hamstring muscles, these injuries often being associated with activities such as soccer.

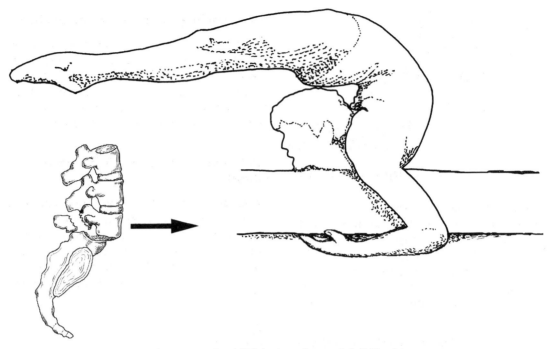

Figure 9.5   Spondylolysis and spondylolisthesis.

9.3.3   Spondylolysis and spondylolisthesis

Activities that put excessive strain on the back, particularly hyperextension, can cause these injuries (Figure 9.5).

They are particularly prevalent in gymnasts, butterfly swimmers and children involved in weight training. Spondylolysis is a stress fracture of the vertebra and spondylolisthesis the movement of one vertebra out of alignment with another. This usually occurs at vertebra L5, which moves forwards relative to L4 resulting in pinched nerves and pain.

9.3.4   Osgood–Schlatter's disease

Osgood–Schlatter's disease primarily occurs in young teenage boys (Figure 9.6).

It is an overuse injury cause by the repeated pulling of the patellar tendon at its site of attachment to the tibia in the process of knee extension. This site of attachment is relatively weak since it is part of the epiphyseal growth plate and the repetitive stress causes an apophysitis with associated inflammation, degeneration of the area and pain. The disease is quite often associated with activities such as football where the kicking action greatly

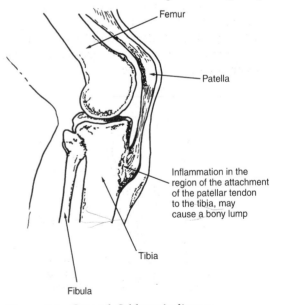

Femur

Patella

Inflammation in the region of the attachment of the patellar tendon to the tibia, may cause a bony lump

Tibia

Fibula

Figure 9.6   Osgood–Schlatter's disease.

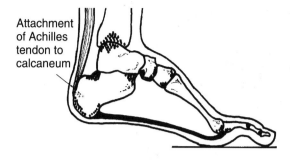

Attachment of Achilles tendon to calcaneum

Figure 9.7 Sever's disease (apophysitis calcanei).

increases the amount of stress experienced at the site of patellar tendon attachment. Other activities such as jumping or basketball, which involves a considerable amount of jumping, can also induce this condition, although it occurs in runners as well. Upon healing a permanent bony lump develops.

9.3.5 Sever's disease (apophysitis calcanei)

Sever's disease (Figure 9.7) is an apophysitis of the calcaneum at the insertion of the Achilles tendon.

It is caused by repeated explosive movements such as jumping or sprinting where the tendon causes excessive tension at its attachment to the immature bone in the region of the epiphyseal plate. The disease is therefore very similar to Osgood–Schlatter's, which occurs at the knee.

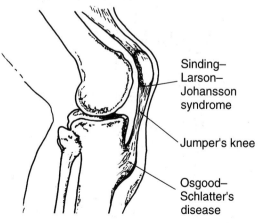

Sinding–Larson–Johansson syndrome

Jumper's knee

Osgood–Schlatter's disease

Figure 9.8 Sinding-Larson–Johansson syndrome.

9.3.6 Sinding-Larson–Johansson syndrome

Repetitive explosive and jumping activities can cause an excessive amount of stress to be placed on the patellar tendon just below the patella. This can cause an apophysitis at the inferior pole of the patellar tendon with associated inflammation and pain (Figure 9.8).

9.3.7 Thrower's elbow (Little Leaguer's elbow)

Whereas tennis elbow is more common among older individuals, the similar condition of 'thrower's elbow' is more common among the young. In particular it is prevalent among young baseball pitchers, hence its common name of 'Little Leaguer's elbow' (Figure 9.9).

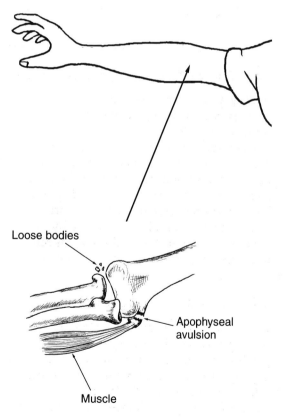

Loose bodies

Apophyseal avulsion

Muscle

Figure 9.9 Thrower's elbow (Little Leaguer's elbow).

It is an overuse injury caused by pronating the elbow while throwing. The muscles involved in this throwing action attach to the medial epicondyle of the humerus in the region of its epiphyseal plate; hence the area is relatively weak and vulnerable to apophysitis. Overuse causes inflammation and pain when throwing. Thrower's elbow is prevalent among javelin throwers, cricketers, golfers and baseball pitchers.

9.3.8 Scheuermann's disease

Scheuermann's disease is a rounding of the back (kyphosis). The onset of this condition may be related to activities such as cycling with racing handlebars that are set too low, rowing, weight training and long-distance running. It is a hereditary trait, which causes a number of the vertebrae to become wedge-shaped because of a reduced amount of growth on the anterior side of the vertebral body.

9.3.9 Chondromalacia patellae

Chondromalacia patellae (Figure 9.10) is more common among females and particularly among female endurance runners.

It is caused by a roughening of the back of the kneecap (patella) as it passes over the

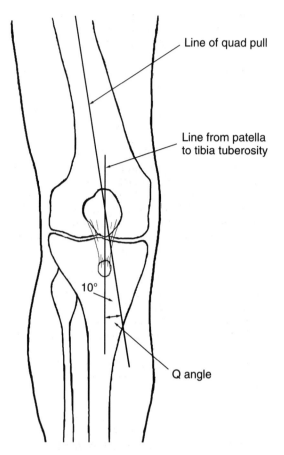

Figure 9.11 Q angle.

femur during the flexion and extension movements of the knee. In females who possess relatively wide hips the angle of pull of the patella across the kneecap (Q angle) is more acute (Figure 9.11), which can cause a certain amount of friction as it passes over the femur resulting in inflammation and degeneration of the dorsal surface.

9.4 FURTHER READING

Anderson, S.J. (1991) Acute knee injuries in young athletes. *Physician and Sportsmedicine*, **19**(11), 69–76.

Caine, D.J. and Broekhoff, J. (1987) Maturity assessment a viable preventive measure against physical and psychological insult to the young athlete. *Physician and Sportsmedicine*, **15**(3), 67–79.

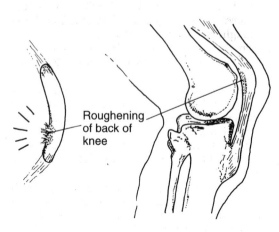

Figure 9.10 Chondromalacia patellae.

Caine, D.J. and Lindner, K.J. (1985) Overuse injuries of growing bones: the young female gymnast at risk? *Physician and Sportsmedicine*, **13**(12), 51–64.

Carmichael, D. (1986) What every adult should know about children and sport. *Sports Coach*, **10**(3):41–45.

Clain, M.R. and Hershman, E.B. (1989) Overuse injuries in children and Adolescents. *Physician and Sportsmedicine*, **17**(9), 111–123.

Commandre, F.A., Taillan, B., Gagnerie, F. et al. (1988) Spondylolysis and spondylolisthesis in young athletes: 28 cases. *Journal of Sports Medicine and Physical Fitness*, **28**(1), 104–107.

Dalton, S.E. (1992) Overuse injuries in adolescent athletes. *Sports Medicine*, **13**(1), 58–70.

Gerbino, P.G. and Micheli, L.J. (1995) Back injuries in the young athlete. *Clinics in Sports Medicine*, **14**(3), 571–590.

Gerrard, D.F. (1993) Overuse injury and growing bones: the young athlete at risk. *British Journal of Sports Medicine*, **27**(1) 14–18.

Goldberg, B. (1989) Injury patterns in youth sports. *Physician and Sportsmedicine*, **17**(3), 174–186.

Gray, M. and Young, J. (1986) Weight training and the prepubescent athlete. *Journal of Applied Research in Coaching and Athletics*, **1**(3), 201–211.

Hay, M.C. (1980) Sports injuries in childhood and adolescence. *Sports Coach*, **4**(4), 26–33.

Hayes, J.M. and Masear, V.R. (1984) Avulsion fracture of the tibial eminence associated with severe medial ligamentous injury in an adolescent. *American Journal of Sports Medicine*, **12**(4), 330–333.

Inoue, G., Kuboyama, K. and Shido, T. (1991) Avulsion fractures of the proximal tibial epiphysis. *British Journal of Sports Medicine*, **21**(1) 52–56.

Ireland, M.L. and Hutchinson, M.R. (1995) Upper extremity injuries in young athletes. *Clinics in Sports Medicine*, **14**(3), 533–569.

Jenkins. N.H. and Mintowt-Czyz, W.J. (1986) Bilateral fracture separations of the distal radial epiphysis during weight lifting. *British Journal of Sports Medicine*, **20**(2), 72–73.

Kozar, B. and Lord, R.M. (1983) Overuse injury in the young athlete: Reasons for concern. *Physician and Sportsmedicine*, **11**(7), 116–121.

Kujala, U.M. and Orava, S. (1993) Ischial apophysis injuries in athletes. *Sports Medicine*, **16**(4), 290–294.

Legwold, G. (1982) Does lifting weights harm a prepubescent athlete? *Physician and Sportsmedicine*, **10**, 141–144.

Maddox, B. (1994) Over-use injuries in children. *Physiotherapy in Sport*, **17**(3), 11–15.

Maffulli, N. and Pintore, E. (1990) Intensive training in young athletes. *British Journal of Sports Medicine*, **24**(4), 237–239.

Micheli, L.J. and Fehlandt, A.F. (1992) Overuse injuries to tendons and apophyses in children and adolescents. *Clinics in Sports Medicine*, **11**(4), 713–726.

Micheli, L.J. and Klein, J.D. (1991) Sports injuries in children and adolescents. *British Journal of Sports Medicine*, **25**(1), 6–9.

Micheli, L.J. (1995) Sports injuries in children and adolescents: questions and controversies. *Clinics in Sports Medicine*, **14**(3), 727–745.

Outerbridge, A. R. and Micheli, L. J. (1995) Overuse injuries in the young athlete. *Clinics in Sports Medicine*, **14**(3), 503–516.

Paletta, G.A. and Andrish, J.T. (1995) Injuries about the hip and pelvis in the young athlete. *Clinics in Sports Medicine*, **14**(3), 591–628.

Pappas, A.M., Zawicki, R.M. and Goldberg, B. (1991) Baseball: too much on a young pitcher's shoulders? *Physician and Sportsmedicine*, **19**(3), 107–117.

Roemmich, J.N. and Rogol, A.D. (1995) Physiology of growth and development: its relationship to performance in the young athlete. *Clinics in Sports Medicine*, **14**(3), 483–502.

Rowland, T.W. and Walsh, C.A. (1985) Characteristics of child distance runners. *Physician and Sportsmedicine*, **13**(9), 45–53.

Russell, K. (1986) Competition and the growing child: stress or distress? in, *The Growing Child in Competitive Sport*, (ed. G. Gleeson), Hodder & Stoughton, London, pp. 145–156.

Sahlin, Y. (1990) Sports accidents in childhood. *British Journal of Sports Medicine*, **24**(1) 40–44.

Schmidt-Olsen, S., Jorgensen, U., Kaalund, S. and Sorensen, J. (1991) Injuries among young soccer players. *American Journal of Sports Medicine*, **19**(3), 273–275.

Smith, A.D. and Tao, S.S. (1995) Knee injuries in young athletes. *Clinics in Sports Medicine*, **14**(3), 629–650.

Smith, A.D., Andrish, J.T. and Micheli, L.J. (1993) The prevention of sport injuries of children and adolescents. *Medicine and Science in Sports and Exercise*, **25**(8 Suppl.), 1–7.

Speer, D.P. and Braun, J.K. (1985) The biomechanical basis of growth plate injuries. *Physician and Sportsmedicine*, **13**(7), 72–78.

Stanitski, C.L. (1989) Common injuries in preadolescent and adolescent adults. Recommendations for prevention. *Sports Medicine*, **7**(1), 32–41.

Stanitski, C.L. (1993) Combating overuse injuries. A focus on children and adolescents. *Physician and Sportsmedicine*, **21**(1), 87–106.

Vines, G. (1988) Is sport good for children? *New Scientist*, **21 July**, 46–51.

Welford, R. (1989) Injuries in children's sport. *Practitioner*, **233**(1475), 1246–1249.

Yde, J. and Nielsen, A.B. (1990) Sports injuries in adolescents' ball games: soccer, handball and basketball. *British Journal of Sports Medicine*, **24**(1), 51–54.

(1981) Injuries to young athletes (position statement). *Physician and Sportsmedicine*, **9**(2), 107–110.

10. The effects of overtraining on endocrine and immunological function

10.1 INTRODUCTION

The large volumes of training being undertaken by many sports performers have obvious implications for the incidence of overuse injuries. However, in addition to this, excessive amounts of training can also adversely affect a number of the body's physiological systems and in particular the endocrine and immunological systems. The issue of overtraining and its effects upon these systems, as well its potential for causing 'staleness' and 'burnout', is therefore a topic the practitioner should be aware of.

The physical stresses experienced by the body during normal physical activity represent a temporary disturbance of the body's homeostatic state. This will include:

- an increased use of oxygen;
- an increased production of carbon dioxide;
- an increase in the acidity of various body fluids;
- a rise in body temperature;
- an increase in the use of energy stores;
- general circulatory changes.

In response to these stresses and the general demands of the activity a number of endocrine-related changes are observed in the body before, during and after exercise, an obvious example of which is the secretion of adrenalin (epinephrine) in response to anxiety and the physiological stresses of the activity. Rises in various other hormones such as growth hormone (GH), glucagon, testoster-one, antidiuretic hormone (ADH), aldosterone and thyroxine are also observed, whereas the levels of circulating insulin decline. In the context of these changes in the levels of circulating hormones a number of differences are noted between trained and untrained individuals. In general, there is a smaller change from the resting levels in trained individuals, which is believed to be related to the trained individual experiencing less physiological stress because their body is more adapted to the activity. Indeed, if the responses are related to relative exercise intensities rather than absolute levels the differences are greatly reduced. For example, if a fit and unfit individual were asked to run at the same speed for a couple of miles the changes in the unfit individual would be of a greater magnitude because they would be finding the exercise more difficult than the fit individual and would therefore be experiencing greater physiological stress. However, if both individuals were asked to run the distance at 70% of their maximum speed, this would produce the same level of physiological stress in each of them, even though the fit individual would be running faster. In this situation the magnitude of the hormonal responses is likely to be more similar.

In the highly trained sports performer, overtraining in the form of excessive amounts of training over a period of weeks or months can affect the normal hormonal responses to exercise. This can have an adverse effect upon the endocrine system, which results in the suppression of some hormones and elevated levels of others. This in turn may affect the immune system, resulting in temporary immune suppression and hence an increased vulnerability to minor illnesses. Therefore, whereas exercise in general may benefit the immune system, excessive amounts may adversely affect it and go some way towards explaining why many top performers appear to be particularly vulnerable to mild viral infections such as colds, flu and sore throats.

10.2   THE EFFECTS OF OVERTRAINING ON ENDOCRINE FUNCTION

The research evidence on the topic of overtraining and the endocrine system is complex and can be contradictory. This is probably because of the large number of factors involved, for example:

- the type of exercise;
- the absolute and relative exercise intensity;
- the duration of the exercise;
- the nutritional status of the individuals
- the fitness of the individual and their level of performance;
- anatomical and morphological factors;
- psychological factors.

In females, overtraining has been associated with menstrual dysfunction such as oligomenorrhoea and amenorrhoea. In these conditions the exact relationship between overtraining and irregular or absent periods is complex. The factors that contribute towards these conditions are believed to include:

- low levels of body fat or a loss of body fat, which may have a direct effect and/or work indirectly via a reduction in oestrogen levels;
- mental stress associated with high levels of training and competition – this may again have a direct effect or work indirectly via an increase in the levels of certain stress hormones;

- physical stress associated with high levels of training and competition, which again may be a direct effect or work via changes in the levels of various stress and anabolic hormones;
- alterations in the levels of various sex hormones such as oestrogen, luteinizing hormone (LH), follicle stimulating hormone (FSH), progesterone (P), gonadotrophin releasing hormone (GnRH) and testosterone (T), all of which may be affected by the previously mentioned factors;
- an increase in the level of hormones such as cortisol, adrenalin and prolactin, each of which may again be influenced by the above factors.

In summary, much of the research has looked at endurance runners and swimmers, where there is increase in menstrual dysfunction with training volume. In these subjects the observed hormonal abnormalities include:

- elevated progesterone and LH levels in the follicular phase, accompanied by depressed FSH levels;
- depressed FSH in the luteal phase;
- a suppressed LH surge or pulse which would normally stimulate ovulation.

These findings suggest that the cause of these hormonal changes may be related to alterations in the release of GnRH from the hypothalamus, which normally regulates these hormonal cycles. The basis of this is complex because of the number of interactions between the various hormones involved. However, the explanations put forward include:

- increased levels of stress hormones – cortisol, adrenalin, noradrenalin (norepinephrine) and prolactin – which interfere with GnRH;
- increased basal levels of testosterone, which could suppress the LH surge;
- depressed levels of oestrogen and progesterone, which may be related to a low level of body fat.

In both males and female, overtraining has been shown to increase the levels of various stress hormones (cortisol and adrenalin) and reduce the level of anabolic hormones such as growth hormone and testosterone. In males this suppression may again work via the pituitary gonadal hormonal axis with the stress hormones inhibiting the production of LH, which normally maintains testicular function and hence testosterone production. In cases of chronic overtraining the reduced LH levels could result in the suppression of testosterone, which could then affect the individuals capacity to train, make the necessary physiological adaptations to training and repair any micro- or macrotrauma caused by training, as well as reducing libido.

In summary, the general suppression of the anabolic hormones, and in particular testosterone, can be linked with a decline in athletic performance and the onset of 'staleness'.

10.3 IMMUNOLOGICAL IMPLICATIONS OF OVERTRAINING

While some evidence supports the idea that mild or moderate levels of exercise can promote the immune system and thereby reduce the risk of infections a number of pieces of research have indicated that overtraining can cause a temporary suppression of the immune response, which can increase the individual's susceptibility to infection. The immunological responses to exercise are complex and when studying the area it is important to differentiate between the immediate responses to an acute bout of exercise, the long-term effects of training and the effects of chronic overtraining.

10.3.1 The responses to an acute bout of exercise

During a bout of exercise the number of circulating white blood cells (leukocytes) increases and then returns to normal within minutes or hours after the exercise has ceased, the exact

response depending upon the intensity and duration of the exercise. The rise in circulating leukocytes appears to occur rapidly and has been detected within 10 minutes of the commencement of exercise. This elevated leukocyte level appears to be maintained for at least 15 minutes after the exercise has ceased and in some cases of prolonged exercise they may remain elevated for more than 3 hours. However, contrary to this, other pieces of research have indicated that during prolonged exercise the number of circulating white blood cells may, after an initial increase, start to decline and can fall below resting levels even before the exercise has stopped.

Most of the observed increases in circulating white blood cells are reported to be due to relatively large increases in the number of neutrophils, while smaller fluctuations are observed in the numbers of B and T cells (lymphocytes). However, before considering the possible implications of this on the immune system it is also necessary to consider the effects of the exercise upon the activity of the lymphocytes, which in some research has been shown to be reduced following strenuous exercise, along with the activity of the phagocytic leukocytes. Hence, despite the greater numbers of circulating lymphocytes the immune response may in fact be impaired, thereby reducing the individual's ability to cope with infections and minor illnesses. However the precise implications and possible significance of these transient changes are still, however, an area of debate. Some research also suggests that, during strenuous exercise, there is a decline in the ratio of helper to suppresser T cells, although whether this is maintained for long after the exercise and if it has any significance is unknown.

10.3.2 The effects of chronic overtraining

As indicated above, single bouts of exercise have been shown to elicit an immunological response, the implications of which are unclear. However, in addition to this, a number of other observations have been made concerning the immunological function of sports performers who are overtraining. These concern the general condition of their immune system and an apparent suppression of its responsiveness. For example, the resting levels of lymphocytes in highly trained athletes appear to be lower than in more sedentary individuals. Studies have also associated declines in antibody levels with overtraining, but here again the implications of these findings are uncertain. Some authorities believe this general suppression in immune response to be related to the increased levels of the stress hormones cortisol and adrenalin, although research is continuing in this field. Despite the lack of conclusive and unequivocal research in this topic, the findings to date do go some way towards explaining the apparent susceptibility of top sports performers to viral infections and minor illnesses. Another factor under consideration in this context is the role of the amino acid glutamine. This is used by the cells of the immune system as a source of energy, but may become depleted during strenuous exercise, thereby having the potential to inhibit immune function. Further areas of research that have produced results indicating an alteration in immune function include the influences of psychological stress and the effects of altered levels of thyroid hormones, growth hormones and sex steroids.

10.4   THE RISKS OF TRAINING WITH A VIRUS

In addition to the possible effects of overtraining upon general immunological function it is important for performers and coaches to be aware of the risks associated with training while suffering from a viral infection. The personality and determination of some individuals involved in sport make them reluctant to miss even one training session, even though they are ill. Training in this condition is unlikely to have any benefits and actually conveys a number of risks. Unfortunately, there is a belief among some individuals that if they are ill then exercising will help them to 'sweat it out'. In reality this is a dangerous practice, although most people appear not to suffer from any long-term consequences most of the time, which falsely reassures them that it is OK. In this context the practitioner must try to dispel these misconceptions and inform those involved in sport of the risks.

One of the most extensively documented effects of exercising with a virus is in the case of poliomyelitis, where exercise increases the severity of the complications and paralysis. Research would indicate that when it occurs the paralysis is most commonly present in the exercised limbs, for example the arms of canoeists. However the common practice of immunization against this disease means that is not a concern for most athletes. Indeed for most exercising individuals the main risk of exercising with a virus is associated with viral myocarditis, which can cause permanent damage to the heart, arrhythmias and in some cases fatalities. In Sweden, a number of sudden deaths among elite orienteers have also been attributed to myocarditis caused by *Chlamydia pneumoniae*. The risk of such outcomes make it imperative that the sports performer and coach should be aware of the risks of exercising with an upper respiratory tract infection. Another possible consequence of exercising with a virus is an increased risk of myalgic encephalomyelitis (ME), although the details of this condition and its association with strenuous exercise require further research before firm conclusions can be drawn about it.

Following a viral illness the sports performer may continue to underperform and a number of 'postviral fatigue syndromes' are being recognized. It is therefore important for the performer to realize that if s/he persists with training while ill rather than taking a few days off, it may cause him/her to require a more prolonged absence from training and in some cases the consequences may be long-term or even permanent.

10.5 SUMMARY

While some of the evidence is contradictory it is apparent that the practitioner should be aware of some of the wider issues associated with overtraining. The common reaction of a sports performer or coach to a series of performances that are below par is often to increase the amount of training. However this is quite likely to have adverse effects, as the real cause of the underperformance is overtraining, so that a lessening of the training load or even a complete rest from training would be far more effective. Indeed, many performers notice a significant improvement after a few weeks rest or tapered training. This improvement should not come as a surprise but even so many are reluctant to ease off when they are performing badly.

Another problem that may be associated with overtraining is a depletion of the muscles' glycogen stores. Adequate stores of glycogen are essential for strenuous exercise but may be depleted by regular training and a failure to eat sufficient amounts of carbohydrate, which is needed to replenish these stores. The inclusion of rest or recovery days will enable the rapid replenishment of these stores, if accompanied by a diet that is high in complex carbohydrate, and should enable the individual to train hard when required. To reduce the risk of overtraining and glycogen depletion regular rest days should be scheduled into a training programme and are advocated by many coaches. In summary, planned rest days on a regular basis can prevent a number of the physical and mental problems associated with overtraining such as burnout, staleness, overuse injuries and endocrine and immunological dysfunction.

10.6 FURTHER READING

Asgeirsson, G. and Bellanti, J.A. (1987) Exercise, immunology and infection. *Seminars in Adolescent Medicine*, 3(3), 199–204.

Booth, R.J. (1993) Exercise, overtraining and the immune response: a biological perspective. *New Zealand Journal of Sports Medicine*, 21(3), 42–45.

Budgett, R. (1990) Overtraining syndrome. *British Journal of Sports Medicine*, 24(4), 231–236.

Csillag, C. (1992) Sweden: deaths among orienteers. *Lancet*, 340.

Cumming, D.C., Brunsting, L.A., Strich, G. et al. (1986) Reproductive hormone increases in response to acute exercise in men. *Medicine and Science in Sports and Exercise*, 18(4) 369–373.

Eicher, E.R. Infection, Immunity and Exercise. *Physician and Sportsmedicine*, 21(1), Jan. (1993) 125–135.

Fitzgerald, L. (1991) Overtraining increases the susceptibility to infection. *International Journal of Sports Medicine*, 12(Suppl. 1), S5–S8.

Fry, R.W., Grove, J.R., Morton, A.R. et al. (1994) Psychological and immunological correlates of acute overtraining. *British Journal of Sports Medicine*, 28(4), 241–246.

Fry, R.W., Morton, A.R., Garcia-Webb, P and Keast, D. (1991) Monitoring exercise stress by changes in metabolic and hormonal responses over a 24-h period. *European Journal of Applied Physiology and Occupational Physiology*, 63(2/4), 228–234.

Fry, R.W., Morton, A.R and Keast, D. (1991) Overtraining syndrome and the chronic fatigue syndrome, part 1. *New Zealand Journal of Sports Medicine*, 19(3), 48–52.

Fry, R.W., Morton, A.R and Keast, D. (1991) Overtraining in athletes: an update. *Sports Medicine*, 12(1), 32–65.

Hackney, A.C., Sinning, W.E. and Bruot, B.C. (1988) Reproductive hormonal profiles of endurance-trained and untrained males. *Medicine and Science in Sports and Exercise*, 20(1) 60–65.

Hondras, M.A., Steinke, N. and Brennan, P.C. (1988) Suppressed phagocytic function in conditioned athletes. *Chiropractic Sports Medicine*, 2(4) 111–114.

Horgan, F. and Kerstetter, T. (1983) Reduced prolactin response to exercise in amenorrheic athletes. *Journal of Sports Sciences*, 1, 227–234.

Jakeman, P.M., Weller, A and Warrington, G. (1995) Cellular immune activity in response to increased training of elite oarsmen prior to Olympic competition. *Journal of Sports Sciences*, 13(3), 207–211.

Keast, D., Cameron, K. and Morton, A.R. (1988) Exercise and the immune response. *Sports Medicine*, 5, 248–267.

Kuipers, H and Keizer, H.A. (1988) Overtraining in elite athletes: review and directions for the future. *Sports Medicine*, **6**(2), 79–92.

Lehnmann, M., Gastmann, U., Petersen, O. *et al.* (1992) Training-overtraining: performance and hormonal levels after a defined increase in training volume versus intensity in experienced middle- and long-distance athletes. *British Journal of Sports Medicine*, **26**(4), 233–242.

Nash, H. L. (1986) Can exercise make us immune to disease? *Physician and Sportsmedicine*, **14**(3), **250–253.**

Parry-Billings, M., Blomstrand, E., McAndrew, N and Newsholme, E.A. (1990) A communicational link between skeletal muscle, brain and cells of the immune system. *International Journal of Sports Medicine*, **11**(Suppl. 2), S122–S128.

Roberts, J.A. (1986) Viral illness and sports performance. *Sports Medicine*, **3**(4), 296–303.

Roberts, J.A., Wilson, J.A. and Clements, G.B. (1988) Viral infections and sports performance – a prospective study. *British Journal of Sports Medicine*, **22**(4), 161–162.

Russell, J.B., Mitchell, D., Musey, P.I. and Collins, D.C. (1984) The relationship of exercise to anovulatory cycles in female athletes: hormonal and physical characteristics. *Obstetrics and Gynecology*, **63**(4), 452–456.

Sander, M. and Rocker, L. (1988) Influence of marathon running on thyroid hormones. *International Journal of Sports Medicine*, **9**, 123–126.

Semple, C.G., Thomson, J.A. and Beastall, G.H. (1985) Endocrine responses to marathon running. *British Journal of Sports Medicine*, **19**(3), 148–151.

Sharp, J.C.M. (1989) Viruses and the athlete. *British Journal of Sports Medicine*, **23**(1), 47–48.

Sharp, N.C.C and Koutedakis, Y. (1992) Sport and the overtraining syndrome: immunological aspects. *British Medical Bulletin*, **48**(3), 518–533.

Sharp, C. and Parry-Billings, M. Can exercise damage your health? *New Scientist* 15th August (1992) 33–37.

Shephard, R.J and Shek, P.N. (1994) Potential impact of physical activity and sport in the immune system – a brief review. *British Journal of Sports Medicine*, **28**(4), 257–255.

Simon, H.B. (1984) The immunology of exercise. *Journal of the American Medical Association*, **242**(19), 2735–2738.

Verde, T., Thomas, S and Shephard, R.J. (1992) Potential markers of heavy training in highly trained distance runners. *British Journal of Sports Medicine*, **26**(3), 167–175.

Wesslen, L., Pahlson, C., Friman, J. *et al.* (1992) Myocarditis caused by Chlamydia pneumoniae (TWAR) and sudden unexpected death in a Swedish elite orienteer. *Lancet*, **340**, 427–428.

Index

Page numbers in **bold** type refer to figures; those in *italic* to tables